WAITING
FOR BEBÉ

WAITING FOR BEBÉ

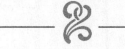

A Pregnancy Guide for Latinas

LOURDES ALCAÑIZ

Preface by Faustina Nevarez, M.D., OB-GYN
Illustrations by Stanley and Mark Coffman
Translated by José Nicholson

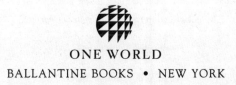

ONE WORLD
BALLANTINE BOOKS • NEW YORK

A One World Book
Published by The Random House Ballantine Publishing Group

Copyright © 2003 by Lourdes Alcañiz

Lourdes Alcañiz text translated by José Nicholson

All rights reserved under International and Pan-American Copyright
Conventions. Published in the United States by The Random House Ballantine Publishing
Group, a division of Random House, Inc., New York, and simultaneously
in Canada by Random House of Canada Limited, Toronto.

One World and Ballantine are registered trademarks and the One World
colophon is a trademark of Random House, Inc.

www.ballantinebooks.com/one/

Library of Congress Control Number: 2003102990

ISBN 0-345-45211-9

Text design by Helene Berinsky

Cover design by Monica Benalcazar
Cover photo © Rick Gomez/CORBIS, Inc./CorbisStockmarket

Manufactured in the United States of America

First English Edition: June 2003

10 9 8 7 6 5 4 3 2 1

We talk without words
And then I sing you to sleep
With the murmur of my blood
And the beating of my heart.

Gioconda Belli

To all Latino women soon to have in their arms
a little piece of their soul.

CONTENTS

ACKNOWLEDGMENTS

Before I wrote books, I thought the phrase that usually starts one off—
"This book wouldn't have been possible without the help of . . ."—was
some kind of conventional formula, the same as saying "Sincerely yours"
or "Kind regards" at the end of a letter. But after working for nearly two
years on this book, I can assure you there is no truer phrase than that one.
I really do want to thank all the people without whom this book wouldn't
have been possible.

First, this book wouldn't have been possible without the help of Dr.
Faustina Nevarez. Even though she's one of the busiest women in southern California (Dr. Nevarez is chief of the Department of Obstetrics and
Gynecology at the Kaiser Medical Center in Los Angeles), she still found
the time to patiently look over my work and come up with some magnif-
icent suggestions on how to make the book better. Thanks, Tina, for all
the hours you dedicated to this project.

This book wouldn't have been possible without the help, warmth, and
professionalism of my literary agent, Judith Riven, and my editor, Elisa-
beth Kallick Dyssegaard. It also wouldn't have been possible without the
valuable information many people have passed on to me along the way.
Among them are Mariana Rapp of the Hispanic Prenatal Care National
Hotline, Nicky Colbert of the National Partnership for Women and
Children, Jean Aadmodt of the Maternal and Child Bureau of Health Resources and Services Administration, Joe Luchock of the Health Insurance Association of America and Roberto Cervilla of Herbs of Mexico.

This book wouldn't have been possible without the help of my family and friends: my dear uncle, Dr. José Conde Hernández, who shared his knowledge as a medical professor and M.D. and answered my wacky questions at all hours of day and night; my mom, Lourdes March, who patiently looked over all the lists of *hierbitas y comidas*, herbs and foods; my dear friend Nelda Mier—journalist, doctor, social worker—who showed me the light with her suggestions and her caring critiques; and my friend Caroline Traiser, who never got to see the book become a reality. Thanks also to *mis compañeros de profesión y de risas*, my professional and laughter colleagues, journalists Jairo Marin and Luis Beltran, and to my friend Vanessa Willoughby, who so generously devoted many hours to this project.

But above all, this book wouldn't have been possible without the help, support and understanding of my husband Donaldo, the rock who always keeps me steady during the storm, and without the patience of my life's dearest treasures, Adriana and Patricia, who had to share their mother with a computer for months on end. They are the real inspiration for this book.

FOREWORD

Since I finished my residency in obstetrics and gynecology in 1984, I have been blessed and privileged to assist families in one of the most important events in their lives. Likewise, I feel privileged to have assisted with the development of this book. It has been a journey of exploration in medicine and the childbirth process as well as an exploration of the subtle yet unique approaches to our Latina heritage. Beyond being a guide to health care, pregnancy and childbirth, *Waiting for Bebé* presents childbirth through the eyes of Latinas in America.

Both my children were born while I was in medical school in the '70s. It was a time when everyone strived to keep the process as natural as possible. Twenty-five years later, as a physician and head of a busy department in a tertiary-level hospital in Los Angeles, I have more respect for the wisdom of nature but am also aware of the realities of what is natural. As women, we are fortunate to live in the twenty-first century in a country where childbirth is safer than at any other time in the history of humankind. Some of this we owe to modern technology, but it is also important that we keep technology's limitations in mind.

Lourdes Alcañiz is an excellent researcher and writer. Our collaboration was most effective; we viewed the process of reproduction from our personal interpretations as women, mothers and Latinas.

There is no other pregnancy book currently available for Latinas that presents such a sweeping scope on childbirth—medical, technical, clinical, personal and cultural viewpoints. The efforts to transcend and coalesce the different Latino, American and medical cultures into a cohesive, negotiable, understandable and workable whole is a struggle all pregnant Latinas face. It is our hope that *Waiting for Bebé* will facilitate this understanding and empower the reader to negotiate from a position of knowledge through the basic and intimate process of childbirth.

Faustina Nevarez, M.D.
Chief of Obstetrics and Gynecology at
Kaiser Los Angeles Medical Center, California

INTRODUCTION

I live far away from the majority of my family. So do many Latinas in the United States. It's tough not being able to participate more often in grand family reunions with children of all ages and sizes, wonderful food and music from the homeland. There are few things in this life as *el calor de la familia*, the warmth of the family, to give us that special feeling of knowing where we come from and who we are; the feeling of being with *nuestra gente*, our people.

Still, after years of being away from the family, it seems we adapt and become accustomed to a few visits here and there and some phone calls. Even though I still cry at the goodbyes, I thought I'd overcome the need to be so close to my family. I was in for a surprise.

When I got pregnant, I had my adoring husband and my friends in southern California, but I began to miss my mom, my aunts and my cousins like never before. We spoke on the telephone often, but it was not the same. I had so many questions, so many fears and doubts and so many new emotions every day that I didn't know what to do with them. The Latina in me missed the afternoon visits from friends and relatives, the food, the advice on how to deal with nausea, the stories other women in my family told about their pregnancies. More than anything I missed the comfort and caring mothers-to-be are showered with in Latino families. I read a lot of books about pregnancy and they did help me to understand what was going on a little better, but I didn't find in them *la voz amiga y de confianza*, the friendly and trusting voice I was looking for.

A few months later I was diagnosed with gestational diabetes. As I began to do some research on the problem I had developed, I discovered that Latina mothers-to-be are three times as likely to suffer from diabetes during pregnancy as the rest of the population. And that wasn't all I found out: There's a whole series of illnesses that affect us Latinas during pregnancy more than everyone else. Some have genetic causes; others are due to social factors. Those illnesses range from problems with the gallbladder to certain types of hepatitis. However, I couldn't find a single book among the dozens packed on the pregnancy shelves in the bookstores that dealt specifically with the problems and situations pregnant Latinas face. Even if I had had my family close to me, I still wouldn't have known about all these illnesses; all this information was as new to them as it was to me.

What I hope to do with this book is provide that *voz amiga y de confianza*, the friendly, caring voice I was looking for—but a voice that will also give you the most up-to-date and accurate medical information about the health problems that affect pregnant Latinas.

Here you'll read about all kinds of aspects of Latina pregnancy, from how to find prenatal care if you don't have health insurance to which herbs can be harmful to you and your baby. You'll get tips on how to handle a doctor who doesn't understand our culture and how to create a healthier and more nutritious menu for your pregnancy using Latino foods. You will find out about the physical and emotional changes you and your baby and even your partner are going through. Each pregnancy chapter has a special section dedicated to dads-to-be. If they don't have enough time to read the entire book, these short sections will help them understand in a few minutes what you're going through physically and emotionally. You'll also learn what you can expect during labor, delivery and afterward. The Contact List at the end of the book provides all kinds of telephone numbers and addresses where you can go to get help or more information.

This is the book I would have liked to read during my first pregnancy. Thanks to my research and what I learned after the birth of my older daughter, my second pregnancy and delivery were much easier and healthier. That's the information I want to share with you, *de una madre latina a otra*, from one Latina mother to another, as we do in our families.

Le deseo lo mejor—I wish you the best in this special time of your life, when the word *familia* takes on a whole new, deeper meaning.

Hollywood, Florida, summer 2002

1

Getting Ready for Bebé

Every time my mother peels an apple, a tomato or a peach, she buries the peels in her garden. Well-nourished soil, she says, yields healthy plants. And she must be right because there's always disputes among our neighbors and family to see who gets the leftover *calabacitas* or zucchini my mom doesn't need. She's certainly got the best garden in the neighborhood.

The equivalent of this secret for a woman who wants to become pregnant is folate or folic acid, a balanced diet and prenatal visits. If you're thinking about having a baby, one of the best things you can do is prepare your body for pregnancy. And if you're already pregnant, it's never too late to start giving your baby the best possible care. The information in this chapter will help you achieve a healthy pregnancy for both you and your baby.

Taking care of yourself before conceiving is very important because some of the most critical moments of a baby's development take place during the first weeks of gestation, when you probably don't even know you're pregnant. In fact, this advice applies to all women of childbearing age, since half the pregnancies in the United States are unplanned.

What you eat and do is as important as what you don't eat and don't do. The beginning of the pregnancy is when the baby is most vulnerable to what you send to him or her through your blood. At this time the structure that will become the nervous system, spinal column and brain is starting to shape. Home remedies and some drugs could affect this development. So can certain illnesses you may contract.

Being healthy during pregnancy is crucial for the baby and for you too. From an embryo that starts half as small as the dot on top of this *i* you will grow a whole little human being inside yourself. The work the body of a pregnant woman does while resting has been compared to climbing a mountain. Starting as healthy as possible will help you make this work much easier. It's a very good idea to see your obstetrician/gynecologist before you get pregnant. And make an appointment for your partner to see his general physician; that way both of you will know that everything's the way it should be. Many Latinos don't know they have diseases such as diabetes and high blood pressure, which can affect the pregnancy.

And don't forget to get your spirit ready. Fill your heart with *todo el amor*, all the love you can. Your baby will benefit from it as much as from the folate and vitamins you will give him or her through your blood. *La verdad*, truth is, I think the secret to the success of my mom's garden is the love and care she pours on it every day.

NUTRITION

Eating healthy is always important, but if you are planning to have a baby or are already pregnant, a balanced diet should be one of your priorities. This is not only because you will feel much better, but because once pregnant you will be the one deciding your baby's menu every day. Prenatal vitamins are only a complement to your diet. There is nothing that can substitute for healthy nutrition. Every day you should eat fresh vegetables, fruits, grains, proteins (meats, poultry, fish or eggs) and dairy products. In Chapter 3 you will find the types of foods and portions recommended during pregnancy. If you are not pregnant yet you can start this diet, subtracting around 200 calories.

FOLATE OR FOLIC ACID

Folic acid is a member of the B complex group. Our body uses folic acid to make red blood cells and proteins such as DNA. These are required for a baby to develop normally. A lack of folic acid can cause defects in what is called the fetal neural tube, which is the structure the baby's nervous system grows from. One of the most common defects produced by a lack of folic acid is spina bifida, where the spinal column is not closed at its end.

This doesn't mean that if you haven't taken folic acid before getting pregnant, your baby is going to have a defect. Millions of healthy babies have been born even though their mothers didn't take folic acid pills. But today we are aware of the causes of these birth defects, and we know that taking folic acid is one way to reduce the chance they will occur. Since the U.S. Centers for Disease Control and Prevention began their campaign to promote the use of folic acid a few years ago, the number of babies born with these birth defects has dropped by 19 percent.

You can find folic acid in green leafy vegetables (such as spinach and Swiss chard), citrus fruits (like oranges and lemons) and legumes (beans and lentils) as well as in fortified breakfast cereals. In its natural state, or as it's found in these foods, folic acid is called folate. Folic acid is the same vitamin, but made artificially. Our bodies process folic acid more easily than folate, and that's why it's a good idea to take it in pill form before and during your pregnancy.

The recommended dosage for women who plan to get pregnant or who are already pregnant is 400 micrograms daily (0.4 milligrams daily). Most health stores carry folic acid pills in these concentrations, but unless your doctor prescribes it, you shouldn't take more than 1,000 micrograms of folic acid a day. Along with folic acid, you can take a vitamin pill, or you can take a vitamin pill that already contains folic acid. Once you are pregnant, your doctor will prescribe a vitamin pill made especially for pregnant women.

WEIGHT BEFORE PREGNANCY

The closer you are to your ideal weight, the easier the pregnancy will be. If you are very overweight, it's advisable to lose as much as you can before getting pregnant because you will gain weight during pregnancy. Two of the most common illnesses for Latinas during pregnancy, diabetes and hypertension, are related to obesity. Various studies show that obese Latinas suffer more complications during pregnancy than those who are at normal weight.

Being overweight doesn't mean carrying a few extra pounds, it means being excessively fat. A visit to your obstetrician/gynecologist will help you determine your health status and whether you should lose weight. For women who are under their ideal weight it is more important to put on a healthy number of pounds during the pregnancy than to gain weight beforehand.

Foods to Watch Out For

Some foods can contain bacteria or toxic substances that may not be harmful to you but can be harmful to the baby. Watch out for them before and during the entire pregnancy.

Soft Latino Cheeses

Listeria is a bacteria that lives in certain types of soft cheeses and can pass through the placenta and infect the baby.

There are a few types of Latino cheeses that can be contaminated, such as *queso blanco, queso fresco, queso de hoja, queso crema* and *asadero*. The list also includes other cheeses such as Feta (sheep's or goat's milk cheese), Brie, Camembert or cheese with blue veins such as Roquefort or blue cheese. To destroy the bacteria you should cook these cheeses until they boil or, better yet, use hard cheeses instead.

Sometimes you can find unwrapped cheeses in some *tiendas del barrio*, neighborhood shops or minimarkets, sitting next to raw sausages and meats. Take a close look at where these cheeses were before you buy anything because they might have contaminated nearby foods.

Ceviche and Other Raw Foods

Bacteria and parasites like raw foods. It's where they can multiply quickly without being disturbed. That's why health authorities advise women who are thinking about getting pregnant not to eat raw fish, meat, eggs or milk and juices that haven't been pasteurized. Ceviche, chorizos (cured sausages), *jamón serrano* (cured ham), sushi and carpaccio are more likely to have bacteria or parasites growing in them. It's also a good idea to thoroughly wash raw vegetables before eating them.

Contaminated Fish

The Food and Drug Administration has advised pregnant women and women who are thinking about getting pregnant to avoid several types of fish: tuna, shark, swordfish, king mackerel and tilefish. These fish can have high levels of mercury, which could harm the fetus's nervous system. Although fish is an excellent source of nutrients, before and during pregnancy you should eat it just two or three times a week (see page 47).

Liver

Animal livers have a lot of vitamin A—that's good for you. But at the same time, the liver contains a lot of the hormones and antibiotics the animals are given, so it's better to limit the amount of liver you eat.

Artificial Sweeteners

Watch out for two of them: cyclamate and saccharin. Instead, sweeten your drinks with or drink sodas that contain aspartame, which is found in the brands Equal and NutraSweet. Because all these artificial sweeteners are chemical compounds, it's a good idea to use them in moderation. Don't use more than four packets of artificial sweetener a day or drink more than two artificially sweetened sodas daily.

Preservatives

Prepackaged meals contain a lot of preservatives (you know, those unpronounceable ingredients on the back of the box). How they exactly affect your unborn baby is not known, so the best thing to do is to avoid them.

Coffee

I've got a friend who drinks seven cups of coffee a day, not American coffee but the boiled, strong coffee we Latinos like. She even drinks a cup before going to bed and she claims *que duerme como un tronco*, she sleeps like a log!

Not everyone is immune to caffeine; babies are definitely not. Caffeine is a stimulant that passes through the placenta, the organ that filters to your baby what you eat or drink. So you might want to start substituting decaffeinated coffee for regular or reducing the number of cups you drink every day. Some studies indicate that a couple of cups of coffee a day during pregnancy aren't harmful. Caffeine is also found in tea, chocolate and colas as well as in Latino drinks such as *mate* or *guaraná*.

Herbs

Herbal remedies are used by a lot of us Latinas; they've been proven successful over thousands of years in our cultures. But not all herbs are safe to use during pregnancy. For example, herbs that help with cramps and to regulate menstruation relax the uterus and could cause bleeding and miscarriage. There are others that stimulate contractions (see page 61).

WHAT TO QUIT

Drinking, smoking or handling toxic substances is not a good idea, even if you may not have noticed any changes in your body after having a few alcoholic drinks, smoking a couple of cigarettes or using certain chemical products. But when you're thinking about getting pregnant, what might not seem harmful to you could have consequences for the baby.

Alcohol, Tobacco and Drugs

Latina women smoke less than any other ethnic group in the United States; we don't drink much either, which is very wise during pregnancy. Tobacco interferes with fetal development because it constricts the blood vessels of the placenta; as a result, the baby gets less oxygen and nutrients and grows less than it should. The toxins found in tobacco pass through the mother's blood into the baby.

Alcohol also crosses the placenta, and if you drink regularly during pregnancy, it can cause fetal alcohol syndrome, which results in a whole range of problems from birth defects to mental retardation. The same is true for drugs such as cocaine, heroin or marijuana. There is no safe amount of these drugs for the baby.

Lead

Lead is a metal found in certain products such as paint. Lead can be inhaled from things such as paint dust or it can get into your body through the foods you eat. It then accumulates in your bones.

A recent study showed the mental development of babies born to mothers with high levels of lead in their bones is slower compared to children born to mothers with significantly lower levels. In addition to mental retardation, lead can cause problems in the nervous system and in the kidneys, and some blood disorders such as anemia. Children absorb much more lead than adults.

Even though you may not currently be working with lead-based products, you may have in the past and the metal may have already accumulated in your bones. The lead level in your body is measured through a blood test, and certain treatments can help to reduce those levels. Ask your doctor for a blood test if you think that you might have been exposed to high levels of lead. The products you should take most care with are:

- *Digestive remedies*. Some traditional Latino products to help with digestive problems have high levels of lead in them. For example, *greta*, a yellow-gray powder, is nearly pure lead. Other remedies you should stay away from include *alarcón, azarcón, coral, liga, María Luisa* and *rueda*.

- *Paints*. This is the most common source of lead poisoning. In 1950 the federal government limited the amount of lead that could be added to paints, and in 1978 the levels were reduced again. Still, houses built and painted before 1950 may have high levels of lead in them. The maximum level of lead allowed today in paints is 600 ppm (parts per million). When paint begins to chip and peel away from the walls, the dust that comes along with it contains lead. You can breathe it in or perhaps get it on your hands and fingers and ingest it inadvertently. If you think you may have high-lead paint in your house, call the telephone number in the Contact List (page 361). In the meantime, don't sand, scrape or burn any of the paint because you may expose yourself to very high levels of lead. Also, vegetables grown in gardens next to houses with lead-based paints may also have absorbed the metal. You can have your soil tested for lead as well.

- *Water*. The water pipes in many older houses are made of lead. When the pipes corrode, the metal begins to mix with the water that flows through them. The lead especially concentrates in the water sitting in the pipes overnight. Let the water run for about 30 seconds before you use it for the first time in the morning. You can have your water tested as well (see page 361).

- *Ceramics and crystal*. Some ceramic or crystal items are decorated with paints that contain lead. If the glaze on pottery appears chalky, don't use it for eating or drinking, or for storing food or cooking, because it may contain lead. In particular, acidic foods (lemons, salsas) and hot drinks can easily pick up the lead from these containers. Don't put them in the microwave oven. Take a close look at the color of the ceramics. The ones painted yellow, orange, red, green, light blue or black may have lead in them. Ceramics sold for "decoration only" should never be used for cooking.

- *Soldered food cans*. In 1996 the United States federal government prohibited the sale of foods in cans soldered with lead. Other countries may not have passed similar laws, so avoid cans when traveling abroad unless you are sure that they are not soldered.

- *Sweets*. Some candies imported from Latin America may have a high lead content because of the wrapping used. The Food and Drug Administration put out a warning about some lollipops and individually wrapped candy imported from Mexico and the Philippines. Several children were poisoned in the United States after eating them.

- *Cosmetics*. *Kajal*, *khol* and *surma* are Middle Eastern cosmetics, used as eyeliners, that have a high lead content.

There are also some professions that might cause lead contamination. Jobs that expose you to lead include work with automobile batteries or radiators, work with melted metals, paint removal, construction or remodeling of old buildings or bridges, or a shooting gallery. If your partner works with materials that could contain high levels of lead (paints, batteries, radiators, melted metals), make sure he leaves his clothes outside the house and takes a shower before coming into contact with you or your children.

Lead poisoning symptoms are difficult to detect. You may feel irritable or tired, or you may not feel anything at all. Talk to your doctor or the National Lead Information Center (see Contact List) if you think you or someone in your family may have been contaminated by lead.

Mercury

This metal is found in fish such as shark, swordfish and king mackerel and also in certain imported cosmetics. A few years ago, there were several cases of women poisoned by mercury after using a beauty cream imported from Mexico. It's difficult to know if a cosmetic bought in another country contains mercury or lead unless it's analyzed in a lab.

WORKPLACE SAFETY

Examine your workplace if you are thinking about getting pregnant. Watch out for chemicals and strenuous physical activity.

- *Beauty salons*. There is a higher rate of miscarriages among women who work with hair coloring and other products for forty hours a week in an enclosed beauty salon or beauty school. Try to make sure your workplace is well ventilated.

- *Cleaning services*. Some industrial cleaning and dry cleaning products release fumes that shouldn't be breathed. Use gloves and make sure the area you're working in is well ventilated.
- *Factories, printing and photography labs*. Some of these places use chemical products that are particularly dangerous during pregnancy, including arsenic, cadmium, carbon monoxide, DDT, lead, lithium, mercury, toluene, nicotine or vinyl chloride. These are only a few examples. Find out the names of the chemicals you're working with and talk to your obstetrician/gynecologist about them.
- *Teachers*. Educators need to be careful about coming into contact with sick children, especially if you haven't been vaccinated for rubella. Wash your hands often and don't eat children's leftovers.
- *Jobs that require heavy lifting*. Extreme physical exertion can cause problems, especially in the first three months of pregnancy.

If you find yourself having to do one of the jobs listed above, your employer might be obligated, depending on the size of your company, to give you a position that puts you and your baby at lesser risk during pregnancy (see page 27).

OVER-THE-COUNTER AND PRESCRIPTION DRUGS

Pharmacies in Tijuana and other Mexican border cities do a booming business. Not only do they have local customers, but lots of people cross the border from the United States to buy prescription drugs they can't buy at home without a prescription. The drugs sold at these border pharmacies range from antibiotics and birth control pills to thyroid and diabetes remedies and tranquilizers.

When you don't have medical insurance, going to a doctor and buying the medicines they prescribe isn't cheap, and sometimes it seems easier to try a few tablets of the leftover drugs in the medicine cabinet, or even borrow some from a cousin, aunt, neighbor or friend who assures us she's taken these pills for the same problem and *fueron una bendición*, they were a blessing. But taking drugs this way can cause trouble, and during a pregnancy this is altogether not a good idea.

There are many drugs that can cross the placenta and affect the baby, and some of them can cause birth defects. So during your nine months of pregnancy, your gynecologist should be the one who decides which medicines you take. Something as simple as an aspirin is not considered safe during pregnancy, especially in the last three months, because it can cause bleeding and postpone your due date.

There is a drug that's popular in Latino stores known as "Mexican aspirin" that you should be aware of. Metamizole (trade name Dipyrone) is an analgesic that's been banned in the United States, but it's sold in Mexico. In certain Latino markets in the United States you can still buy it. This medicine kills white blood cells, which are the ones that defend your body against infection. Just recently, several people, including children, have been hospitalized with serious infections after taking it.

What follows is a list of medicines that can cause birth defects. Talk to your doctor before you stop taking a prescribed medicine. Also keep in mind that this list is only a guide. If you're worried about what drugs you're taking, call your doctor or the Teratology Information Service (see Contact List), an institution that keeps track of drugs and other substances that are harmful to babies. Below you will find the generic names of these medicines, since the brand names vary by country.

- *ACE (angiotensin-converting enzyme) inhibitors:* Drugs prescribed, among other things, to control high blood pressure, such as benazepril, captopril, enalapril, ramipril, etc.
- *Acne and psoriasis medication:* Isotretinoin, etretinate
- *Antibiotics:* Tetracycline, doxycycline, streptomycin
- *Anticoagulants:* Warfarin
- *Anticonvulsants:* Used for treating epilepsy. Phenytoin, carbamazepine, trimethadione, paramethadione, valproic acid, etc.
- *Antidepressants:* Lithium
- *Antimetabolites and anticancer drugs:* Aminopterin, busulfan, cytarabine, methotrexate, etc.
- *Antirheumatics:* Penicillamine
- *Antithyroid drugs:* Used to treat thyroid gland dysfunction, such as propylthiovracil, tapazole
- *Hormones:* Androgens (male hormones), DES (diethylstilbestrol)
- *Leprosy complications:* Thalidomide

If you are taking oral contraceptives or shots, you should wait to get pregnant until you've completed two to three menstrual cycles without this form of birth control. If you get pregnant right away, it will be difficult to figure out exactly when you conceived. Knowing the date of conception is important to see if the baby is growing normally. Also, it's difficult to predict the birth date if you don't know when the pregnancy began. A difference of two to three weeks can be crucial at the end of your pregnancy to determine if your labor should be induced because you are overdue.

DIABETES AND CHRONIC ILLNESSES

There are some chronic illnesses that can have an effect on pregnancy and the baby. Diabetes, a very common disease among Latinos, is one of them. If you are a diabetic and your sugar levels aren't under control, you have a greater chance of having a miscarriage or a baby with a birth defect. Asthma can also affect the amount of oxygen your baby receives, and high blood pressure increases the chances you'll have a complicated pregnancy. But don't stop treating these illnesses without first talking to your doctor.

If you are taking drugs for a chronic illness, such as diabetes, hypertension, epilepsy, asthma, depression or a thyroid problem, you should *not* stop taking those medicines the moment you find out you're pregnant. Consult your doctor first.

If you have a chronic illness, the effect of stopping the medication could be worse than the medicine itself. You should make an appointment with your doctor as soon as possible and find out what's the best way to treat your illness during pregnancy. Many women who have chronic illnesses are able to keep them under control and have successful pregnancies.

IMMUNIZATIONS

There are some infectious diseases, such as rubella, that could cause complications during pregnancy. It can be determined through a blood test if you are immune against some infectious diseases or not. Vaccines exist for some of them, but it's not advisable to get pregnant until three months after the vaccination.

Vaccinations are useful if you work in an environment where these diseases may appear, such as in institutions with children or groups of people who have not been vaccinated themselves. Some of these vaccinations are required for immigration (see page 158) and also for travel to certain countries.

Generally, vaccines that contain live virus are not recommended just before or during pregnancy.

Hereditary Diseases

Genetic tests allow doctors to determine the likelihood you or your partner will pass on a hereditary disease to your baby. Hereditary diseases include sickle cell anemia (which affects some Latinos of Caribbean origin), cystic fibrosis and hemophilia. If these types of illnesses or others exist in your family, a genetic analysis can show the statistical likelihood of their being passed on to your children (see page 115).

Pets and Toxoplasmosis

Maria García, a Latina mother-to-be, has a Chihuahua she loves. Before getting pregnant, Maria allowed Pancho to lick her face during his moments of rambunctious happiness. But when she got pregnant, this ritual started worrying her—Pancho's mouth was in a lot of places during the day. During the following months, she wouldn't let Pancho lick her and she washed her hands every time she touched the dog.

It's a good idea to maintain a more hygienic relationship with your pets if you're thinking about getting pregnant, especially if there are cats in the house. Cats can spread a disease called toxoplasmosis through their feces. This illness doesn't have any symptoms in the mother, but it can infect the fetus during the first three months of pregnancy. So, it's better for another member of the family to *encargarse de la tarea*, take on the chore of changing the cat litter. It's possible that a mother-to-be who's lived for a long time with cats has already built up defenses against this disease, in which case it wouldn't infect the baby. A blood test can tell you whether you've had toxoplasmosis, but it's not 100 percent accurate.

But don't worry, pet lovers—all you really need to do is stay away from the cat feces and wash your hands well after petting the animals. Toxoplasmosis can also be contracted by eating raw meat or fish, ceviche or sushi, or certain types of cured but uncooked meat, such as chorizos, and through dirt-contaminated vegetables that haven't been washed well.

X Rays and Dental Care

Before you actually start trying to conceive, it's better to be done with any routine medical procedure that require X rays, anesthesia or chemical products. If you need X rays, ask always to be covered with a lead apron that keeps the radiation from reaching your body. Many dentists and radiologists use this protection regularly. If you are pregnant and you already had an X ray, chances are everything will be all right (see page 143), but talk to your obstetrician/gynecologist anyway.

The hormones produced during pregnancy can affect your gums—they could bleed and feel more sensitive. A teeth cleaning is a good way to prepare your gums for the changes they'll be going through. Once you are pregnant, it is recommended that you go to the dentist for at least one more cleaning.

Exercise

Physical exercise before and during pregnancy is beneficial, as long as your doctor approves. Sports that include contact or falling (boxing, karate, water skiing, horseback riding, etc.) can be dangerous, more so if you are not used to them. However, walking, swimming and even aerobic exercises will help you get in shape. You will find some helpful exercises in Chapter 3.

Hot Tubs and Saunas

When your body's temperature is raised to high levels, the baby's body is also heated. In the first weeks of pregnancy, the baby is building the structures it needs to survive and continue to grow. So during that time it's not a good idea to take extended hot baths or sit in Jacuzzis or saunas. Some studies have shown that sustained temperatures higher than 102.6 degrees Fahrenheit (39.2 degrees Celsius) can cause birth defects in laboratory animals. Avoid exposing yourself to high temperatures during the first three months of pregnancy.

You can still take a relaxing warm bath—these studies are based on truly hot baths, where the body heats up to more than 102 degrees Fahrenheit and stays that way for more than ten minutes. Just be sure to check the water temperature before you go in. Electric blankets aren't recommended for the same reason. Also, talk to your doctor if you've got a high fever.

AND DAD?

Your husband's sperm will be healthier and stronger for their long journey if he doesn't drink, smoke, do drugs or take other toxic substances. The temperatures of saunas and Jacuzzis are not good for the health of sperm either. Ideally he should have a routine checkup before you start trying to conceive, especially if he has a chronic illness such as diabetes or if he's taking any medications.

THE SECOND CHILD

When is the best time to begin planning to have a second child? There are many couples who don't have to think about this question because their second child is a *sorpresa,* a surprise. (Sometimes the first was too!) But for those who want to think ahead, there are all kinds of things to consider. Some say it's better to have children close together because if they're nearly the same age they'll have more in common. Others would rather the first child be several years older than his siblings so that he won't need as much attention when the new baby arrives.

But according to the experts, the most important factor in determining when to have a second child is how quickly the mother recuperates from the first birth. Studies show that from eighteen months to five years between siblings is ideal. It is not recommended that you get pregnant less than six months after having a baby since 70 percent of such pregnancies have a spontaneous rupture of the amniotic sac, and there's a 30 percent greater chance of developing complications.

Of course, many families whose children are separated by only a year find it's not a problem for them or the kids, except for the number of *pañales,* diapers, around the house. But if you want to keep risks to a minimum, separating children by two to five years appears to be the best option.

AFTER LOSING A BABY

Losing a baby is a very hard and sad experience for a couple, especially for the mother. Even if the pregnancy was lost during the first weeks, the presence of a baby is very real for many women. Getting well emotionally is just as important as recovering physically (see page 181). Take your time. You are the only one who knows when you will be emotionally ready to try again.

Your doctor is the best person to consult as to when your body is ready to get pregnant again. Generally, it's recommended you wait at least three months to allow the interior lining of the uterus to rebuild itself.

PRENATAL CARE

You might be thinking: "These recommendations and precautions are all very well, but I'm already pregnant!"

When there's time to plan, preparing yourself for pregnancy is great. But the truth is, life doesn't always go according to plan. For many of us, finding out we're expecting is a total surprise. During my first pregnancy, I had to read the pregnancy test instructions three times to make sure that the two little pink lines on the test strip meant I was in fact going to have a baby. *No lo podía creer*, I just couldn't believe it.

In any supermarket or pharmacy you will find home pregnancy tests that can detect if you're pregnant, even just a few days after conception. When a woman is pregnant her body produces a hormone called beta-HCG, or Beta Human Chorionic Gonadotropin, and that's what these tests detect. If the test results are positive, there's a 99 percent chance you are pregnant (see page 138).

By that time, the first stages of fetal development have already taken place. But relax—that doesn't mean that if you've drunk several herb infusions or several cups of coffee or even if you've had a couple of alcoholic drinks, you've hurt your baby. What a positive pregnancy test does mean is that now it's time to take care of yourself and, most important of all, that it's time to ask for an appointment with the doctor as soon as possible.

Lilliam Martinez and her husband, Sergio, spent years preparing for the trip of their lives: a vacation in Italy. Just a few days before they were scheduled to leave, Lilliam *se sentía diferente*, felt a little strange. She thought perhaps it was the excitement of the upcoming trip, but just in case (and also because deep down she suspected the real reason she was feeling "strange") she made an appointment with her doctor. Her physician couldn't tell for sure if she was pregnant, since it was still too early to hear the baby's heartbeat. Lilliam considered canceling the trip, but her doctor told her that wasn't necessary. She just needed to take care of herself.

Lilliam followed her doctor's instructions to the letter. From the beginning, she assumed she *was* pregnant. She took with her a pregnancy book and the prenatal vitamins her doctor had prescribed for her. These vitamins turned out to be a very good idea. The European tour was organized by a travel agency and it proved difficult to follow an appropriate diet. "There was always wine on the table, but never milk," Lilliam remembered. During the tour stops, she and her husband looked for shops to buy fresh fruit. When they returned to the United States, the doctor confirmed the news: Lilliam was pregnant and everything was going well. Lilliam's precautions helped her baby during its first weeks and gave Lilliam the peace of mind of knowing that she'd done all she could to give her baby a healthy start to life.

Not all of us make it to the doctor so quickly. Sometimes, when it's the second child, we think we know the routine and don't rush to make an appointment. Others will wait at least three months, when there is less risk for a miscarriage. After all, in the past women didn't go to the doctor until they had gone at least two months without a period. Also, in our culture a pregnancy is a symbol of *buena salud*, good health, and why would you need to go to the doctor if you are healthy?

Truth is, there are many reasons to ask for an appointment with the doctor as soon as possible. Medical and technological advances of the past few years now make it possible to detect and treat problems that in the past were discovered only after it was too late. The statistics show the earlier a woman gets prenatal care, the fewer the problems that develop later in pregnancy. For example, one of the diseases that affects Latinos more than other ethnic groups is diabetes. If this disease is not under control before and during pregnancy, it can have serious consequences for mother and child. Only a doctor can perform the tests to determine if you're diabetic. High blood pressure is another enemy of Latinas. High blood pressure increases the chances of getting preeclampsia, which, along with gestational diabetes, is one of the illnesses most commonly associated with pregnancy. When these conditions are detected and treated in time, the risks for you and your baby are reduced dramatically.

But the most common problem we Latinas have is actually getting medical attention. Many of us don't have medical insurance to pay for it.

One of every three Latinos lacks health coverage. However, the lack of an insurance policy doesn't necessarily mean you have to go without prenatal care. Several state and federal programs offer free or very low cost prenatal care. The following chapter will help you find a doctor and medical insurance for you during your pregnancy, and if you've already got insurance, it will help you to determine if it's the right type.

2

⁂

Health Insurance and Cultural Differences

Health care in the United States is among the most costly in the world, and that includes health care for pregnant mothers and their babies. If you don't have health insurance, you can expect to pay between $2,500 and $10,000 to have a baby, and that's if nothing goes wrong! Heaven forbid if you need special attention from your doctor during your pregnancy or delivery—that can make the bill go through the roof. Health insurance coverage isn't cheap either. The annual health insurance cost average for one person is around $4,000, and family coverage is even more expensive.

So without a doubt, having a baby in this country is *bien caro*, very expensive. Despite that, it is possible to get medical attention during your pregnancy without having to declare bankruptcy—even if you don't have health insurance. In this chapter you'll learn what health insurance options you have depending on your budget and circumstances. The Contact List at the end of the book has names, addresses and telephone numbers of institutions and organizations that can offer you more information about health insurance or help you find coverage close to home if you aren't covered already.

HEALTH INSURANCE AND PREGNANCY

Most health insurance policies give access to medical services in exchange for a monthly payment. This coverage may include pregnancy care or not. There are several ways to obtain a health insurance policy that will pay for your pregnancy and birth, but it's much cheaper, not to mention easier, if you are covered before you become pregnant.

One way to get covered is through the company where you or your husband work. This is called group coverage, and it has several advantages:

- It costs less than an individual policy purchased directly from the insurance company because the employer pays part of the bill.
- The rest of the family can be included in the coverage.
- A physical exam is generally not required before being insured.
- The majority of policies, although not all of them, cover maternity costs.
- Pregnancy and delivery costs will be covered even if you are already pregnant when you or your husband join the company (coverage usually gets activated two or three months after being hired and in some places immediately).
- If you change jobs while you're covered by a company policy, federal law guarantees your pregnancy will not be considered a "preexisting condition." Even if your new employer has a different health insurance plan, the new policy has to cover your pregnancy (although you may have to wait one or two months before the new policy takes effect). The health insurance administrator at your or your husband's job can clear up any confusion you may have about how and when insurance coverage applies to you.
- If you lose your job or get another without insurance, you are usually allowed to keep the insurance through a program called CO-BRA, and pay yourself what the company had paid—at least for a while (see page 22).

Unfortunately, many companies don't offer health insurance coverage to their employees, especially if there are few workers—which, by the way, are precisely the kinds of businesses where most of us Latinos work. If you work for a small company, own your own business or work as an independent contractor it's possible you won't have any coverage at all. In this case, if you are not already pregnant, you have two options:

- Obtain health coverage through a union (if you belong to one) or through a professional association that in some cases may even offer group coverage to its members.

• Buy an individual policy, which means that you will buy your health coverage directly from the insurance company.

With an individual policy you will have a waiting period (generally twelve months) before the insurance company will pay for maternity costs. Another possibility if you don't want to wait that long is to pay a higher monthly premium when you become pregnant. Keep in mind that insurance policies and laws vary from company to company and from state to state. It's a good idea to study your insurance policy—especially the fine print—*antes de firmar nada*, before you sign anything. In the pages that follow, you'll find a list of important questions to ask before buying an insurance policy that will cover your prenatal care and delivery.

TYPES OF INSURANCE

Below is a description of the types of insurance you'll find in the United States, whether your medical coverage comes through your employer or you have purchased it as an individual policy. However, finding individual health coverage once you are pregnant is very difficult because your pregnancy will be considered a preexisting condition. Insurance companies know that they will have to pay for your medical attention, and this is not a good deal for them. However, some insurance companies do not have such rules; much depends on the state in which you are trying to buy coverage. You can find out what laws apply in your state through the National Association of Insurance Commissioners (see Contact List). For coverage while pregnant see page 22.

HMO Insurance
HMO stands for "health management organization." With HMO coverage you pay a monthly premium, and in exchange you receive medical services when you need them from health professionals who are members of your HMO. HMOs establish contracts with the hospitals and doctors who will care for you. The group of hospitals and doctors is called a network.

With HMO coverage you select, or are assigned, a primary care physician, who is the person you'll see first in case of illness or an accident. The primary care physician is also the one who will decide if you need to see a specialist. When you're pregnant, an obstetrician/gynecologist or midwife will become your primary care physician.

There is another kind of HMO called "integrated health care organization." Here doctors work exclusively in offices and hospitals that belong only to that HMO (i.e., Kaiser Permanente). When you belong to such an organization you don't need to go first through a primary care physician. You can choose the obstetrician/gynecologist that you want to see.

On each visit, you may need to make what's called a co-payment. This is usually between $5 and $10 that you pay out of your own pocket. If your plan also covers prescriptions, you can buy prenatal vitamins and other medicines you'll need during your pregnancy for a reduced price (usually between $5 and $10 too).

HMOs tend to be the most economical options of all the traditional insurance choices. The monthly cost for a family is between $200 and $500. If the coverage is offered through your employer, it can be cheaper. Prices also vary according to your age and physical condition.

When you decide to choose an HMO, it's important to know which specialists and hospitals are in its network. Some HMOs are cheap, but their network of doctors and hospitals is limited. You should also make sure the hospital where your doctor delivers babies or where you'd like to deliver is included in your HMO's network.

PPO Insurance

PPO stands for "preferred provider organization." With this type of insurance, you choose the specialist you want to go to, instead of having to first go to your primary care physician for a referral. Along with this greater freedom and flexibility comes greater costs; your monthly premiums are higher and you may have to deal with other expenses such as deductibles and coinsurance.

The deductible is the amount you're required to pay every year out of your own pocket before the insurance coverage begins to pay a percentage of the costs. The higher the deductible, the less you'll pay on your monthly premium. Deductibles range from $100 to $300 for an individual to $500 for a family.

You'll also have to pay the coinsurance. PPOs generally pay for 80 percent of your medical bills; you pay the other 20 percent, called coinsurance. Some but not all insurance policies will cover 100 percent of the delivery expenses.

If you choose a doctor from within the PPO's network, you'll reduce your costs. It's more expensive—but permitted—to choose an out-of-network doctor.

Much like HMOs, when you are covered by a PPO policy through your or your husband's employer, the insurance will usually cover 80 percent of all prenatal care and delivery costs from the beginning of your pregnancy. However, if you buy your PPO coverage directly from an insurance company, there could be a waiting period before the pregnancy expenses are covered or you may have to pay extra fees when you become pregnant. The monthly premiums for PPOs begin at $350 for a couple without children.

POS Insurance

POS stands for "point of service." This type of coverage is similar to the PPO policies. The difference between the plans is that POS coverage includes a primary care physician who coordinates medical services for you, much like in an HMO plan.

Fee for Service

Under a fee-for-service plan, a monthly installment is required. You choose the doctor or hospital you want to go to and your insurance company pays a percentage of the bill, as long as the service is included in the list of covered procedures. Therefore, you'll want to make sure pregnancy procedures are covered and under what circumstances. Deductibles and copays are also part of these plans.

PREGNANCY COVERAGE AND TERMINATION OF EMPLOYMENT

What happens if you lose your job once you've become pregnant or as you're planning to get pregnant? There are laws that will protect you in the following circumstances.

Losing Your Job While Pregnant

A federal law known as COBRA (Consolidated Omnibus Budget Reconciliation Act) requires businesses with group health plans and at least twenty employees to continue medical coverage for you and your family for eighteen months after you've lost your job. The law also says after the death of the employee who was covered or after a divorce, the family can continue to receive medical coverage for another three years. If you decide to use this option, you have to tell your company within sixty days of leaving the job. Keep in mind that your cost will go up because the company isn't responsible for paying its part any longer—you pay for everything.

COBRA Coverage Ends During Your Pregnancy

If after eighteen months of receiving COBRA insurance you or your husband still haven't enrolled in another health plan, HIPAA (Health Insurance Portability and Accountability Act) takes over. This law doesn't guarantee you'll be able to continue with the same health insurance coverage you had before, but it will prohibit insurance companies from denying you coverage just because you're pregnant. Nevertheless, if you're pregnant at the time HIPAA goes into effect, you'll likely have to pay for a more expensive policy.

COBRA Option Is Not Offered in Your Company

If COBRA doesn't apply to your company because it has fewer than twenty employees, you can also search for coverage under HIPAA and convert your group policy into an individual one. And as before, the insurance company you choose must cover you even if you're pregnant, but again, the policy might be more expensive.

PREGNANCY WITHOUT HEALTH INSURANCE

There are several options for having a baby without health insurance. You can choose to get a prenatal package from a private doctor or midwife, or to receive free medical attention from a state program. However, many Latinas earn too much to qualify for Medicaid but can't pay the high costs of an individual insurance policy. If this is your case, you have a few options.

Neighborhood Clinics

These are private, not-for-profit clinics that offer medical attention to uninsured patients. Some three thousand of these clinics are spread across the fifty states and Puerto Rico. You just need to inform them of the number of people in your family and your household income. That information allows the clinic to decide how much to charge you. Costs range from nothing to the full fee that the clinic charges. Prices vary depending on the clinic and the state, but an entire pregnancy package could be around $2,000 to $3,000. These clinics make arrangements with certain hospitals for deliveries. You can get more information by calling 1-888-ASK-HRSA.

Family Planning Clinics

These local organizations offer the most basic and necessary services to people in the community: pregnancy tests, prenatal care, family planning and general medical attention.

A good way to start looking for a community or family planning clinic near you is to call the National Hispanic Prenatal Care Hotline at 1-800-504-7081. It is a nonprofit organization dedicated to helping pregnant Latinas. They will help you find prenatal care near you and will also answer, in English or Spanish, questions you may have about your pregnancy. The only information you need to give is your household income and the zip code where you live. That's it. In the Contact List at the end of the book, you'll find other telephone numbers and addresses to help you find prenatal care in your area.

State Child Health Insurance Program (SCHIP)

SCHIP is a federal program that covers the medical costs of uninsured babies and children. In some states, this program also covers prenatal services and the rest of the family. Even if SCHIP in your state doesn't cover prenatal care, it's still a good program to keep in mind because your babies can be enrolled as soon as they're born. Dial 1-877-KIDS-NOW to be connected with the program in your state.

Other State Programs

Some states offer other options for pregnancy health coverage along with federal programs such as Medicaid or SCHIP. These programs cover people who earn too much to obtain Medicaid and too little to pay for a private policy. A program called Healthy Families exists in many of the states with a large percentage of Latinos. You will get information about what program works in your state and how to subscribe by calling 1-800-311-BABY.

Medicaid

One of the most-used resources pregnant women turn to is Medicaid, the federal program established to help uninsured people. Medicaid pays the entire cost of prenatal care and delivery for women whose household incomes fall below a certain level. The cutoff income is 133% of the federal poverty level for that year.

For example, in 2003, the federal poverty level for a couple was $12,120. A woman who together with her husband earns $16,120 or less (133% of $12,120) has access to the maternity health services covered by Medicaid. Remember, the poverty level is higher the larger the family is, and inflation causes the figure to go up every year.

The federal Medicaid limit (133% of the poverty level) is the absolute minimum established by the federal government. But states can be more generous if they so choose. In reality, many have established the Medicaid qualifying level at 185% of the poverty level. Using the same example, that means that in 2003 a family of two qualified for Medicaid services with a household income of $22,422 or less.

In some states, such as California or Illinois, the figures are even higher (200% of the federal poverty level), which would raise the cutoff income to $24,240. See the Contact List at the end of the book for more information on how to apply for Medicaid in your state.

Many pregnant women use Medicaid. In California, Illinois and Texas, some 40 percent of all deliveries are paid for by Medicaid. A recent study showed there are many more women who could be using free Medicaid services.

Many states offer their Medicaid services through HMOs. Medicaid has an agreement with the HMOs to provide the following services:

• Prenatal care with an obstetrician/gynecologist or midwife
• Blood and urine tests
• Amniocentesis
• Prenatal and delivery education, advice on breastfeeding and baby care
• Delivery care including natural birth centers
• Tubal ligation
• Care for you and the baby up to sixty days after birth (with some exceptions)
• In some cases, transportation to your doctor's visits

Depending on the state in which you live, the services may vary.

If you want to have an epidural during delivery to reduce the pain, check beforehand to make sure the anesthesiologist will accept a Medicaid payment. In the past, there have been some anesthesiologists who have refused to administer an epidural if they weren't paid in cash. This isn't the norm, but unfortunately it's a situation that recurs because some anesthesiologists work independently from the hospital.

In most states, Medicaid coverage is granted almost immediately and the household income level is determined later. The application forms are in English and Spanish, and you'll find Spanish-speaking operators on many Medicaid hotlines.

WIC

WIC (Women, Infants and Children) is another federal program that offers healthy foods and nutrition advice to pregnant women with few resources, women who are nursing, babies and children younger than five. The food is free and obtained through coupons redeemed at authorized supermarkets. Each state has its own rules and regulations governing the household income limits to qualify for WIC. In general, a family of four whose household income is less than $34,040 a year (2003 figures) can expect to qualify for this help. You can obtain information about how to qualify for the program by dialing 1-703-305-1747.

Paying from Your Pocket

Another option is to pay directly for the services of an obstetrician/gynecologist or a midwife. But keep in mind that if there is any complication such as a C-section or if any special treatment is needed, the cost can be very high. The following prices will give you an idea; however, they vary a lot depending on the doctor or midwife and the state and city where you live.

- *Obstetrician/gynecologist.* They offer packages that include prenatal and delivery care. The cost is between $3,000 and $7,000. You have to add the hospital bill ($2,000 to $4,000) as well as the fee for the anesthesiologist ($800 to $3,000), if you use one.
- *Midwife.* Their services are around $2,500 plus the fee for using the hospital or birthing center to deliver. Birthing centers offer prenatal care and delivery packages that run between $3,000 and $5,000 with midwife services included.

MEDICAL COVERAGE FOR YOUR NEWBORN

Most federal insurance programs cover a baby for a brief time following birth. Later they allow you to add your child into the program you're using. Under this system, if your baby needs urgent medical attention after birth, those costs are covered by the government. It's important to know ahead of time what steps you need to take to register your newborn with your insurance carrier, because if you don't fulfill the proper requirements, you could end up paying the bills. With so many things to do after your baby is born, it's easy to forget paperwork like this.

If you're going to include your baby in a PPO-type insurance plan, where you need to pay deductibles for each member of the family, remember you will have to pay a deductible for your baby as well.

If you don't have an insurance policy to include your baby in, the federal SCHIP program is available to you. It covers all medical expenses for your baby, and your other children, for free.

MATERNITY LEAVE AND
WORKPLACE DISCRIMINATION

If you are working, your boss will probably be on the list of people to tell the good news. When and how to tell him or her? For some mothers this could be a difficult moment (see page 173).

Manuela Guardia decided to show her employer a printout of her recent sonogram; they say that *una imagen vale más que mil palabras*, a picture is worth a thousand words. When her boss finally understood that he was looking at the next maternity leave at his company, he barely managed to murmur a not very enthusiastic "Congratulations." Then again, in Manuela's case her boss had been presented with the same news by five employees in two months.

Although creative, this is not the best way to tell your boss. The formal approach might work better for you. However, it's very possible your employer won't react to the news of your pregnancy with champagne and confetti. The first thought that usually passes through a boss's head is "Great. Now I need to find a substitute for three months." Not every boss is that way, but unless your boss is also your husband, keep in mind he likely won't be as *feliz y entusiasmado*, happy and enthusiastic about your pregnancy as you are.

No matter how your boss takes the news, the law is on your side. The Federal Pregnancy Discrimination Act prohibits any form of discrimination against pregnant women in companies that have at least fifteen employees. This means that just because you are pregnant or trying to get pregnant:

- You can't be fired.
- You can't be denied a promotion.
- You can't be forced to take your maternity leave (if you still want to work and are able to do so).
- You can't be denied employment just because you are pregnant.
- You will have all these rights whether you're legally married or not.

This law also spells out that a pregnancy must be considered just like any other illness or temporary medical condition. So, if your workplace offers lighter, easier jobs to employees when they're not feeling well, your boss should offer you the same when you're pregnant, especially if your normal workload includes carrying heavy boxes or other materials, spending hours on end on your feet or other types of strenuous physical activity. Just like someone with a temporary illness, you've got the right to use sick days and be paid for them.

Some states, including California, New Jersey and New York, offer disability pay to employees who can't work because of medical problems, including pregnancy. Depending on the type of work you are doing (see page 8), your doctor can give you a medical leave for temporary disability.

If you think you're suffering from workplace discrimination because of your pregnancy, this is what you should do:

- Write down where and when the discrimination occurred, what was said and who said it.
- Talk to your supervisor or the head of the human resources department at your company and ask about the rules for someone who's got temporary medical problems. Remember, if you find your pregnancy is being treated differently from other temporary illnesses, that's discrimination.
- Talk to your workmates who've been pregnant and find out how they were treated.

- You can file a complaint through a union if you're a member, or through the human resources department. A lawyer can help you through the process, but complaints must be made within 180 days from the moment the discrimination occurred. The Equal Employment Opportunity Commission is another source of information as you begin to formulate your complaint. (See the Contact List.)

In accordance with the Family and Medical Leave Act, you have the right to take as much as twelve unpaid weeks off from work to care for your newborn, adopted baby or foster child. There are some restrictions to this law: you must have worked for a company with at least fifty employees for at least twelve months and put in 1,250 hours a year (about 25 hours a week). The Labor Department can give you more information (1-800-959-3652).

Companies with fewer than fifty employees are not required by law to give you a maternity leave. In this case your doctor can provide you with temporary disability for a few weeks before and after your delivery date. There are five states (California, Hawaii, Rhode Island, New Jersey and New York) where you can receive part of your salary while you are not able to work due to temporary disability related to your pregnancy. This law doesn't prevent your employer from firing you if the company is going through layoffs. However, you can't be fired just because you are on pregnancy-related temporary disability. This is discrimination and a violation of the Federal Pregnancy Discrimination Act.

Some companies outside of the five states listed above have their own programs to cover temporary disability. If your company does not offer maternity leave, find out how it treats other temporary disabilities, such as a heart attack or surgery. Your pregnancy has to be treated the same way.

QUESTIONS FOR INSURANCE COMPANIES COVERING YOUR PREGNANCY

It's important to know what your options are before you choose an insurance company to cover you during your pregnancy. Even when you already have a plan, the rules and regulations covering pregnancy are confusing. The following list of questions can help you choose the right health coverage for you, or figure out exactly what your plan covers now:

- Is maternity coverage part of this plan? Does this plan have a written list showing what medical services are covered as part of maternity?

- Which medical services during pregnancy are not covered?

- Can I switch to another obstetrician/gynecologist or midwife if I'm not satisfied? How many times can I change?

- Which tests will the insurance pay for during my pregnancy (genetic, diabetes, preeclampsia, fetal stress, etc.)?

- Are medications included in this plan?

- Is the hospital where I want to deliver included in the plan?

- Will this plan cover deliveries in birthing centers or at home? Are the services of midwives covered?

- Are there any forms to fill out or procedures to follow before being admitted to the hospital?

- Is the hospital anesthesiologist included in the insurance plan's network, or will those charges have to be paid separately?

- What types of anesthesia are covered?

- How long can I stay in the hospital after a normal birth and after a cesarean?

- Is prenatal education covered? How about education on delivery and nursing? Are breast milk pumps included in this coverage? What other types of equipment needed at home are included?

- What are the rules regarding high-risk pregnancies?

- How long will the baby be covered after it's born?

- What is this plan's quality of service rating? (You can find this out yourself through the National Committee for Quality Assurance; see page 362.)

You should carefully read all documents explaining what services are covered by your policy and get any questions you have answered. Don't worry about how simple your question may seem. Don't be fooled by a promotional brochure. That's not the same as the fine print found on the official insurance policy paperwork. Most insurance companies provide toll-free telephone numbers you can call to get your questions answered.

❧

DOCTORS AND CULTURAL DIFFERENCES

A nurse walks into the waiting room reading off the clipboard she's carrying. The nine women in the waiting room and their six partners look in her direction.

"Luisa Martinez," the nurse calls out, without looking up from the clipboard.

Luisa hurriedly gets up from her seat and walks toward the half-open door. The nurse tells her to sit in a different chair, where another nurse takes her blood pressure; then Luisa is shown to a scale, where she is weighed. Next, Luisa is given a plastic cup and sent to the bathroom to give a urine sample. Then the first nurse gives Luisa a disposable gown and tells her to go to examining room number four, take her clothes off and change into the gown. Luisa follows the instructions and waits sitting on the examining table. The examining room doesn't have much in it, only a stool, a table with medical instruments on it and a tiny sink. The door is ajar and Luisa can hear the doctor's voice. Ten, fifteen, twenty minutes go by, and still no doctor. Luisa *se siente mareada,* feels a little dizzy. She hasn't eaten breakfast because her stomach's upset. Also, her husband was not able to come with her to the appointment, and she misses him. All she wants to do is see the doctor to make sure everything is fine with her pregnancy. Luisa gets up and peeks out the door. She sees two of the other women who were with her in the waiting room. They're also sitting in examining rooms, wearing disposable gowns. The doctor walks from one examining room to the other, giving instructions to the nurses.

Luisa returns to the examining table, sits down and waits another ten minutes. Finally the doctor shows up. He says hello without looking up and takes her chart from the pocket on the door.

"Good afternoon. What can I do for you?"

Luisa hesitates. She doesn't feel very good about this doctor; there's something about him that makes her feel uncomfortable. She thinks he could be a little *más simpático,* more friendly, chat a little bit after making her wait for so long.

"I think I'm pregnant. The home test was positive," she says.

"Date of last period?" the doctor asks.

Luisa answers all the questions. The doctor tells her to lie down and gives her a pelvic examination. He tells her that her cervix is closed, then he calls a nurse, orders a blood test for Luisa and writes a few lines on her chart.

"Any questions?"

The truth is, Luisa has thousands of questions. This is her first pregnancy and she's a little scared. But this doctor *tan apresurado*, with this hurried, unfriendly bedside manner, doesn't seem to be the one to ask.

"We'll see you in a month," the doctor says.

He gives Luisa a prescription for prenatal vitamins and says goodbye without even a handshake.

Luisa gets dressed holding back tears. This is the doctor her insurance plan has assigned her. He's got a good reputation and the insurance company said he's efficient. But Luisa can't even imagine coming back to this man month after month after month. And the thought of him delivering her baby is unbearable.

The health insurance system in the United States doesn't leave much time for developing the patient-doctor relationship Latinos are used to. Doctors have to see a huge number of patients to profit from their practices. But time isn't the only problem. The style of doctors not familiar with Latino culture can be shocking for us. What's considered efficient in Anglo and other cultures is sometimes interpreted as indifference or even *mala educación*, rudeness, in Latino culture.

In the traditional Latino way, a nurse takes the patient to the doctor's office individually. The doctor welcomes the patient and her companions with a friendly handshake and then sits down behind a desk so that they can talk for a little while. Then the doctor will begin to inquire about the reason for the visit, and finally he/she will do an exam, generally in a different room, if that's necessary. Afterward, the patient returns to the desk at the office, where the doctor will discuss the diagnosis and give instructions on what to do and what to take. When it's time to go, the doctor will stand up, shake hands with the patient and her companions and say goodbye.

Especially for first-generation Latinos, the doctor-patient relationship is considered a personal, intimate one. The more distant style some doctors in the United States have can be interpreted as a sign of indifference. Add to that the system of multiple examining rooms, and the feeling is that of being rushed and having no personal interaction whatsoever.

But it's important to remember when going to see a doctor from a different culture that the more distant style doesn't mean *que usted no le importa*, that he/she doesn't care or that he/she won't give you excellent medical advice and service.

In the United States, most doctors are not Latinos, so there's a good chance yours won't be. Of course, this does not mean that all doctors from other cultures have a cold style or even that all Latino doctors are warm and friendly. However there are certain general cultural differences.

- Efficiency is held in high regard in American culture. From that point of view, a non-Latino doctor might think a friendly conversation at the beginning of your visit that doesn't have anything to do with your medical condition might be a waste of your time.

- Most of us Latinos feel more comfortable with less physical space between us.

- Touching the person you're speaking with isn't so common among non-Latinos.

- Smiling or looking another person in the eyes while talking is not that common among non-Latinos either. The absence of all these physical signs of communication could be interpreted—consciously or unconsciously—by a Latino as a *falta de interés*, lack of interest on the part of the doctor.

- Confidentiality is another value traditional American doctors revere. Many patients prefer to make decisions about their health on their own and demand confidentiality from their doctors. We Latinos are different; we might like to include family members on our visits to the doctor as well as when we make decisions about medical treatments.

- Latinos are comfortable using home remedies such as herbs or other traditional, spiritual beliefs to help us feel better. Doctors with a different cultural background might not understand or share these beliefs and customs. All these cultural differences can create *malentendidos*, misunderstandings, and make the doctor-patient relationship a difficult one.

In other words, for many Latinos establishing a personal relationship is the key to feeling comfortable with a doctor. I have to admit I'm one of them, especially when I'm pregnant, because I'm sensitive about everything. When I'm going to have a baby, I need my doctor to pamper me a little more than usual and answer all my questions patiently. I consider *un trato amable y amistoso*, a warm, friendly exchange with my doctor, part of my prenatal care.

The minute my friend Ana Maria Ceballos found out she was pregnant, her top priority was finding a Latino doctor. She prefers a doctor who shares certain cultural values.

> "I like the treatment I get from Latino doctors better. *Me siento más cercana*, I feel closer to a Latino doctor, and I need that during my pregnancy. Besides, what would happen if in the middle of my delivery I am suddenly unable to express myself clearly in English? I need someone who can understand me *en todo momento*, at all times. With a Latino doctor I feel I have one hundred percent understanding. I don't want to put myself in a situation where I know I am going to feel tense."

If a personal relationship with your doctor during your pregnancy is important to you, you may feel more comfortable with a Latino doctor. Although finding a Latino obstetrician/gynecologist is no guarantee of perfect medical treatment, you will at least have found someone familiar with your culture. Don't forget that he/she will be taking care of you in one of the most important moments of your life.

Unfortunately, Latino doctors are scarce in the United States, compared to the ever-growing Hispanic population. Still, it is possible to find a Latino doctor who will be included in your health insurance plan.

- If you've already got health insurance, call the customer service telephone number to get a list of Latino doctors.
- Search for Hispanic last names in the service provider list your insurance company distributes to customers. HMOs usually allow patients to switch doctors once or twice, until you feel comfortable.
- Search through the yellow pages for doctors with Hispanic last names.
- Find a community clinic that offers services in Spanish.
- Call the American Medical Association or the American College of

Obstetricians and Gynecologists (see Contact List) to help you find a Latino doctor in your area.

If for whatever reason you can't find a Latino doctor close to home, the following ideas might be helpful as you try to establish an open line of communication with your obstetrician/gynecologist.

- Before going to the doctor, write down a brief list of questions and concerns you have regarding your pregnancy, starting with the most important.

- Be on time, though you'll usually have to wait. The nurse will appreciate your respect for the office schedule.

- Remember your doctor usually has a predetermined amount of time to spend with you (usually ten to fifteen minutes). If there's not a problem, he/she will try to stick to the schedule.

- It's important to *not* interpret a doctor's distant style as a lack of interest. Instead, think of it this way: the doctor only has a limited amount of time with you and he/she wants to get as much information from you as he/she can.

- Ask! Don't hold anything back. The doctor won't interpret your questions as a *falta de confianza*, lack of confidence in his/her diagnosis or treatment.

- If for any reason you're not comfortable with the doctor's treatment or diagnosis, tell him/her and explain why. Don't sit quietly because *tiene que mostrar educación,* you think that's the polite thing to do. Perhaps there's something the doctor doesn't know about you.

- If there is a medical problem and your family is going to participate in the decision of what to do about it, explain to the doctor that in our culture, important decisions are made by the entire family. Remember, Anglo doctors are more accustomed to dealing with patients who favor privacy.

- If you or any of your relatives don't speak English or you don't feel comfortable speaking English with your doctor, when you make an appointment ask if there's an interpreter available. Bilingual staff members are common in many hospitals and clinics, and according to the law, if the institution receives federal funding, it must provide you with an interpreter.

And more than anything else, tell your obstetrician/gynecologist everything you consider relevant to your pregnancy. Don't assume that he/she already knows. You are dealing with somebody who has a different cultural perspective. The more information you can give him/her about your expectations, the more attention you will get.

3

※

A Healthy Pregnancy

A positive pregnancy test brings lots of questions and concerns to the mind of a pregnant woman, and nutrition is one of the most common. You might be asking yourself questions like "What should I eat now?" Maybe you are watching what you eat, trying not to gain too much weight. Or maybe you're saying to yourself—as I did during my first pregnancy—"Hooray! Now I can eat whatever I like!" In my case, first the morning sickness and then the diabetes forced me to abandon that idea pretty quickly.

WEIGHT GAIN DURING PREGNANCY

Unfortunately for those of us who enjoy eating, the ideas that some of our grandmothers, mothers and aunts had about *comer por dos*, eating for two (or even for three) during a pregnancy have been disproved by doctors a while ago. Of course, there will always be exceptions to the rule, because some mothers do indeed need to gain weight to ensure a healthy pregnancy. But the average weight a woman should gain during her pregnancy is:

- 28 to 40 pounds if you're below your recommended weight
- 25 to 35 pounds if you're at your recommended weight
- 15 to 25 pounds if you're above your recommended weight

These guidelines were established ten years ago by the American College of Obstetricians and Gynecologists. Nowadays some doctors think that this is too much weight to gain; depending on your personal circumstances, your doctor might give you figures closer to 18 to 20 pounds.

However, more important than the amount of weight you gain is how you gain your weight. The recommended pattern is to gain three to four pounds during the first trimester and then three to four more pounds for each month until delivery. Often the weight gain is even greater during the final months, because that's when the baby's growth is greatest.

You can achieve this rate of weight gain by eating around 150 extra calories a day during the first trimester and between 300 and 350 extra calories a day during the second and third trimesters. To give you an idea of how much more food that is, you can get 150 calories from one yogurt and a piece of fruit, and 300 calories from half a cup of beans and one tortilla.

The 25 pounds the average woman gains during a pregnancy are spread out more or less like this:

- Baby—8 pounds
- Placenta—1.5 pounds
- Amniotic fluid—2 pounds
- Breasts—2 pounds
- Uterus—2.5 pounds
- Fat, blood volume and water retention—8 pounds

If you're already a little overweight when you get pregnant, remember that the numbers on your scale are going to go up almost every time you step on it. Weight-loss diets during pregnancy are not a good idea. When you lose weight, your body secretes ketones, a chemical that's harmful to the fetus and can affect normal fetal development. If you suffer from obesity, your doctor will tell you what kind of diet you should follow during your pregnancy.

NUTRITION DURING PREGNANCY

"The very same day I found out I was pregnant, I began to throw up like crazy," says Vicky Ferrer, mother of a little girl, describing her not-so-pleasant memories of pregnancy. "Anything will trigger it. *Me hablaban y vomitaba*, just a person would talk to me, and I'd vomit. *Nada*, nothing helped. And it got even worse when I didn't eat. In fact, the only things that would make me feel even a little bit better were *frituras*, fried foods. Everything I ate had to be fried; otherwise I'd throw it up. Every half an hour I had to put something fried in my mouth, or else a wave of nausea would come over me."

Dana Morales, who is now three months pregnant, cannot tolerate certain smells. "If after having breakfast I smell a cigarette or a sweet perfume, *me descompongo*, I feel sick to my stomach. Any strange smell gives me nausea. If it wasn't for this, I wouldn't have any problem. Also, I can only eat salty things. I don't like sweets anymore."

If you are going through the first weeks of your pregnancy, it's very possible that you are having trouble with morning sickness and eating, or maybe *le tomó manía*, you can't stand certain foods or smells, or like Vicky, you can only eat certain things.

The nausea most women suffer during the first months of pregnancy can put an end to the most healthy nutrition plan. Who wants to eat a nice bowl of vegetable soup when merely the smell of a kitchen sends you running to the bathroom? Fortunately, your body has a sufficient amount of nutrients in reserve during the first trimester so the baby can still grow according to schedule. (See page 152)

When this stage goes away (and it almost always does, but unfortunately there are women who experience nausea during the whole pregnancy—my heart goes out to them), remember that 300 extra calories a day is what your body needs from now on. But just as important as the number of calories you eat in a day is the nutrition you get from them.

---

§

The key to healthy eating while you're pregnant is in the quality, not the quantity, of the foods you eat.

Eating healthy foods is one of the best things you can do for your baby during pregnancy because every day, the menu you choose to follow is the same one your baby's eating from. Eating well isn't just good for the baby, it's also good for you. As it grows, your baby draws not only on the nutrients you pass on to him or her from the food you eat, but also from your bones and muscles. These nine months are like a marathon for your body; in addition to performing its normal functions, it has also got to nourish and grow a little person inside you. The better the food you eat, the more likely it is you'll cross the finish line in good shape.

The following diet provides between 1,800 and 2,200 daily calories, depending on the number of portions you eat. It has the right amount of protein, carbohydrates and fats a pregnant woman needs.

1,800 TO 2,200 DAILY CALORIES

- 7 to 9 servings of cereals, grains and breads (carbohydrates)
- 3 to 5 servings of vegetables (3 daily servings of vegetables rich in vitamin A or C)
- 2 to 3 servings of fruit (2 daily servings of fruit rich in vitamin A or C)
- 4 servings of milk (milk, yogurt, cheese, etc.)
- 3 to 4 servings of protein (meat, fish, eggs, etc.)
- 2 to 3 servings of fat (1 serving = 1 teaspoon of oil, butter, mayonnaise, etc.)
- 6 to 8 glasses of liquids (not more than one soda a day)

For example, on an 1,800-calorie diet you can eat:

- ½ cup rice and 1 medium-sized potato
- 1 slice of whole-wheat bread, 2 corn or flour tortillas, ½ cup cereal and 3 crackers
- 1 cup raw vegetables (lettuce, tomato, carrots, etc.) and 1 cup cooked vegetables (broccoli, spinach, peppers, beets, etc.)
- 2 medium-sized fruits (grapefruits, apples, melons, peaches, etc.)
- 2 glasses of milk, 1 yogurt and 1 ounce of cheese
- 2 eggs, 3 ounces of meat or fish and ½ cup beans
- 2 teaspoons of oil or butter
- 1 soda, 1 cup of coffee or tea and 6 glasses of water

This is only an example. Using the following tables, you can create a menu that suits your tastes. I find it easiest to count my portions with an exchange table like the one below. Exchange tables group together different kinds of foods with similar nutritional values that you can combine to vary your diet. You can find very detailed lists at bookstores. This one (see page 42) is adapted from the one published by the American Diabetes Association and the Mexican System for Exchange Foods.

So for example, to choose your carbohydrates go to the list, choose a food that you like and check the serving size. A carbohydrates serving could be:

- ½ cup breakfast cereal
- 1 corn tortilla
- 1 medium-sized potato
- ½ cup rice
- ½ cup pumpkin
- 6 crackers

If you are eating seven daily servings of carbohydrates, you could eat these six foods or some other six you choose. You can also choose two or more servings of one food, but in order to have nutritional variety it is better to choose different types. You choose proteins, dairy products, vegetables, fruits and fats the same way.

During pregnancy, it's important to choose from certain categories of fruits and vegetables every day. They contain vitamins and minerals necessary for you and your baby's health. Also, some foods already have fats included in their preparation or composition, so when you eat them, they will count toward your fat serving for that day. Other prepared foods will include servings of carbohydrates, protein and fat all rolled into one. You'll also find the exchange portions for fast foods.

Even though this appears a little confusing at first, within a week you'll be an expert on nutritional exchanges. It's an efficient and healthy system for controlling what you eat that you can also follow when you're not pregnant.

Note: One ounce equals 28 grams.

Carbohydrates (6–11 Daily Servings)

It's best to vary your carbohydrates as much as possible, choosing from the different categories. Choose daily one serving of grains, another of cereals and another of starchy vegetables. Whole-wheat breads and corn tortillas are better options than white-flour ones.

BREADS AND TORTILLAS
- *Arepa* without cheese—½ *arepa*
- Bagel—½ bagel
- Bread, white, whole-wheat, pumpernickel—1 slice
- Buns for hot dogs or hamburgers—½ bun
- English muffin—½ muffin
- Corn bread—1 2-inch square (+ 1 fat)
- Corn tortilla (yellow, blue or black corn)—1 6-inch tortilla
- Croutons—1 cup (+ 1 fat)
- White or whole-wheat tortillas—1 7–8-inch tortilla
- *Gordita*—½ *gordita*
- Jalapeño bread—1 small slice (+ 2 fats)
- Low-fat bread—2 slices
- Pancake—2 4-inch pancakes (+ 1 fat)
- *Pupusas* (no filling)—½ *pupusa* (+ 1 fat)
- Sweet bread (*media noche*)—½ slice
- Taco shell—1 6-inch piece (+ 1 fat)

CRACKERS
- Animal crackers—6 crackers
- Crackers filled with cheese or peanut butter—3 crackers (+ 1 fat)
- Graham crackers (2½-inch squares)—3 crackers
- Melba toast—4 slices
- Round appetizer crackers—6 crackers (+ 1 fat)
- Saltine crackers—6 crackers
- Whole-wheat crackers, no fat—3 crackers

SNACKS
- Fig bars—2 pieces
- French fries—10–15 fries (+ 1 fat)
- Nuts—4 halves (+ 1 fat)
- Plantain chips—12 pieces (+ 2 fats)
- Popcorn (already popped), no fat—3 cups
- Potato chips, no fat—12–18 chips

- Pretzels—¾ ounce
- Refried flour *chicharrón (chicharrón de harina enchilado)*—1 ounce (+ 1 fat)
- Rice cakes—2 4-inch cakes
- Tortilla chips—6–12 chips (+ 2 fats)

CEREALS
- Breakfast cereal, no sugar—½ cup
- Cereal bar—1 bar (+ 1 fat)
- Cheerios—½ cup
- Corn flakes—½ cup
- Flour for cooking—3 tablespoons
- Granola (no fat)—¼ cup
- Muesli—¼ cup
- Oats—½ cup
- Oat flakes—½ cup
- Pasta—½ cup
- Puffed cereal—1½ cups

GRAINS
- Beans—⅓ cup
- Chickpeas—½ cup
- Corn, yellow or white—½ cup
- *Gandules*—⅓ cup
- Lentils—½ cup
- Rice (cooked), white, brown or wild—½ cup

STARCHY VEGETABLES *(Choose at least two times a week)*
- Pumpkin—½ cup
- Sweet potato—½ cup

OTHER STARCHY VEGETABLES
- *Chayote*—½ cup
- *Jícama*—½ cup
- Mashed potato—½ cup
- Mixed vegetables (corn, peas and other vegetables)—1 cup
- Peas—½ cup

- Potato, boiled or roasted—1 small
- Yucca—½ cup

Vegetables (3–5 Daily Servings)

In general, vegetable servings are equivalent to 1 cup raw and ½ cup cooked. A serving of vegetable juice such as tomato or carrot juice is ½ cup. You should eat at least one serving of raw vegetables every day. Vegetables high in vitamins A and C are orange, red, yellow or dark green. Vitamins A and C are important for a healthy pregnancy, so it's recommended that you eat vegetables with these colors every day.

VEGETABLES RICH IN VITAMIN A *(Choose one a day)*
- Carrots
- Red peppers
- Tomato, *jitomate, jitomatillo*
- Salsa—¼ cup
- Squash

VEGETABLES RICH IN VITAMIN C *(Choose one a day)*
- Asparagus
- Broccoli
- Brussels sprouts
- Dark green lettuce
- Endives
- Green beans
- Green peppers
- Green tomato
- *Nopalitos*—1 cup, raw or cooked
- Spinach
- Swiss chard

OTHER VEGETABLES
- Alfalfa sprouts
- Artichokes
- Beets—¼ cup, cooked or raw
- Cabbage, green or purple
- Cauliflower

- *Chilacayote*
- Cucumber
- Eggplant
- Hearts of palm—2 pieces
- *Maguey* or yucca flowers—¼ cup
- Mushrooms
- Onion—¼ cup cooked or 1 medium-sized raw
- Pumpkin flowers
- Soy sprouts
- Turnip
- *Verdolaga*
- Watercress
- *Xoconostle*—3 pieces

Fruits (2–4 Daily Servings)
One serving of fruit equals:

- One small to medium-sized piece of fresh fruit
- ½ cup canned fruit or fruit juice
- ¼ cup dried fruit

As is the case with vegetables, you need to eat fruits with a high vitamin A and C content.

FRUITS (*Choose two daily*)
- Apricots, dried—8 halves
- Apricots, fresh—4 whole
- Grapefruit—½ grapefruit
- Mandarin—2 small
- Mango—½ fruit
- Melon (cantaloupe)—1 cup, cubed
- Nectarine—1 medium
- Orange—1 medium
- Orange or grapefruit juice—½ cup
- Papaya—1 cup, cubed
- Peach—1 medium
- Peach, dried—2 halves
- Strawberries—1¼ cups

OTHER FRUITS
- Apple juice—½ cup
- Banana—1 small
- Berries—¾ cup
- Blackberries—¾ cup
- Cherimoya fruit—⅓ medium
- Cherries—12 pieces
- Dates, pitted—3 pieces
- Fresh pineapple—¾ cup
- Grape juice—⅓ cup
- *Mamey*—⅓ medium
- *Maracuyá*—3 pieces
- Medlar—25 pieces
- Prunes—2 small
- Prunes, dried—3 pieces
- Raisins—2 tablespoons
- Raspberries—1 cup
- Tamarind, pulp—⅓ cup
- *Tecojote*—2 pieces
- *Tuna*—2 pieces
- Watermelon—1 slice or 1¼ cups

Dairy Products (4 Daily Servings)

Milk and yogurt are great sources of calcium. Cheeses will give variety to your dairy servings, but some of them have lots of calories and there are others that you should avoid during pregnancy (see page 4), unless you cook them first.

MILK AND YOGURT
- Evaporated milk—½ cup (+ 1 fat)
- Nonfat yogurt—1 cup
- Powdered milk—½ cup (+ 1 fat)
- Kefir, *jocoque*—1 cup
- Skim or 1 percent milk—1 cup
- Soy milk—1 cup

- Whole milk—1 cup (+ 1 fat)
- Yogurt, frozen, nonfat, no sugar—½ cup
- Yogurt, frozen, with fat and sugar—¼ cup (+ 1 fat)
- Yogurt, nonfat, or low-fat, fruit-flavored and aspartame-sweetened—1 cup
- Yogurt with fruit—1 cup (+ 2 carbohydrates)

LESS FATTY CHEESES
- Cottage cheese—¾ cup
- Feta—1 ounce
- *Fresco* (fresh Mexican cheese)—1 ounce
- *De hoja*—1 ounce
- Mozzarella—1 ounce
- *Oaxaca*—1 ounce
- *Panela*—1 ounce
- Parmesan, grated—2 tablespoons
- White Mexican cheese (*queso blanco*)—1 ounce

FATTY CHEESES
- American—1 ounce
- *Asadero*—1 ounce
- Blue cheese—1 ounce
- Brie, Camembert—1 ounce
- Cheddar—1 ounce
- *Chihuahua*—1 ounce
- *Cotija*—3 teaspoons
- Cream cheese—1 ounce
- Monterey Jack and jalapeño pepper—1 ounce
- Provolone—1 ounce
- Swiss—1 ounce
- Yellow cheese—1 ounce

Proteins (3–4 Daily Servings)

Some sources of protein have a high fat content. So if you don't need to gain weight quickly, it's better not to eat these foods more than once or twice a week. One serving of meat or fish is 3 ounces.

LESS FATTY MEATS AND FISH
- Beef
- Chicken or turkey without the skin
- Fish (salmon, sardines, tilapia, hake, etc.)
- Lamb
- Shellfish
- Shrimp

FATTY MEATS
- Bacon
- Bologna
- *Carnitas*
- Ham
- *Machaca*
- *Menudo*
- Pork
- Salami
- Sausage
- Turkey or chicken with the skin

FOODS THAT CAN BE USED AS PROTEIN SERVINGS
- Beans, lentils, etc.—1 cup
- Cottage cheese, low-fat or nonfat—¾ cup
- Eggs—2 large
- Low-fat cheese—3 ounces
- Low-fat yogurt—1¼ cups
- Tofu—1 cup

Fats (3–4 Daily Servings)

Fats such as lard, oil, mayonnaise, cheese sauces and others are some of the most tasty things on the menu . . . but they're also full of calories. So if you're trying to watch your weight during your pregnancy, you should cut back on fatty foods. Limit but don't eliminate them, because fats are also necessary for a healthy pregnancy. You can always choose to cook with vegetable oils such as olive oil or margarine instead of animal fats such as lard and butter. This is good for your cholesterol count as well.

FATS

- Alfredo sauce—1 teaspoon
- Avocado—⅛ (1 ounce)
- Blue cheese—½ tablespoon
- Caesar dressing—1 teaspoon
- French dressing—1 teaspoon
- Grated coconut—2 tablespoons
- Guacamole—2 teaspoons
- Hollandaise sauce—1 tablespoon
- Lard—1 teaspoon
- Margarine—1 teaspoon
- Mayonnaise—1 teaspoon
- Nuts—4 halves
- Oil (avocado, coconut, corn, olive, etc.)—1 teaspoon
- Olives—8
- Peanuts, toasted, with chile—2 teaspoons
- Peanut butter—1 teaspoon
- Ranch dressing—½ tablespoon
- Sour cream, nonfat—3 tablespoons
- Sour cream, whole—2 tablespoons

Liquids

During pregnancy, the volume of your blood will increase considerably. That's why it's doubly important to drink the recommended eight glasses of water a day. It's not a really pleasant thought if you're already waking up twice in the middle of the night to go to the bathroom, or if you have to stop at a gas station on the way home from work. But besides giving your baby what he/she needs, drinking more water helps you avoid retaining water in your legs, a common complaint among pregnant women. Even though it may not seem to make much sense, the more water you drink, the more water you eliminate from your body. Of your eight glasses of liquid a day, one can be a soda and another can be coffee or fruit juice.

Prepared Foods

Here you will find the serving equivalents for many of the prepared foods available in your supermarket. All you have to do is count the carbohydrates, proteins and fats you see in parentheses toward your daily serving count.

- Bean burrito—1 medium (2 carbohydrates, 1 protein, 2 fats)
- Bean soup—1 cup (1 carbohydrate, 1 protein)
- Chili con carne—1 cup (2 carbohydrates, 2 fats, 2 protein)
- *Chimichanga*—5 ounces (2 carbohydrates, 1 protein, 2 fats)
- Enchilada, beef or chicken—10 ounces (3 carbohydrates, 1 protein, 1 fat)
- Soft tacos—2 (3 carbohydrates, 2 proteins, 2 fats)
- Spaghetti or pasta, canned—½ cup (1 carbohydrate, 1 fat)
- Stuffed chile—1 medium (1 carbohydrate, 1 protein, 1 fat)
- *Tamales*—6 ounces (1 carbohydrate, 2 fats)
- Vegetable soup, canned—1 cup (1 carbohydrate)

Fast Foods

- Burger, regular—1 medium (2 carbohydrates, 2 proteins)
- Hot dog with bun—1 medium (1 carbohydrate, 1 protein, 1 fat)
- Pizza, thin crust—¼ 10-inch pizza (2 carbohydrates, 2 proteins, 1 fat)
- Pizza, pepperoni, sausage, etc.—¼ 10-inch pizza (2 carbohydrates, 2 proteins, 2 fats)
- Subway sandwich—1 6-inch sandwich (3 carbohydrates, 1 vegetable, 2 proteins, 1 fat)
- Taco, fried shell—1 6-ounce taco (2 carbohydrates, 2 proteins, 2 fats)
- Taco, soft—1 3-ounce taco (1 carbohydrate, 1 protein, 1 fat)

You might have noticed that in all these food tables there are not a lot of sweets. That's right. Those little delicacies don't have a lot of nutritional value for your baby, and if, like many of us, you have a tendency toward diabetes, sweets will make this disease much worse (see Chapter 4). But let's be real. If there is not a health problem, who doesn't want some sweets here and there? Here you have a list for those *momentos dulces*, sweet moments. As you can see, the amounts are little because the calories are big. You can exchange sweets for carbohydrates, subtracting the fats from your daily allowance.

Desserts

- *Ate*—½ ounce
- Brownie—2-inch square (+ 1 fat)
- *Buñuelo*—·1 medium (+ 1 fat)
- *Cajeta*—2 teaspoons
- Cake—1-inch square (+ 1 fat)
- Chocolate chip cookies—3 pieces (+ 1 fat)
- Chocolate or vanilla milk—1 cup
- Chocolate syrup—1 tablespoon
- *Churro*—1 medium (+ 1 fat)
- Cinnamon rolls—1 roll
- Coffee creamer—1½ tablespoons (+ 1 fat)
- Condensed milk—1 tablespoon
- Doughnut covered with sugar—1 ounce (+ 1 fat)
- Filled cookies, Oreo type—2 cookies (+ 1 fat)
- Frozen yogurt, no fat, no sugar—½ cup
- Fruit pie—1 thin slice (+ 1 fat)
- Ice cream with fat and sugar—¼ cup (+ 2 fats)
- Ice cream, no fat, no sugar—½ cup
- Jams—1 tablespoon
- *María* cookies—5 pieces
- Peanut *palanqueta*—½ piece (+ 1 fat)
- *Piloncillo*—2 teaspoons
- Sweet bread—1-inch square (+ 1 fat)

VITAMINS

One of the first things your doctor will prescribe for you is prenatal vitamins. There's a little controversy over whether they really make any difference. But while the debate continues, it seems as though an extra vitamin pill doesn't do any harm, especially to cover for those days where your diet isn't as healthy as you'd like it to be. Nevertheless, it's extremely important not to take too many vitamins because a vitamin overdose can cause birth defects. Vitamin supplements, even if they are made from herbs, and especially those known as "megavitamins," are not recommended during pregnancy. The vitamins sold with a doctor's prescription tend to be more appropriate for pregnancy than the ones sold over the counter. If you do buy over-the-counter vitamins, look for the ones made for pregnant women.

Vitamins in pill form are a good complement to a healthy diet. But the best way to get the vitamins you need is through the foods you eat. The list that follows details which vitamins are most important for pregnant women and the foods they're found in.

Folate or Folic Acid

Ideally folic acid should start to be taken three months before getting pregnant (see page 2), but if you have just discovered that you are going to have a baby, you should take it anyway. Lack of folic acid in pregnant women is related to birth defects in the spine and nervous system of the fetus.

Folate or folic acid is found in oranges, green leafy vegetables, beans, peas and fortified breads, and breakfast cereals.

Vitamin A

Vitamin A is very important for the growth and development of the baby's teeth and bones. However, when taken in excessive amounts, it can cause problems in the fetus. You must take care with certain medicines (such as Retin-A) that can increase the level of vitamin A in your bloodstream. Also, make sure you are not taking a vitamin or herbal supplement that contains more than 5,000 IU of vitamin A. In addition to increasing the risk of birth defects, an overdose of this vitamin can make you sick to your stomach and give you headaches.

Vitamin A is found in fatty fish, egg yolks, liver, butter, cheese, green vegetables such as broccoli and spinach, carrots, and fruits such as mangoes and peaches.

B Vitamins

The vitamins that form the B group include B_1 (thiamine), B_2 (riboflavin), B_3 (niacin), B_5 (pantothenic acid), B_6 (pyriodoxine) and B_9 (folic acid). These vitamins are key to many stages of your baby's growth and development. For example, B vitamins help with the creation of red blood cells and the development of the nervous system. Not enough vitamins from the B group seems to make a mother feel more nauseous during pregnancy.

There are B vitamins in milk, meat, fish, cheese, dried fruits, grains, cereals, potatoes, avocados, oranges, grapefruit, pineapple, mushrooms and tomatoes.

Vitamin C

Vitamin C is needed to maintain healthy muscles and a strong immune system (what the body uses to fight off infections). Vitamin C is eliminated from the body almost immediately, so you have to eat foods rich in vitamin C several times a day. These include oranges, grapefruit, lemons, strawberries, papaya, broccoli, green peppers and tomatoes. Milk, eggs and fish are also good sources.

Vitamin D

This vitamin helps with the absorption of calcium and therefore helps to build strong bones and teeth for the baby as well as protecting yours. A vitamin D deficiency can cause rickets in newborns. Good sources are fortified milk and dairy products such as cheese and butter, as well as eggs, and fish such as sardines, salmon and herring.

Vitamin E

Vitamin E is key to good neurological development and helps to prevent cellular deterioration. It's been proven to help prevent miscarriage, and in high doses (administered by a doctor only), it can control preeclampsia or high blood pressure during pregnancy.

Vitamin E in its natural form is found in avocados, broccoli, spinach, sweet potatoes, asparagus, tomatoes and blackberries.

Vitamin K

This vitamin is needed for the formation of certain proteins and therefore for the healthy development of your baby. It also helps your baby's blood clot normally. Newborn babies don't have this vitamin in their bloodstreams yet, so doctors will give them a shot of it in case they have some internal bleeding during birth. Vitamin K is passed to the baby through mother's milk. Green leafy vegetables, fruits and nuts contain vitamin K.

MINERALS

Minerals are as important as vitamins for a healthy pregnancy. In fact, during pregnancy, a mother's ability to absorb some minerals increases.

Calcium is critical for mother and baby. It is necessary for the formation of strong teeth and bones. If a baby doesn't get enough calcium through your diet, it will begin to drain it from your bones. That's why it's important for a mother to increase the number of calcium-rich foods she eats during pregnancy and while she's nursing. Some good sources of calcium include milk and milk products, sardines and green leafy vegetables such as spinach and broccoli. If, like many Latinas, you have lactose intolerance and can't digest milk or dairy products, you'll have to take calcium supplements.

Sodium (salt) is another necessary mineral. In the past doctors recommended limiting sodium intake to prevent fluid retention during pregnancy, but now, because we know that a pregnant woman's blood volume increases so dramatically, scientists say a moderate amount of sodium in the diet is beneficial.

Iodine is usually present in small amounts in the body, but during pregnancy this mineral is in greater demand. The thyroid gland needs iodine to make the hormones necessary for the mother's body to function properly. For the first three months of pregnancy the fetus doesn't have a thyroid gland and gets its iodine from the mother. That's why it's important to use iodized salt.

Other minerals important during pregnancy are iron, phosphorus, magnesium and potassium found mainly in green leafy vegetables, grains and eggs.

EXERCISE DURING PREGNANCY

Studies say two of every five Latinas don't exercise regularly. Maybe. *Hay tanto que hacer,* we've got too much to do during the day and when we get home, there's only more: things to take care of, make dinner . . . you know the routine. So when all that's finished, many of us will probably like to spend time *en familia,* with our families rather than alone in the gym lifting weights or doing aerobics. Nevertheless, exercising during pregnancy is an investment that will pay off in the long run, provided you have your doctor's seal of approval.

Although now is not the time to join a soccer team, in moderation exercise does nothing but help. In case you were a serious athlete before you got pregnant, you can still continue to play your favorite sports if you're careful. Activities where you can fall or bump into something, such as skiing or horseback riding or even cycling, aren't a good idea if you're not used to them. But there are other sports you can practice that will help you through your pregnancy.

During her second pregnancy Laura Suito exercised regularly. "With this baby I walked and swam a lot. I walked around the mall or in places with air-conditioning *para no acalorarme,* so I would not get overheated. I strolled a lot with my husband, and I swam up to the last week. This delivery was much easier than the first one."

Again, before beginning any physical activity, you must talk to your doctor about what's appropriate. Women who have had several spontaneous abortions or premature births or who have heart disease may be advised not to take up too much exercise when they're pregnant. If you suffer from diabetes or hypertension during pregnancy, you ought to talk to your doctor about what type of exercise is appropriate and how long you should do it, because that will influence your illness.

The benefits of regular and moderate exercise during pregnancy have been scientifically proven. They include:

- Reducing the back pain that's so common during pregnancy
- Reducing fatigue
- Improving circulation and alleviating swollen legs and constipation
- Reducing mood swings
- Making delivery less exhausting
- Controlling diabetes or hypertension

❧

The goal of exercising is to improve your muscle tone and endurance. Don't work out until you drop or sweat profusely.

Your body will tell you if you're pushing too hard. If you feel dizzy, too hot, too cold or nauseous or if you have any other symptom that makes you feel ill, you ought to stop exercising immediately and talk to your obstetrician/gynecologist about it. Drink water before, during and after exercising. Wear comfortable clothing in layers so that you can remove a piece if you get too hot as your workout progresses. And don't forget to wear comfortable shoes that support your feet and your body properly.

Twenty minutes of exercise three days a week is enough to keep yourself in shape during pregnancy.

The Best Workouts

It's good to warm up before you work out and cool down afterward. Choose some light exercises such as rotating your shoulders and neck and other stretches. These exercises facilitate blood flow to your muscles in order to get them ready for more strenuous activity, and they will help you avoid injuries.

Swimming

It's one of the best exercises for the pregnant woman. Floating in the water helps you to forget how much extra weight you're carrying around. *Créame que,* believe me, when you get to the eighth and ninth months your joints will appreciate the break. In the water, you can exercise your arms and legs without the extra weight of pregnancy. And if you go with your partner, you can make swimming a nice and different activity for the two of you to share.

Walking

Along with swimming, walking is one of the best exercises a pregnant woman can do. Walking only twenty minutes at a time, three times a week, will help you feel less tired and will cut down on the swelling in your legs. The idea is to walk at a brisk pace, but one at which you can still maintain a conversation. If you can't continue to talk while you walk, slow down. One way to make this exercise a little more interesting is to put on headphones and walk a *ritmo latino,* to the rhythm of your favorite salsa beat. Or you can turn your walk into a family outing before or after dinner. It won't hurt the rest of your family to get out of the house either.

In addition to these exercises, there is another series of activities that will help prepare your body for childbirth and ease back pain. Below you'll find some of the basic movements, but you can find more in books, videos and even classes at the gym for pregnant women.

Leg Lift Crawl

This will strengthen the muscles of your back and abdomen. On hands and knees, lift your left knee and bring it forward, toward your elbow. Then push your leg back slowly, as if you were kicking. Do this exercise to a count of six and repeat it from six to twelve times with each leg.

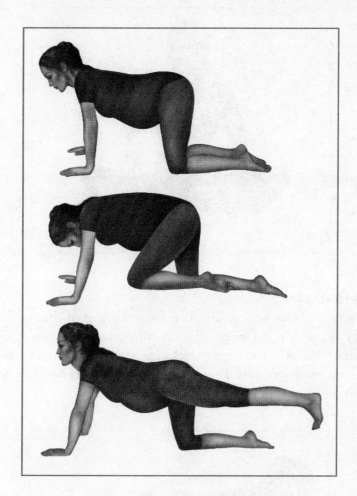

Pelvic Strengthening

An ideal posture to strengthen the muscles in your thighs and lower back. You can sit like this on the floor to read or watch TV. Sit on the floor with your knees bent, your ankles crossed and your back straight. That will help you through the nine months of pregnancy and during delivery.

In order to improve the muscular tone in your thighs when you have to be semiseated to push, put your heels together and bring your heels as close to your body as you can. Then count to five and return to the original position. Repeat the exercise from six to twelve times.

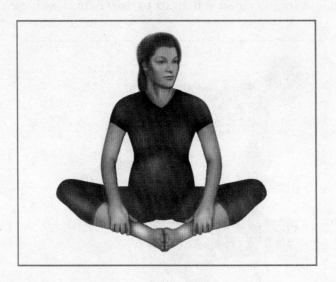

Pelvic Rocking

This is one of the best to alleviate lower back pain during the last months of pregnancy. Get on all fours with your back straight. Slowly arch your back as if you were stretching like a cat. Contract your buttocks muscles as you arch. Then return to the starting position. Repeat this move eight times.

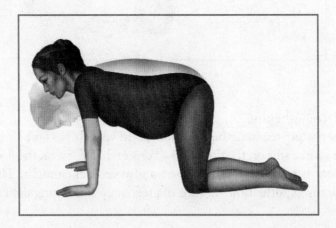

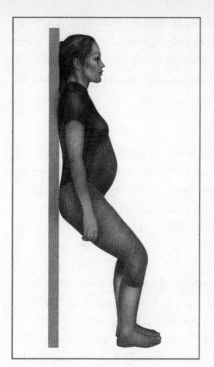

Back Press

Stand with your feet about 10 inches from a wall. Bend your knees and press your lower back against the wall to a count of twelve. Repeat this exercise ten times. It will ease your back pain and will strengthen the muscles of this area.

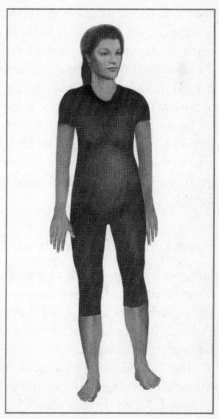

Pelvic Tilt

According to research, this exercise helps with round ligament pain (see page 215). Standing with your feet together, raise a straightened leg vertically 1½ to 2 inches. This will make your hip tilt around 30 degrees. Count slowly to six and repeat the movement ten times with each leg, four times a day (morning, noon, dinnertime and bedtime) as well as every time you feel pain.

Kegel Exercise

Kegels are one of the exercises most recommended to pregnant women before and after delivery. They help to strengthen the muscles of the pelvis and vagina. The best way to understand how to do a Kegel exercise is to interrupt your urine flow while you're peeing. The muscle you're using to stop urination is the one the Kegel exercise focuses on. Once you've figured out how to do a Kegel exercise, you can do it anywhere: while you're driving or reading or before falling asleep. You should do thirty to forty a day.

Breathing and Relaxation Exercise

Learning how to breathe deeply will help you relax during your pregnancy and delivery, especially if you plan to use breathing techniques for birth.

Lying on your bed or sofa, close your eyes and begin to breathe in slowly through your nose. Concentrate on your stomach while you breathe and try to take in as much air as possible. Use your abdominal muscles to breathe deeply, filling your lungs all the way to the bottom. Imagine a string pulling up on your belly button as you inhale. Next, breathe out all the air you've taken in through your mouth. Concentrate solely on breathing and try to leave your mind blank. Repeat this exercise for ten minutes or longer. You can also play some soft music to help you relax.

Beginning with the fourth month of pregnancy, it's not a good idea to spend a long time lying on your back, because you can put pressure on the arteries that supply your baby with oxygen (see page 192). Instead, try doing this exercise leaning back against a pillow or sitting upright in a comfortable chair.

HERBS DURING PREGNANCY

Long before the first medical school was established in the United States, Latin America had its own indigenous schools where the medicinal benefits of herbs were taught. By 1552 the effects on the human body of more than 1,200 herbs had already been documented, and many of these same herbs are used today.

The Latino tradition of using medicinal herbs has remained intact through the centuries. In fact, in the United States, the demand has even increased due to the fact that a big percentage of Latinos do not have health insurance. A high number of Latinos—as many as 80 percent, according to some studies—use home remedies to treat health problems such as diarrhea, conjunctivitis or indigestion. Unfortunately, home remedies aren't always innocuous, especially when you're pregnant.

For example, mugwort and rue, two herbs used to treat *empacho*, an upset stomach, stimulate bleeding and could cause abortions. Not all herbs have the same effects in all women, but if you've had miscarriages in the past, you should be careful with these types of herbs. Herbs for constipation stimulate intestinal muscles and can provoke uterine contractions, and there are diuretic herbs that are as strong as a pill. Diuretics can cause dehydration and affect your kidneys, one of the critical organs for your baby's well-being. After delivery you should be careful with herbs that pass through your milk since they can cause diarrhea or other problems for your baby.

These home remedies are especially dangerous during the first three months of pregnancy, when the baby is forming its organs and basic structures. If you're thinking about getting pregnant, or even if you're in your childbearing years, I would recommend you talk to your doctor before taking any home remedy. If you get pregnant unexpectedly, you won't know until you miss your first period, and your baby will already have been growing for several weeks.

Some people believe herbs can't be harmful because they are natural products. Nothing could be further from the truth. Herbs make up part of many of the prescribed and over-the-counter drugs sold in pharmacies today. Herbs that are taken in concentrated form—in pills or tablets—are even more potent.

During my pregnancies, I took special care to watch which herbs I used. But in my last one, I was ten days past my due date and desperate to have the baby, so I decided without telling my doctor to try a home remedy *para ver si ya*, to speed things up. Only a couple of hours after taking this home remedy, I began to have wild contractions. They took me completely by surprise and eventually led to the birth of my daughter. Although in my case the herbs did achieve the desired effect, *me dan escalofríos*, I get chills every time I think about what would have happened if I'd taken those herbs at the beginning of my pregnancy for any of the other ailments they treated.

I don't mean to say all herbs are off-limits during pregnancy. In fact, below you will find some that have beneficial effects for the mother-to-be. But aside from these you should be aware of the effects of certain herbs and home remedies during your pregnancy.

What follows is a list of herbs that are considered to be the most dangerous to a pregnant woman. The list of herbs pregnant women should not take is much more extensive, so please, talk to your doctor.

Beside each herb you'll find its Latin name and then its Spanish name, as well as its possible effects on pregnancy. You will also find some of its uses, but keep in mind that these are traditional uses and in the majority of the cases they have not been proved through scientific studies.

Remember also that herbs and prescribed drugs don't mix well. Some herbs can increase the effect of certain medications, while others counteract the effect of prescribed drugs or cause undesired side effects.

English Name	Spanish Name	Latin Name	Effects on Pregnancy	Uses According to *Boticarios* or Herbalists
Aloe vera	*Sávila, alcíbar, aloé vera*	*Aloe barbadensis*	Stimulates bleeding. Stimulates intestinal muscles and can stimulate uterine contractions. Passes through mother's milk.	Strong laxative and diuretic. Burns and skin irritations.
Angelica	*Angélica*	*Angelica archangelica*	Stimulates bleeding.	Rheumatism, colds, cramps, colic and fever. Diuretic and expectorant (for coughing).
Arnica	*Árnica*	*Arnica montana*	Stimulates bleeding.	Treats bumps and bruises and mouth and throat inflammation.
Barberry	*Agracejo, bérbero*	*Berberis vulgaris*	Stimulates uterine contractions and bleeding.	Liver and gum problems. Laxative.
Bearberry, uva-ursi	*Gayuba, aguavilla*	*Arctostaphylos uva-ursi*	Reduces amount of blood flow to the uterus.	Uric acid, kidney stones and cystitis. Is a very strong diuretic.
Bitterwood, quassia	*Hombre grande, amargo*	*Quassia amara*	Stimulates uterine contractions.	Intestinal parasites, upset stomach, diarrhea. Treats alcoholism.
Black cohosh	*Hierba de la cinche, cimífuga negra*	*Cimicifuga racemosa*	Stimulates bleeding. Passes through mother's milk.	Relaxant, treats premenstrual syndrome, colds and diarrhea.
Bloodroot, red root	*Sanguinaria, raíz colorada, litospermo*	*Sanguinaria canadensis*	Stimulates bleeding. Passes through mother's milk.	Bronchitis, pneumonia, skin fungus.
Blue cohosh	*Cimífuga azul*	*Caulophyllum thalictroides*	Stimulates uterine contractions.	Colic and menstrual and gastrointestinal problems.
Borago	*Borraja*	*Borago officinalis*	Passes through mother's milk.	Reduces fever. Depurative, antirheumatic and expectorant.
Buckthorn	*Arraclán, frágula*	*Rhamnus frangula*	Stimulates intestine and could cause uterine contractions.	Diuretic and laxative.

English Name	Spanish Name	Latin Name	Effects on Pregnancy	Uses According to *Boticarios* or Herbalists
Calamus	*Cálamo aromático*	*Acorus calamus*	Passes through mother's milk.	Asthma and respiratory problems.
Cascara buckthorn	*Palo bañón, cáscara sagrada, ladierno*	*Rhamnus purshiana*	Stimulates uterine contractions. Passes through mother's milk.	Laxative. Gallbladder stones and liver problems.
Cassia	*Chacara, canafistula*	*Cassia fistula*	Stimulates intestine and could cause uterine contractions.	Purgative. Urinary problems.
Cinchona	*Quina roja*	*Cinchona ledgeriana*	Stimulates uterine contractions.	Malaria, poor digestion, colds, headaches. Appetite stimulant.
Coltsfoot	*Fárfara, uña de gato, pata de mula*	*Tussilago farfara*	Passes through mother's milk.	Respiratory problems, diarrhea.
Comfrey	*Consuelda, sinfito*	*Symphytum officinale*	Passes through mother's milk. Toxic for the baby.	Bumps and bruises, swelling and gastro-intestinal disorders.
Corn smut	*Cuitlacoche*	*Ustilago maydis*	Stimulates uterine contractions.	This fungus makes the corn cob kernels expand as they fill with spores. It's a delicious Mexican favorite, but you should be cautious about how much you eat during pregnancy. It's dangerous in concentrated drops. It's used to improve circulation and to treat menstrual problems.
Damiana	*Damiana*	*Turnera diffusa*	Stimulates bleeding.	Upset stomach, aphrodisiac, hormonal problems.
Devil's claw	*Garra del diablo, uña del diablo*	*Harpago-phytum procumbens*	Stimulates uterine contractions.	Anti-inflammatory, analgesic. Kidney problems.
Dong quai	*Dong Quai*	*Angelica sinensis*	Stimulates bleeding.	Pollen allergies and menstrual problems.
Ephedra	*Popotillo, canutillo, efedra, Ma huang, te mormón*	*Ephedra vulgaris*	Reduces amount of blood flow to the uterus. Passes through mother's milk.	Allergies. Diuretic and stimulant. Reduces appetite.

English Name	Spanish Name	Latin Name	Effects on Pregnancy	Uses According to *Boticarios* or Herbalists
Eucalyptus	Eucalipto	Eucalyptus globulus	Stimulates bleeding. Passes through mother's milk.	Colds, congestion, fever. Expectorant.
European pennyroyal	Poleo-menta	Mentha pulegium	Fetal abnormalities.	Colic and menstrual delay.
Gingko biloba	Gingko	Gingko biloba	Passes through mother's milk.	Circulation and memory loss.
Goldenseal	Sello de oro, botón de oro, hidraste	Hydrastis canadensis	Stimulates uterine contractions.	Vaginal fungal infections.
Groundsel	Matarique	Senecio vulgaris	Stimulates bleeding. Passes through mother's milk.	Migraines, asthma, nausea and menstrual problems.
Horehound	Marrubio, masto	Marrubium vulgare	Stimulates bleeding.	Lung congestion, works well with fever. Expectorant.
Hyssop	Hisopo	Hyssopus officinalis	Stimulates bleeding.	Chest congestion, flu, intestinal parasites.
Licorice	Orozuz, regaliz	Glycyrrhiza glabra	Passes through mother's milk.	Anti-inflammatory and diuretic. Treats ulcers and emotional instability.
Maidenhair	Culantrillo, avenca, adianto	Adiantum capillus-veneris	Stimulates bleeding and uterine contractions.	Throat irritation and rheumatism.
Mallow	Malva	Malva sylvestris	Passes through mother's milk.	Mouth and throat irritations. Stimulates breast milk but could have effects on the baby.
Manacan	Manaca	Brunfelsia uniflorus	Stimulates bleeding and uterine contractions.	Lung congestion, works with fever. Expectorant.
Mayapple, American mandrake	Mandrágora, podófilo	Podophyllum peltatum	Fetal abnormalities. Stimulates uterine contractions. Stimulates bleeding. Very toxic.	Laxative. Intestinal parasites.
Milk thistle	Arzolla, cardo lechero, cardo de María	Silybum marianum	Stimulates bleeding.	Liver problems and poisoning. Antidepressant.
Mugwort	Estafiate	Artemisia vulgaris	Fetal abnormalities. Stimulates bleeding. Passes through mother's milk.	*Empacho*, upset stomach, colic, diarrhea and parasites. Stimulates and regulates menstrual cycle.
Myrrh	Mirra	Commiphora myrrha	Stimulates uterine contractions. Passes through mother's milk.	Gum problems and infections.

English Name	Spanish Name	Latin Name	Effects on Pregnancy	Uses According to *Boticarios* or Herbalists
Osha	*Chuchupate, perejil de campo, levístico*	*Ligusticum porteri*	Stimulates bleeding. Passes through mother's milk.	Viral infections. Diuretic and expectorant.
Rhubarb	*Ruibarbo*	*Rheum palmatum*	Stimulates bleeding. Passes through mother's milk.	Constipation and diarrhea, tract diseases. Arthritis and skin problems.
Rue	*Ruda*	*Ruta graveolens*	Stimulates bleeding. Passes through mother's milk.	*Empacho*, upset stomach, cramps. Disinfectant and diuretic. Menstrual problems.
Sarsaparilla	*Zarzaparrilla*	*Smilax officinalis*	Stimulates bleeding. Passes through mother's milk.	Depurative, anti-inflammatory, for rheumatic and kidney problems.
Senna	*Hojasenn*	*Cassia angustifolia*	Stimulates uterine contractions. Passes through mother's milk.	Strong laxative.
Shepherd's purse	*Bolsa del pastor*	*Capsella bursa-pastoris*	Stimulates uterine contractions.	Stops any kind of bleeding.
Tansy	*Tanaceto, hierba lombriguera*	*Tanacetum vulgare*	Fetal abnormalities. Stimulates uterine contractions and bleeding. Passes through mother's milk. Very toxic.	Intestinal parasites, rheumatism, kidney problems and colds.
Thuja	*Tuya*	*Thuja occidentalis*	Stimulates uterine contractions and bleeding. Passes through mother's milk. Very toxic.	Muscle pain and rheumatism.
Wild yam	*Dioscorea*	*Dioscorea villosa*	Stimulates uterine contractions.	Muscle relaxant. Reestablishes female hormonal balance. Treats irritable bowel.
Wormseed, Mexican tea	*Epazote, ambrosía*	*Chenopodium ambrosioides*	Stimulates bleeding and intestine and could cause uterine contractions. Passes through mother's milk.	Dysentery, intestinal parasites and upset stomach. Laxative.
Wormwood, Mexican tea	*Ajenjo, aluinos*	*Artemisia absinthium*	Fetal abnormalities. Stimulates bleeding. Passes through mother's milk.	Calms cramps and muscular pain, diarrhea, liver and gallbladder problems, intestinal parasites and menstrual delay.

Common Herbal Infusions

Some herbs are very common in the kitchen. In small amounts, they're a delicious condiment for the foods we eat and are usually harmless. Nevertheless, during pregnancy, it's not a good idea to take high concentrations of these herbs or infusions because they can cause bleeding or contractions. Some of these herbs include:

- Basil
- Chamomile
- Eucalyptus
- Marjoram
- Mint
- Nutmeg
- Oregano
- Parsley
- Pennyroyal
- Rosemary
- Saffron
- Sage
- Thyme
- Wormseed

One example of a high concentration is pesto, an Italian sauce that contains a lot of basil; it is not recommended if you have had miscarriages in the past. Infusions of watercress, carrot seeds or parsley aren't recommended either.

HERBS THAT TRADITIONALLY HAVE BEEN USED DURING PREGNANCY

There are many herbs that have been used in pregnancy by many women with good results. However, keep in mind that this is not medical information but just advice and traditions from *boticarios o yerberos*, herbalists. Talk to your obstetrician/gynecologist before taking anything, because each person can react differently to herbs.

Red Raspberry Tea (Hojas de frambuesa, *Rubus idaeus*)

This is one of the best herbs for women in the last weeks of pregnancy. It's a uterine tonic that strengthens the muscles of the uterus and pelvis. Don't drink this herb in the first months of pregnancy, especially if you've got a history of spontaneous abortions, because it can cause uterine contractions. Pour one cup of boiling water over two spoonfuls of dried red raspberry leaves and let it stand for ten to fifteen minutes. Two or three cups daily during the last six weeks of pregnancy will help you prepare for delivery.

Squaw Vine (Squaw Vine, *Mitchella repens*)

It's also a tonic that prepares the uterus for delivery. In the weeks previous to your due date you can use it along with the red raspberry tea. Squaw vine also soothes nipple irritation during breastfeeding. You can rinse your nipples with the infusion.

Add two teaspoons in two cups of boiling water. Cover and let it stand for half an hour. You can drink from one to three cups a day.

Nettle Tea (Ortigas, *Urtica dioica*)

Nettle contains a lot of iron and calcium, two of the minerals pregnant women most need. Also, it helps to reduce the pain of hemorrhoids and leg cramps. It's prepared in the same manner as the red raspberry tea and you can drink two cups a day.

Ginger (Jengibre, *Zingiber officinale*)

Ginger helps to ease the discomfort of nausea. One study done several years ago with pregnant women proved its effectiveness. Ginger can be taken in capsules or in tinctures, but always in moderation. High levels of ginger in the body can lead to spontaneous abortions. Talk to your doctor before using it.

FOLK HEALERS AND SAINTS

I've got a friend who believes in having a good *barrida o limpia*, spiritual cleansing, once a month to wash away all those negative energies that stick to him every day. *Cuidar de su espíritu*, taking care of your spirit when you're pregnant is important, and whatever technique or tradition you follow that contributes to your serenity and inner peace is welcome. Your baby can tell when you are nervous or tense, happy or relaxed.

Folk healers can be a positive influence on your spiritual state if they are careful with their home remedies. *Sobadores* or *hueseros* as well as chiropractors can help with the back pains many pregnant women suffer from, as long as they don't manipulate you too forcefully.

Nevertheless, there is one procedure you should be careful with: turning the baby around to avoid a breech birth. This is for two reasons: first, the only way to be absolutely sure the baby is coming out feet first is through a sonogram, and second, a procedure of this type can cause problems, from breaking your water to causing permanent harm to you or your baby. Some obstetricians/gynecologists, but not all, will do this procedure in the hospital, assisted by technical equipment.

For Catholic Latinas, San Ramón Nonato is *el patrón de las embarazadas y parturientas*, the patron saint of pregnant women and women in labor. San Ramón was never born because his mother died during his delivery around the year 1200. The name Nonato means "not born" in Latin. His story is a moving one, and there are several very appropriate and beautiful prayers for pregnant women (see Contact List). The Virgin Mary as well as her mother, Santa Ana, are also considered protectors of pregnant women.

MENTAL HEALTH

Every Latina knows *la importancia de la familia*, the value of family. Taking care of our husbands, children and other relatives, cleaning the house and making sure guests are entertained (whether they're announced or not) is probably part of your upbringing. Many of us work hard during the day and when we get home, the work continues: cooking dinner, washing clothes, getting ready for tomorrow. We are the family's engine; we make sure everything gets done. Sometimes our own needs end up at the bottom of the list because we feel if we don't fulfill our responsibilities to the rest of the family, we're not being *buenas esposas y madres*, good wives and mothers.

The physical and mental fatigue that comes with pregnancy might keep us from doing so much for others. If that's happening to you, don't blame yourself or feel guilty. You're not being a bad wife, nor are you abandoning your family. If your car has space for four people and you try to fit eight in, you don't think it will go as fast, do you? Well, your body is going through the same thing: it's now working for two instead of just one. Your body needs physical and mental rest. Lying down with your feet up while feeling guilty you haven't prepared tomorrow's lunch doesn't really make much sense. You'll only make yourself more tense. The priority for you now should be your health and that of your baby. Even though you don't believe it, the world will continue to function with wrinkled shirts and frozen dinners.

Your partner might find it difficult to understand how tired you are, and he may even feel a little resentment because you're not paying as much attention to him. Get him to read this book, or at least the "For

Dad" sections in each chapter. On page 315 you'll find a few suggestions on how to handle your life if you feel it's about to implode.

Mental health during pregnancy is as important as physical health. A flexible, positive attitude and a lot of *buen humor*, good sense of humor will help you to enjoy the changes your body is going through and the changes in your role as mother and wife.

4

Diabetes and Pregnancy

During the fifth month of my first pregnancy, I just couldn't get over feeling exhausted. Two hours after getting up in the morning, the only thing I felt like doing was going back to bed. After eating it was worse. I was so tired I could barely think. My husband and friends told me not to worry about it, that feeling tired was just part of having a baby. They told me to try to sleep more. But that didn't work. Even though I'd sleep twelve hours a day, I still felt *muy cansada*, very tired. And that wasn't all. I was constantly thirsty. I began to drink a lot of water, and the more I drank the more I had to use the bathroom, especially at night.

At that time, my job as a news producer for Univision in Los Angeles kept me very busy, and I missed my checkup for that month without scheduling a new one. One day at work after lunch, I went to the parking garage to look for some papers I'd left in the car. When I got in, I was so tired and the seat felt so good, I decided to close my eyes, *solo un momentito*, just for a moment. I couldn't stay long; in fifteen minutes we had to begin planning that evening's newscast.

When I opened my eyes, an hour and a half had passed and the news was about to begin! *Volé*, I flew back up to the newsroom, where my co-workers had been going crazy looking for me. It goes without saying that evening's *noticiero*, newscast, wasn't one of the highlights of my career, but that night I made an appointment with my doctor.

A few days later, I had some tests done to find out what my blood sugar levels were. When the results came back, my doctor called me to say I had gestational diabetes. The doctor's explanations were useless to me at that point. The only thing I could do was cry! *Mi bebé* was in danger and I would have to take insulin shots *por el resto de mi vida,* for the rest of my life! Fortunately, my husband, who's a lot more level-headed than I am, was calm enough to listen to the doctor and figure out exactly what gestational diabetes is and what could be done about it. At work the next day, I found I wasn't alone: three other Univision co-workers had been diagnosed with gestational diabetes, and all gave birth to *bebés sanos y hermosos,* healthy and beautiful babies.

Gestational diabetes is one of the most common complications among pregnant Latinas. This disease, which appears only during pregnancy, affects us much more than the rest of the population, and it gets worse with each pregnancy and with age.

It's not only gestational diabetes that we have to watch for. There are thousands of Latinas who don't even know they have diabetes before they get pregnant. The high blood sugar levels that this disease produces can affect your baby.

WHAT IS DIABETES?

Diabetes is a condition that prevents the body from properly using the food we eat. We eat to supply our body's cells with energy so they can work. Through the digestion process we turn food into glucose. Glucose is the fuel our cells use to keep running. When our cells get the right amount of glucose, we've got enough energy to go about our daily lives.

But in order for our cells to "eat" that glucose, they need some help. That help is insulin. Insulin is produced by the pancreas every time we have something to eat. Imagine insulin as a key that opens a door in the cells to let glucose in. If there is not enough insulin, glucose cannot come in.

People who have diabetes don't produce enough insulin, or if they do, they cannot use it properly. As a result, glucose cannot get inside the cells and it remains in the bloodstream. That excess sugar in the bloodstream can cause various problems. The most common are:

- *Frequent urination.* Glucose needs a lot of water to be flushed out of the body. Diabetics find themselves urinating often, especially at night.

- *Thirst.* The excessive loss of water from frequent urination makes diabetics thirsty. The severity ranges from a little dry mouth to extreme thirst.

- *Fatigue.* The body's fuel can't get into your cells, so, just like a car with no gas, they can't operate properly. No fuel for the body makes diabetics feel tired.

- *Hunger.* Even though diabetics may be eating well, their cells aren't because there is not enough insulin in the bloodstream. The cells feel hungry and keep asking for more food. That's why some diabetics can eat a lot and still lose weight.

- *Tingling in the legs.* Excessive amounts of sugar in the bloodstream can damage nerves. Diabetics need to watch out for cuts or bruises they get on their legs because they may not feel them.

- *Cuts and scratches may take longer to heal.* High levels of sugar in the bloodstream can weaken the body's defenses. The immune system does not work that well, and there is a bigger risk for infections.

- *Blurred vision.* Blood vessels in the eyes deteriorate due to high blood glucose levels.

TYPES OF DIABETES

Although the result for the body's cells is the same—they don't get the food they need—there are several types of diabetes. Their causes are different.

Type I Diabetes
People who have type I diabetes produce very little insulin or none at all. For reasons that are not totally understood, their immune system destroys the insulin-producing pancreas cells. Their symptoms are severe and they need daily insulin shots so their cells can get enough glucose to work. This type of diabetes usually appears in people age twenty and younger.

Type II Diabetes
The majority of diabetics are type II; it is also the most common among Latinos. With type II diabetes, the body is unable to use insulin properly. This condition is known as "insulin resistance." The more insulin the body needs, the less the pancreas is able to produce.

Women who have type II diabetes are generally overweight, don't exercise much, have diabetic relatives and have had gestational diabetes in the past. Type II diabetics can control their problems with diet, exercise and medicines, but in some cases daily insulin pills or shots are needed.

Gestational Diabetes

It only happens during pregnancy. Pregnancy hormones produced by the placenta prevent insulin from working properly, and glucose can't get into the cells. All this sugar in the blood affects the baby (see page 74).

DIABETES BEFORE PREGNANCY

Every year there are more diabetics in the United States, and we Latinos have double the risk of developing it compared with other ethnic groups. Not only that, but there are hundreds or thousands of Latinos who have diabetes but don't know it, and most of them are women. Today, one in every four Latinas has diabetes. The problem with getting pregnant without knowing that you are a diabetic is how that excess sugar in your blood will affect your baby.

During the first weeks of pregnancy the baby's organs are formed, including the heart and what is called the neural tube. This tube gives rise to the baby's brain, spinal column and nerves. At this time, a high blood sugar level can cause birth defects and miscarriages.

By the time a woman discovers that she is pregnant and asks for a doctor's appointment at which diabetes can be detected and treated, six or eight weeks have passed. That's why is so important to go to your doctor regularly if you are of childbearing age and, if you get pregnant, to ask for a prenatal appointment as soon as possible. With appropriate care, you can have a healthy baby. Studies show that if a diabetic mother has her blood sugar levels under control, she's at no higher risk than the general population of having a baby with birth defects.

There is no "high blood sugar numbers" or "almost diabetes." If your blood sugar level is above the normal range, *you have diabetes.*

Type II diabetes, the most common among Latinos, is sometimes considered not so serious since insulin is not needed. But this is not true. If you are a Type II diabetic and your blood sugar levels are high before conception, the risk for your baby is also high.

In addition, if you don't have your diabetes under control, you can have health problems. Diabetic Latinas are twice as likely to have damage to their kidneys or eyes and eight times more likely to develop problems with the circulatory system. These complications of diabetes can get worse during pregnancy if you are not under a doctor's supervision.

GESTATIONAL DIABETES

Gestational diabetes appears only during pregnancy, not before, and occurs because the placenta produces hormones that affect insulin's ability to do its job. After eating, glucose stays in the mother's blood, since it can't enter the cells. On one hand, you are not getting adequate nourishment. On the other, the baby is getting all the sugar excess through your blood.

Inside the womb the baby is attached to the placenta through the umbilical cord. Oxygen and nutrients pass from you to your baby through the placenta.

The Baby's Risks

The consequence of your high blood sugar levels is that the baby will get too fat. It's as if you were feeding your baby cake and candy for breakfast, lunch and dinner. This type of diabetes doesn't lead to birth defects, but it does cause other problems.

Fetus glucose absorption

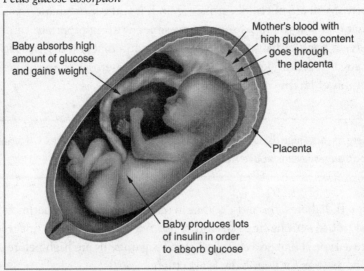

Baby absorbs high amount of glucose and gains weight

Mother's blood with high glucose content goes through the placenta

Placenta

Baby produces lots of insulin in order to absorb glucose

Low blood sugar level (hypoglycemia)

The baby's body has to produce a large amount of insulin in order to process all the sugar that's entering its bloodstream through the placenta. The baby's pancreas automatically produces insulin when it detects glucose in the blood. When the baby is born and the umbilical cord is cut, the supply of glucose from the mother is cut off too. But the baby's pancreas continues to produce a lot of insulin. All the extra insulin works on the small amount of glucose that is left in the baby's blood and quickly consumes it. This leaves the baby with no sugar in its bloodstream, which can lead to unconsciousness. Doctors might have to revive the baby by giving it glucose. Eventually, however, the baby's insulin levels balance out with the amount of sugar in the bloodstream.

Arm paralysis

Babies who have grown too big inside the womb are at risk of getting "stuck" during delivery. The head can go through, but their shoulders are too wide to pass through the mother's pubic bone inside the birth canal. This is called shoulder dystocia. During birth the baby's still breathing through the umbilical cord. When he or she gets stuck, the umbilical cord gets compressed and blood cannot circulate. Babies go blue quickly, and if the obstetrician/gynecologist doesn't do a special maneuver, they could suffer from brain damage in a matter of minutes due to the lack of oxygen. In addition, some nerve fibers in the neck can get damaged. This fibers are part of the nerve that gives movement to the arm (brachial plexus). The result could be a baby with a temporarily or permanently paralyzed arm.

If your obstetrician/gynecologist thinks the baby is too big, he/she will recommend a cesarean. However, is not possible to determine accurately the baby's weight before birth, and sometimes there are surprises.

Future development

Studies have shown that children of diabetic mothers have a greater chance of being overweight. There is even one study that shows that children of diabetic mothers who didn't have their glucose levels under control can have psychological difficulties and coordination problems when they are between six and nine years old.

The Mother's Risks

The first complication caused by gestational diabetes is that you will have an increased likelihood of a cesarean birth or C-section. As with any other type of surgery, this means there could be problems with anesthesia or infection. The recovery time for a cesarean birth is longer than for a vaginal birth, and you can feel very uncomfortable for a few days due to the incision.

The baby's size can be estimated prior to delivery with an ultrasound, but the results can be as much as a pound over or under the baby's real weight. This weight and the room you have inside your pelvic opening will determine if you'll need a C-section (see page 301).

Usually gestational diabetes disappears after birth because the hormones that interfere with the insulin disappear when the placenta is passed. However, after developing gestational diabetes you have higher chances of having it again in your next pregnancy. Mothers, especially Latinas, who have had gestational diabetes have a much greater likelihood of developing type II diabetes as they grow older. More than half of the women who have gestational diabetes will develop type II diabetes in the five to ten years following. For Latinas, especially those with Mexican ancestry, this risk is even higher.

To make sure your diabetes is gone after you deliver your baby, your doctor will probably measure your blood sugar levels six weeks after birth. If your levels are normal after that time, you should check them again every year.

As you can see, diabetes before, during and after pregnancy is a very real enemy for Latinas, but with the right prenatal care you will be fine.

TREATMENT OF GESTATIONAL DIABETES

Hormones produced by the placenta block the proper use of insulin. As the pregnancy moves along, the levels of these hormones increase and it is more difficult for the mother's body to make the right amount of insulin and use it properly.

Between the twenty-sixth and thirty-sixth weeks of pregnancy, these hormones are at their highest levels. That is why during the twenty-eighth week doctors will perform a glucose test, to see if you are having problems processing the sugar in your blood. If the test results are positive, the doctor will do another, more thorough test called the glucose tolerance test. That will confirm if you have gestational diabetes (see page 130). Not all obstetrician/gynecologists perform these tests. However, the American Diabetes Association recommends that all pregnant women who fall into the following categories should take the glucose test.

- Are 25 or older
- Were overweight before they became pregnant
- Have a family history of diabetes, especially their parents
- Are Hispanic, African American, Native American or Asian American

The majority of gestational diabetes cases are controlled through a balanced diet and exercise, but sometimes that is not enough, and you might require insulin shots. Insulin pills are not prescribed during pregnancy because the insulin passes through the placenta to the baby and increases the baby's insulin levels. However, there is good news for needle loathers like me. A new study shows that glyburide, a drug commonly taken to control diabetes, is safe to take in the last six months of pregnancy. Doctors are free to treat pregnant mothers with glyburide now, but the drug's manufacturers need government approval to promote the pill for the treatment of gestational diabetes. The American Diabetes Association has recommended more studies before prescribing the drug to pregnant women, but ask your doctor about it. Maybe in the near future this will be an alternative to needles.

Glucose Monitors

The first step toward controlling glucose levels is measuring them. The most common way is using a glucose monitor. It's a small machine, easy to use, that will allow you to measure your blood sugar levels at home, at work or wherever is convenient.

Glucose is measured through a small drop of blood placed on a measuring strip connected to the machine. This strip is chemically treated and can tell you how much sugar is in your blood.

Of all the inconveniences that diabetes caused during my pregnancy, the most *fastidiosa*, annoying, was having to prick my finger every day to measure my blood sugar levels. I had to test myself at least three times a day. I ended up hating the finger pricks. The truth is, *no duele tanto*, they don't hurt that much (although sometimes I'd prick my finger in the wrong place and it would hurt!). The pain is in having to do it over and over again for several months. There were days when it would take me half an hour before I could actually push the button on the little machine that would send the lancet into the tip of my finger. Despite all that, I was able to squeeze out a drop of blood from my fingers *todos los días,* every day. I knew the consequences of gestational diabetes for my baby and for me.

Along the way I learned some tricks to make the pricking process a little easier to take:

- The sides of the fingertips have fewer nerve endings, which makes the prick less painful, but they've still got enough of a blood flow to make the test successful.

- Washing your hands with warm water right before the prick increases the blood flow to the fingertips and ensures that no bacteria gets into the cut (using alcohol to disinfect the finger before the prick can alter the test results). Remember to wash off any food that may be left on the fingertips before the test, because that could change the results, too.

- Massaging the fingertip before the prick also helps increase blood flow.

- I used one finger each time, both sides, so they had a few days to rest between prickings.

The number of times blood sugar levels need to be tested depends on your glucose levels and whether you need insulin shots. Normally, women with gestational diabetes take the test when they wake up and

Glucose monitor and measurement strip

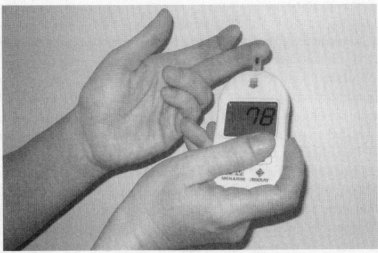

after breakfast, lunch and dinner. If you are taking insulin shots, you might have to test your glucose levels more often. There's some alternatives to pricking your fingertips every day, but they are expensive (see Contact List):

- *Glucowatch*. This is a device that you wear like a watch. It reads blood sugar levels during the day, through your wrist's skin. You will have to prick yourself once a day to adjust the readings to a glucose monitor.
- *Lassete*. It's a little portable laser to make a tiny hole in your finger, instead of using the lancet. In theory you only feel a little pressure.
- *Soft-Tact and FreeStyle*. A machine that extracts the blood and measures the blood sugar level at the same time. You can use it on your arm instead of your finger. It creates a small suction vacuum in your skin where the lancet shoots. The suction brings a small amount of blood to a strip that measures the glucose.

The Readings
The desired glucose readings are measured in milligrams of sugar per deciliter of blood (mg/dL).

- Fasting   Less than 90 mg/dl
- One hour after eating   Less than 140 mg/dl
- Two hours after eating   Less than 120 mg/dl

You will probably be asked by your doctor to keep a record of the results. Some of the glucose monitors have a memory, but I find it easier to have my results at a glance on a notepad. If you need insulin, you should note the quantity and time the shots were given. It helps to write down whether you exercised, if you felt stressed or if you took any type of drug like Tylenol or cold medicine. All these things can affect the test results. Your doctor will review your notes to see if you need adjustments in your diet, exercise or insulin.

Diet
You might be able to keep your gestational diabetes at bay just by changing your diet. If you control what you eat, you will limit the amount of glucose that enters your bloodstream. The more you eat, the more glu-

cose you process and the more that gets passed on to your baby. This isn't to say you have to give up eating altogether. It's just that you will have to pay attention to the amount and the type of food on your plate.

In addition to watching the amount of food you eat, it's important to know which kinds of foods to eat. There are three main groups:

- *Carbohydrates*. Fruits, vegetables and cereals are all carbohydrates. There are two types of carbohydrates: simple and complex. When you have diabetes it is important to be able to tell them apart. The simple ones come from refined products such as sugar, cake, candy, white flour, white-flour tortillas, white bread and pasta. They are digested easily and pass quickly into the bloodstream. As a result, eating simple carbohydrates raises your glucose level almost immediately. If you have gestational diabetes, your insulin will not be able to process the glucose, and so it will be passed on to your baby. Complex carbohydrates—from whole-grain products such as whole-grain bread, whole-grain tortillas, corn tortillas, vegetables, cereals without sugar and grains—take a longer time to digest before they turn into glucose and pass into your bloodstream. Because the process is slower, lower levels of insulin are capable of handling the glucose that goes in the blood. Note that although fruits are a healthy food, they have high levels of fructose, another type of sugar to be wary of.

- *Proteins*. It takes a long time for the body to turn proteins into glucose. Foods high in protein include meats, fish, eggs, milk and cheese. It's a good idea to choose ones low in fat.

- *Fats*. Your baby needs fat for his or her development, but too much fat will cause you to gain weight. Your risk of developing type II diabetes after your pregnancy is bigger if you are overweight. Too many fats are unhealthy because they cause weight gain, and overweight people are more prone to type II diabetes after pregnancy. There are foods rich in fat, like bacon, french fries and avocados, and fats used to cook, such as lard, butter and oil. Some fats are healthier than others; for example, vegetable fats such as olive oil are good for your heart.

If you have gestational diabetes, your doctor will set up a diet for you. Most plans have three small meals and three snacks a day. It's important to pay attention to how much time passes between meals, in order to maintain a constant amount of glucose in your blood. Too little blood sugar is not good either. A small meal every two or three hours is advised. Here's an example of the diet a doctor might recommend. You can check the food lists in Chapter 3 to give variety to your menu:

7 A.M.—Breakfast:	1 scrambled egg
	1 whole-grain tortilla
	1 teaspoon of butter
	Tea or decaffeinated coffee
9 A.M.—Snack:	½ cup of nonfat yogurt or milk
	½ cup of sugar-free cereal or ½ piece of toast
	½ piece of fresh fruit
Noon—Lunch:	3 ounces of meat (or fish or chicken)
	1 cup of brown rice or two whole-grain tortillas
	1 cup of vegetables
	1 cup of nonfat yogurt or milk
	½ piece of fresh fruit
	2 teaspoons of oil or butter
3 P.M.—Snack:	½ cup of nonfat yogurt or milk
	½ piece of fresh fruit
6 P.M.—Dinner:	4 ounces of broiled lean meat or chicken
	1 cup brown rice or pasta or 2 corn tortillas
	½ piece of fresh fruit
	1 cup of vegetables
	1 cup of nonfat yogurt or milk
	2 teaspoons of oil or butter
8 P.M.—Snack:	1 ounce of cheese
	1 small whole-grain tortilla

This diet ensures that your blood sugar levels don't get too high. That allows your insulin to work more efficiently in processing the glucose so your baby will not get too much. Since sugars and refined foods send glucose levels through the roof, you should read the labels on the foods you are thinking of buying to make sure they do not contain these ingredients. Sugar can appear under many names on a food label:

- Corn sweetener
- Corn syrup
- Dextrose
- Disaccharide
- Fructose
- Galactose
- Glucose
- High-fructose corn syrup (HFCS)
- Honey
- Juice concentrates
- Lactose
- Maltose
- Maple syrup
- Molasses
- Natural sweeteners
- Sucrose

The doctor might also recommend that you talk to a dietician, who can create a personalized eating plan.

Insulin

"I can still remember how much I cried that day. Even though I was following my diet to the letter, my sugar levels were not going down. For my baby's health and for mine, my doctor decided to begin giving me insulin shots. When he said it, *mi corazón se paró*, my heart stopped. The pricks to my finger to check my blood sugar levels were bad enough, and now I had to shoot myself up with insulin! The next day, a nurse showed me how to do it. Right away I felt better. The needle was *chiquita, chiquita*, very, very little! In the end, it wasn't as upsetting or as painful as I thought it would be. Besides, it was for *mi bebé* and only lasted a few months."

That's the story of Univision anchor Socorro Cruz. It happened to her; it could happen to any pregnant woman, no matter how closely she follows a special diet. It's still possible your blood sugar levels will not go down. As a result, a doctor may prescribe insulin shots, although you may be able to take insulin in pill form.

There are different types of insulin, depending on how long they take to start acting:

Type of Action	Starts Acting	Maximum Effect	Time It Lasts
Ultrafast	5–15 minutes after injecting	30–90 minutes	3–5 hours
Short-acting	30–60 minutes after injecting	1–2 hours	5–8 hours
Intermediate-acting	1–3 hours after injecting	8–15 hours	18–24 hours
Long-acting	4–8 hours after injecting	8–12 hours	36 hours

You will combine these types of insulin depending on your lifestyle so their maximum effect coincides with the times you are going to eat. For example, you can use an intermediate- or long-acting insulin early in the morning to help you maintain a level of insulin till the afternoon and also help you take care of your lunch. For breakfast you will use a rapid-acting one. To get the right amount of insulin, you need to measure your blood sugar levels.

There are several ways to inject insulin, but the most common is with a needle as a subcutaneous shot (just under the skin). The insulin needle is short and thin, which makes this procedure easier to manage. A good place for the shot is the abdomen. Just take a big pinch of your skin, find a place where the tip of the needle doesn't hurt and inject perpendicular to the skin. To make sure that the insulin is absorbed in the subcutaneous fat you should release the pinch after you finish injecting. Your doctor will show you how to do it, and don't worry—you will not have to do it alone until you feel you are ready.

Exercise

One of the best parts of my pregnancy was going for walks with my husband. They were part of my daily exercise plan. Before I got pregnant, my husband and I always found excuses to avoid exercising: "It's too cold." "It's too hot." "I'll be late for work." But when I found out I had gestational diabetes, there were no more *excusas*. My husband is a morning person and helped me to get up a little earlier every day. After breakfast we'd go out together for a walk in the neighborhood. My glucose level dropped dramatically as my spirits rose. During the last weeks of my last pregnancy, these walks also helped me to get rid of some of the swelling in my legs. I know, it's not easy to walk when you feel like an elephant, but believe me, *vale la pena*, it's worth it.

Exercise helps to control blood sugar levels, both for women who are taking insulin shots and for those who are only watching their diet. Studies show that as little as twenty minutes of exercise three times a week can improve blood sugar levels. Walking, swimming or other moderate exercise is perfect for women with gestational diabetes. But because exercise helps your body to consume glucose, you should ask your doctor's advice before choosing an exercise regimen.

Gestational diabetes is a serious illness, but one that can be overcome with proper medical supervision.

5

Health Concerns for Latinas During Pregnancy

In the last chapter we talked about diabetes, a disease that, because of our genetic makeup, among other reasons, affects Latino women disproportionately during pregnancy. Due to a combination of genetic and environmental factors, we are also likely to suffer from several other illnesses that will affect our pregnancies. For example, if you're of Mexican descent and you are having a hard time with nausea and abdominal pains, gallstones might be the problem. Women of Mexican origin are much more likely to have gallstones. Or if you suffer frequent severe headaches, the reason could be high blood pressure; many of us only learn we've got high blood pressure when we're pregnant. A number of the illnesses described below don't present symptoms until they've reached an advanced state. That's why it's a good idea to get physical checkups before and during your pregnancy.

All the information that follows may be a bit worrisome, but the best way to prevent health problems is to be informed about which ones affect us more, and how. Don't forget that despite all these warnings about the problems we Latinas can suffer, our babies are born as healthy as babies of other ethnic groups in the United States.

HYPERTENSION

Along with diabetes, hypertension is one of the most common complications during pregnancy. This problem affects pregnant Latinas at the same rate as the rest of the population. But nearly half of the Latinas who have hypertension don't know it. So it's common to discover for the first time when we are pregnant that our blood pressure is higher than normal.

Hypertension during pregnancy can be a minor problem or an illness that requires immediate medical attention. Complications of hypertension include preeclampsia, a disease that appears only during pregnancy.

Normal blood pressure is around 120/80 mm Hg (millimeters that the mercury goes up on the measuring device), although during pregnancy normal readings could be a bit higher or lower. These numbers measure the amount of pressure the blood is exerting on the veins and arteries when it flows through your body, pumped by the heart.

The heart is a hollow muscle that contracts to expel blood. The contraction is called the systolic movement; during this phase the blood pressure rises. The first number of the reading measures the blood pressure at its highest point; this is called the systolic or maximum pressure reading. The second number measures the blood pressure in between beats, when the heart is resting (diastole). It's called the diastolic or lowest reading. The cycle from high to low pressure takes less than a second to complete. This is your heartbeat.

Blood pressure readings vary depending on the amount of blood the heart pumps and the capacity of the arteries and veins to stretch in order to allow the blood to pass through the body. It's something similar to what happens when you pump water through a garden hose. The more water that goes in and the less the rubber stretches, the greater the pressure will be.

High blood pressure is when the systolic reading is higher than 140 mm Hg and the diastolic reading is higher than 90 mm Hg.

No one knows for sure why we get hypertension, but it's believed that factors such as diabetes, eating too much salt or having stress contribute to its appearance. High blood pressure is painless and doesn't have many detectable symptoms, but if it isn't treated, the arteries eventually harden because of all the pressure they must withstand. Hardened arteries lead to heart attacks, strokes and kidney failure.

During pregnancy, the volume of the mother's blood increases between 20 and 40 percent. That's because the uterus needs more blood

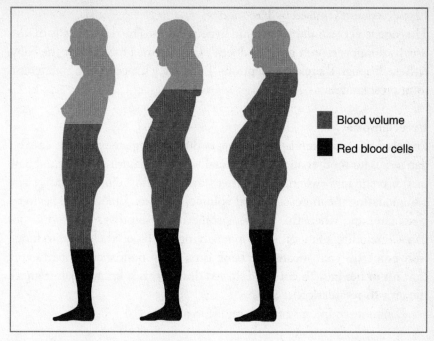

Blood volume

Red blood cells

Blood volume increase during pregnancy

flow to give oxygen and nutrients to the baby. Plus, some of the mother's organs, such as the kidneys, need more blood to work harder. To make room for this extra blood, the arteries and veins relax. But hypertension prevents the arteries and veins from making more space for the extra blood, and depending on how high the blood pressure is, it can mean less blood (and therefore oxygen and nutrients) for the baby and the mother's internal organs.

There are several types of hypertension that can appear during pregnancy. Some women can suffer from a combination of them.

Chronic Hypertension

This is the type of high blood pressure that was present before the pregnancy began and that some of us don't know we have. Generally, there aren't many risks for the baby, but the problem is that it increases the chances of complications such as preeclampsia.

Nonetheless, a mother-to-be with high blood pressure can have normal readings during the first part of the pregnancy, because that's when the arteries and veins are relaxing and expanding to allow room for the increased blood volume.

Hypertension Caused by Pregnancy

This one is very similar to chronic hypertension. The difference is that it usually disappears after birth. It doesn't cause many problems for the baby either, although there are exceptions. Pregnancy hypertension is different from preeclampsia.

Preeclampsia

Preeclampsia or toxemia only appears during pregnancy, and it can be dangerous for mother and baby. It usually shows up during the second half of the pregnancy, when the mother's arteries and veins, instead of accommodating the increased blood volume, contract. Blood could begin to coagulate, and when this happens some of the mother's most vital organs—including the uterus—stop receiving the blood they need to function properly. That means the baby isn't being nourished properly and that his or her growth could be slowed down (this is known as intrauterine growth retardation).

Common symptoms of this condition are:

- A quick rise in blood pressure
- Protein appearing in urine tests (which means the kidneys could be damaged)
- Quick weight gain and swelling of the face and hands due to water retention
- Headaches, stomach pains, nausea, seeing flashes and momentary loss of vision

When a doctor thinks a mother may have preeclampsia, it usually means a trip to the hospital so she can receive close medical attention. Preeclampsia can go from minor to serious in a matter of hours. If it isn't treated, it could become eclampsia, an illness so severe that the mother can have convulsions, she can suffer a stroke, her liver can rupture or the placenta, the organ that gives oxygen and nutrients to the baby, can tear off the uterus wall (a condition known as placenta abruptio).

If you go into convulsions at any time during your pregnancy, someone should immediately call 911 or the emergency services near where you live.

Preeclampsia can be mild or serious, but in the end, the only real cure is the birth of the baby. When it's not too serious, doctors recommend resting on the left side to alleviate the pressure on the main arteries, cutting back on salt or drinking more water. If the symptoms are severe enough, sometimes the doctor will induce labor, even if it results in a premature birth, because the health and life of the mother and the baby could be in danger.

Natacha Rodríguez suffered hypertension problems during both her pregnancies. She didn't know her blood pressure was high before she got pregnant.

"During my first pregnancy, my doctors watched me closely because my blood pressure readings were 140 over 80. Everything was going well until my fifth month, when I began to get this *horrible dolor de cabeza*, terrible, terrible headache. I called my doctor and she sent me to the hospital right away. My blood pressure had jumped to 170 over 100. I didn't have any symptoms of preeclampsia, but they kept me in the hospital for a couple of days of observation.

"Fortunately, everything went well during the rest of my pregnancy, although I was very swollen. *Se me hincharon hasta los ojos*, even my eyes were swollen. After I gave birth, I breastfed my baby for about five months. One day I decided to go to the doctor because I had stomach pains. I thought it was simply *agruras*, too much acid in my stomach. But in reality, I was five months pregnant! Not only that, but my blood pressure had returned to sky-high levels.

"During my next prenatal visit my doctor got worried because my daughter wasn't growing according to schedule; she was about two months behind. I started to take some medicines for my hypertension so my baby would begin to get more oxygen. One month passed, and my blood pressure readings were still too high and I had another severe headache. They quickly checked me into the hospital and I was diagnosed with preeclampsia. I had blood pressure readings of 180 over 110. The drugs finally took effect and my readings went down some. But when I reached the eighth month of my pregnancy, they jumped up again and *mi bebé seguía demasiado chiquita*, my baby still wasn't as big as she should have been. That's when the doctor said not to take any more chances—it was time for Cristina to be born.

"I really got scared. They did a test to see how developed her lungs were and she was born by cesarean section. She weighed five pounds.

The doctors kept a close watch over me while I was in the recovery room and even though I got a little better, my readings were still too high while I was in the hospital. They sent me to a cardiologist who gave me several prescriptions, which I am still taking four years later. I really have to take care of myself because high blood pressure is something that you don't feel. Some days I feel great and when I check it is really high, and other days is the opposite. It's something you don't have control over."

Although preeclampsia isn't too common, the most recent studies show during the last decade the number of cases has increased by 40 percent. The chances that preeclampsia will strike increase when the mother:

- Is older than thirty-five
- Is pregnant with more than one baby
- Is pregnant for the first time
- Suffered from hypertension, diabetes or obesity before the pregnancy
- Has had preeclampsia in previous pregnancies or has a family history of preeclampsia

Why preeclampsia appears and how to prevent it remain a mystery. According to the latest theories, it could be caused by a problem in the placenta implantation. The placentas of women with preeclampsia send a signal to the body through an enzyme saying that the baby is not getting enough blood. This is not true, but the body reacts by sending more blood. The blood pressure goes up and the blood vessels constrict, causing all the problems associated with this disease. Preeclampsia disappears once the baby is born and the placenta is not present anymore.

In summary, hypertension is something that we Latinas have to take very seriously before, during and after pregnancy. The main cause of death among Hispanic mothers after giving birth is hypertension that appears during pregnancy.

Obesity

When it comes to eating healthy foods, we Latinos know what we are talking about. Our foods have more fiber and less cholesterol and we eat more vegetables than the rest of the population. For example, the combination of rice and beans is an ideal dish because it provides proteins with less fat. We're also known for eating lots of fruits and vegetables that are full of vitamins A and C, such as tomatoes, chiles and peaches. Potatoes and corn have a lot of fiber that the body processes slowly, something good for your health. In general, Hispanic women have higher-than-normal levels of folic acid.

So if we eat so well, why is it that obesity rates in the Latino population are so high? According to the 2000 National Health Survey, three of every ten Latinos are obese.

Obesity during pregnancy is pretty uncomfortable and has the potential for many unpleasant consequences. According to several studies:

- Obese women are twice as likely to have a cesarean section.
- C-sections have more risk of complications for overweight women.
- If you were already overweight when you got pregnant, it's three times more likely your baby will be overweight, too, compared to Latinas who got pregnant at a normal weight. A baby who gains too much weight can have problems during birth and later (see page 74).
- Overweight Latinas have a tendency to gain more weight than they need to during their pregnancies.

But before you begin to feel guilty about those *deliciosos tamales*, wonderful tamales you were thinking about preparing this weekend, let me tell you a story about the Pima Indians.

THE THRIFT GENE

For thousands of years, the Pima Indians of Arizona hunted, fished and grew food on their lands. They were in great physical shape, but their survival depended on the cycles of the harvests and Mother Nature. There were times when food was plentiful and there were times when food was scarce. The Pima were forced to change their ways when U.S. farmers redirected their water supply in the late nineteenth century and they began to eat the flour, sugar and lard the government gave them. The prosperity of the post–World War II years put an end to the Pima traditions, because no longer did they need to hunt, fish or farm the lands to survive. Instead, they were able to buy a hamburger and fries for lunch and dinner. Today, 95 percent of the Pima are overweight and they have the highest diabetes rate in the world.

But the most interesting part of this story is that there's another Pima population that lives in a remote part of the Mexican Sierra Madre. That group still hunts, fishes and farms the way their ancestors did—even going hungry at times. Not one of the Mexican Pima Indians was overweight, and only three suffered from diabetes at the time a study was done to compare their health to Arizona Pima Indians.

That contrast forced scientists studying the Pima to consider the existence of a "thrift gene." This gene would allow its carrier to store fat during times of plenty, fat that could be used for survival during times of want. Other studies of the Manitoba Indians in Canada have confirmed the existence of this gene.

There's more. Another genetic study in Germany comparing obese and normal-weight people showed that overweight people had three times the likelihood of inheriting the thrift gene (one from each parent) compared with the people whose weight was closer to normal. Among the women in the study, those who carried the thrift gene were six times more likely to retain their weight after a pregnancy compared with those who didn't inherit the gene.

In other words, we're living in bodies genetically designed to survive periods of hunger, just as our ancestors did. In reality, at least in the Western world, food is plentiful almost all the time. This survival mechanism is turning against us. Even though the studies are still ongoing, it appears we Latinos have a much higher likelihood of carrying copies of the thrift gene than the rest of the population.

Our genetics may be working against us, but that doesn't mean we have to suffer *la maldición del gen*, "the curse of the thrift gene," for the rest of our lives. There are two weapons we can use to fight this gene before, during and after pregnancy, as the Sierra Madre Pima Indians proved: a healthy diet and regular exercise.

With or without the thrift gene, obesity is not a good prospect for Latinas during pregnancy. But the most important thing to remember is that with the help of your doctor, you can control your weight gain through a healthy diet and exercise.

GALLBLADDER DISEASE

"*Me duele el hígado*," "my liver hurts," is a common expression used to describe the general pains we sometimes get in the upper right side of the abdomen. During pregnancy, this phrase gets very real for some Latinas. Women of Mexican descent have a much higher chance of gallbladder disease. The gallbladder is one of the many organs affected by the hormonal upheaval during pregnancy. For women who have normal gallbladders, pregnancy doesn't make much of a difference, but women who have had problems with their gallbladders before getting pregnant can find the process of having a baby only makes the discomfort worse.

Laura García had trouble with hers during her third pregnancy.

"I started feeling discomfort around the fifth month. First it was *como un dolor en la espalda,* like a back pain up there, to the right side. My husband used to give me massages and it felt better. However, later my back hurt worse. Then the gallbladder pain started. Anything I ate gave me a stomachache. I had to cook for myself as if I was a baby, with no fats at all. I couldn't tolerate milk, nor cheeses, chiles or salsa, and only a few eggs. *Hasta después supe,* only later I found that when you have gallbladder problems you can't even touch eggs or *frijoles,* beans. But eight weeks or so before having the baby I started swimming and I started to feel much better."

The gallbladder is a hollow muscle, situated beneath the liver and connected to it on one end and to the small intestine on the other (see illustration on page 99). Its job is to store bile to aid in the breakdown of fats. When the foods we eat enter the small intestine, a signal is sent to the gallbladder to begin contractions in order to send out bile.

Bile is produced in the liver and is made up of bile acids, salts, water and cholesterol, among other things. There are two common ways for gallbladder stones to build up:

• If we eat a lot of fats, it's possible our bile contains a lot of cholesterol. The more cholesterol, the more likely it is that sediments and eventually stones will appear.

• When the gallbladder doesn't contract enough to completely empty and the bile pools in the bottom, stones also form.

The hormones produced during and after pregnancy actually make both circumstances more likely. On one hand, an elevated level of estrogen makes the liver increase the amount of cholesterol in the bile. On the other, pregnancy hormones make the gallbladder enlarge and lose its muscle tone and consequently make it more difficult to empty completely.

Sediments in the bile form stones that can obstruct the drainage tubes to the intestine in the gallbladder. The blockage causes inflammation and infections that show up as pains, nausea, fever, chills and vomiting, or in other words, a gallbladder or biliar colic will happen. It's common to discover during pregnancy there are stones or obstructions in the gallbladder. Three of every ten pregnant women have gallstones, although only a small number of those have colics.

If you're suffering from stomach pains and from nausea and vomiting that don't go away by the beginning of the second trimester, it could have something to do with your gallbladder, especially if you're of Mexican descent.

A simple ultrasound test will show if the problem is there. Even if doctors do find you've got gallstones, if you don't suffer any symptoms, it's better not to do anything because the problem is likely to go away when you give birth. Minor symptoms during pregnancy can be treated, and in the case of extreme colics, there is a low-risk surgery to remove the gallbladder.

There really isn't much you can do to control your increased hormonal production during pregnancy, but a healthy diet and regular exercise can prevent or at least lessen gallbladder problems during pregnancy. High-fat foods (especially animal fat such as lard) are equivalent to a nuclear bomb for your gallbladder. In fact, it is believed that certain foods are directly related to gallbladder problems. In order of danger, they are eggs, pork, onions, chicken and other poultry, milk, coffee, citrus, corn, beans and nuts. Avoid these foods if your gallbladder is sensitive. It will help you reduce the risk of a colic. As the saying goes: *No aprovecha lo comido, sino lo digerido,* "Enjoy what you can digest, not what you can eat."

INFECTIOUS DISEASES

Protecting our babies during pregnancy is a biological instinct. During these nine months, we're more cautious and we often decide what we're going to do based on how the action might affect the baby, whether it's taking a flight of stairs or eating an unusual dinner. Logically, the first thing that passes through our minds when we get sick is "How will it affect my baby?" And if we're talking about an infectious illness, we're likely to worry even more.

Infectious diseases are produced by viruses or bacteria that somehow get into our bodies. The most common are colds or the flu, or diarrhea caused by eating something that's spoiled. Those kind of illnesses don't really threaten the baby. However, there are other infectious diseases that, if left untreated, can affect baby and mother. Some infections are more common among Latinos, and we need to pay special attention to them.

Rubella

Rubella or German measles is an infection caused by a virus. This illness wouldn't be that big a deal if it wasn't for the harm it can do to the fetus if the mother catches it during the first months of pregnancy.

Rubella is spread through the air and takes two to three weeks to incubate once it enters the body. In adults, it appears as a pink rash that begins on the face and makes its way toward the feet. It lasts one to five days and sometimes is accompanied by a slight fever, joint pain and swelling in the lymph nodes behind the ears and at the back of the neck. In children, the symptoms are less noticeable.

Rubella can have different effects on the fetus depending on when the mother is infected.

- During the first trimester the fetus is harmed 85 percent of the time.
- From weeks 10 through 16 the percentage of damaged fetuses is less.
- After 20 weeks of pregnancy it's rare that the baby shows any ill effects.

When rubella attacks the fetus, it's known as congenital rubella syndrome. It can harm nearly all the baby's organs, although deafness and blindness are the most common results. Spontaneous abortions are also common in the first weeks of pregnancy.

But if you've already had rubella in the past or if you've been vaccinated against it, you don't have anything to worry about—you can't get the disease. And if you can't get rubella, neither can your baby, because the virus is transmitted to the fetus only through your blood.

A blood test done in your first prenatal visit detects rubella antibodies, which our bodies produce to fight the virus. When you don't have antibodies it means that you haven't been vaccinated or had the disease, and you'll have to take precautions to make sure you don't come into contact with anyone in your workplace or elsewhere who may have rubella. If your husband or other people you live with haven't been vaccinated, ask your gynecologist about the possibility of them getting a vaccination.

In the 1960s, a rubella epidemic in the United States affected thousands of people. So in 1969, the rubella vaccine became commonplace and the number of cases dropped dramatically. Nevertheless, in many Latin American countries, policies to ensure all children were vaccinated for rubella didn't come into place until the end of the 1990s. As a result, the segment of society in the United States most affected by rubella is Latinos born in Latin America. In fact, 83 percent of the cases of congenital rubella syndrome in past years were seen in Latino babies whose Latina mothers were born in other countries. In the United States, rubella mostly affects people between twenty and thirty-nine years of age, and the outbreaks are most likely to happen at workplaces where several people aren't vaccinated.

In case you decide to get vaccinated before getting pregnant, you should wait at least three months to conceive. The rubella vaccine can't be given once a woman becomes pregnant, and it's not recommended while she's breastfeeding. These days, the rubella vaccine is commonly given to all children once they are a year old and again between four and six years of age. It's given along with the vaccines for measles and mumps and known as MMR (measles, mumps and rubella). There is no risk for you if your other children need this vaccine while you are pregnant.

Measles and Mumps

These two infectious diseases don't harm the fetus, although they can cause premature birth. If during your pregnancy you come into contact with someone who has one of these two diseases, it's possible to determine through a blood test whether you're immune.

In cases where a doctor fears a mother has been infected, she usually is given gamma globulin—extra antibodies that help fight the infection. Sometimes these illnesses appear soon before a baby is to be born and there's a chance they'll be transmitted to the baby in the process. They can be serious for a newborn.

Chicken Pox

It's very rare that a baby will get infected by the mother's blood and develop congenital chicken pox syndrome, even in the first weeks of pregnancy, when the fetus is most susceptible.

Chicken pox is a very contagious infection that's still common, especially among children. Between 85 and 95 percent of pregnant women are already immune to chicken pox, probably because they caught it when they were girls. Still, there is a small percentage of adult women who get chicken pox while they're pregnant. This illness is spread through the air, through the saliva of an infected person or through contact with the rash it causes.

If you haven't yet had chicken pox and someone in your house comes down with it, there's a 90 percent chance you'll be infected, too. A chicken pox antibody treatment helps ease the symptoms. Although the baby most likely won't get it, adult-onset chicken pox is generally severe and painful and can result in pneumonia. One of the most obvious chicken pox symptoms is a rash made up of little red bumps that later turn into small, liquid-filled blisters.

The chicken pox vaccine shouldn't be given during pregnancy. Scientists haven't documented any cases of mothers-to-be getting chicken pox from recently vaccinated children, so don't worry if you have to get another child vaccinated.

Fifth Disease

This illness is very common among children and causes a red rash on the face, arms and legs. Around half of adult women are immune to this disease because they've already had it. However, if you don't have antibodies for this illness and you get infected, there is some risk of miscarriage.

If you work with school-age children or have other children who could become infected, ask your doctor to test you for fifth disease antibodies. If you don't have them, you should avoid contact with infected children because there is no treatment for this illness.

Tuberculosis

Tuberculosis infection usually happens after the baby has been born because of contact with someone who's in the active phase of the disease. Tuberculosis doesn't cause birth defects, and cases of infection from mother to baby are very rare. Pregnancy doesn't make mothers-to-be any more susceptible to the illness either.

At the end of the 1950s in the United States, doctors thought tuberculosis was a disease of the past. But in the last few decades, a great number of people have come down with it. This is an illness that disproportionately affects minorities in the United States, and we Latinos have double the chance of getting it compared with the rest of the population. Cutting down on the number of Latino tuberculosis cases was the goal of a government program called Healthy People 2000. Although there's been a slight improvement, the objectives still haven't been reached.

Tuberculosis is caused by a bacterium called *Mycobacterium tuberculosis*. When these bacteria invade, the body's immune system reacts and "surrounds" the infected cells. The cells remain corralled for years until for one reason or another, the immune system fails, the bacteria win the war and the disease is activated. In some people, the body can rid itself of the bacteria completely, without any complications.

The tuberculosis bacterium is spread through the air, but prolonged contact with someone who's developed the illness is needed for it to pass from one person to another. Some of the symptoms of the disease in its active state include fever, weight loss and night sweats. In extreme cases, a victim might have chest pains, continuous cough and bloody mucus.

To determine if someone is infected with tuberculosis, doctors use the tuberculin test, which consists of a small injection under the skin of the arm. It can be given during pregnancy, because it doesn't present any risks to the mother or baby. If the disease is in its latent or inactive stage, doctors will usually postpone treatment until after the baby is born, as long as there aren't any other complications. But if the tuberculosis does become active during pregnancy, a quick response is necessary, because if left untreated, this disease can have serious consequences for the mother.

The antibiotics used to treat pregnant women (isoniazid, rifampicin) don't harm the fetus and are effective. They require extended treatment periods, sometimes as long as several months. It's important to follow the recommended dosage and treatment schedule, because if you stop taking the drugs prematurely, the bacteria might develop a resistance to the medicine and your illness will return. In fact, one of the reasons tuberculosis is so prevalent today is that current antibiotics don't work against new strains of bacteria that have developed a resistance.

Cytomegalovirus

This is a very common virus among small children in day care or kindergarten and it doesn't cause much trouble in adults.

Although it's rare, pregnant women can pass the virus to the baby if they get infected for the first time during pregnancy. As a result, babies can have hearing or seeing problems and mental retardation. If the baby is infected during or after birth, it doesn't cause any harm.

Hepatitis

Hepatitis is a chronic or acute inflammation of the liver. The most common reason people get hepatitis is a virus that attacks the liver. To date, scientists have discovered seven types of hepatitis (A, B, C, D, E, F and G) that can damage the liver. A and B are the ones that most affect Latinos.

Hepatitis can be transmitted to the baby while it's in the uterus or during or after birth. When it's treated in time, most babies and their mothers respond well. Pregnancy doesn't make hepatitis worse (except in the case of hepatitis E, which isn't common in the United States). That means if a woman who has hepatitis gets pregnant, her pregnancy won't affect the status of her illness.

A healthy liver is essential to good health, and it plays an important role during pregnancy.

The liver is situated just behind the ribs on the right side of the abdomen, and it carries out some of the most complex and varied functions in our bodies. Among other things, it's in charge of:

Gallbladder and liver position

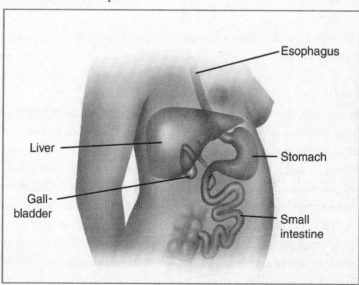

- Removing toxins from the blood
- Making bile, which helps to digest fats
- Storing the glucose, proteins, vitamins and minerals from the foods we eat
- Combating infections

The incubation period for hepatitis is between 45 and 160 days. That means that we could have gotten infected a month and a half to five months ago and didn't feel anything. When the illness is finally activated the following symptoms can appear:

- General malaise
- Loss of appetite
- Upset stomach
- Nausea and vomiting
- Liver pains
- Yellow color in the whites of the eyes and skin
- Light-colored stool

Half of the people who have hepatitis don't show any of these symptoms, but they are still able to pass the disease on to others.

Depending on the type of hepatitis virus you have, the method of transmission varies.

Hepatitis A

Hepatitis A, the most common among the general population as well as among Latinos, is passed orally, after someone comes in contact with human feces that are contaminated with the virus. For example, if infected people don't wash their hands after going to the bathroom, they can contaminate other people or the food or drink they're handling.

A blood test determines whether someone is infected. Usually a good diet and rest are enough to rid the body of the disease in a couple of months. During pregnancy it's common to prescribe a dose of hepatitis A immunoglobulin. Immunoglobulin is hepatitis antibodies that have been drawn from someone who's already had the disease, and they help you fight off the infection.

Babies can contract hepatitis during birth through contact with maternal blood or later by mouth, the same as adults. Usually it is not severe, and they will develop antibodies against the disease to make them immune to it for the rest of their life.

Hepatitis B

Hepatitis B is more serious than hepatitis A and can cause chronic hepatitis, cirrhosis or liver failure. This type of hepatitis is the second most common among Latinos, and it's also one of the easiest to be passed from mother to baby. Generally, this virus infects the newborn during birth, through the mother's blood. But it can also reach the baby before then, during the nine months of gestation. The later in the pregnancy the mother contracts hepatitis B, the more likely the disease is to be transmitted to the baby. During birth, the incidence of infection is high. That's why prenatal blood screenings are used to determine whether the mother is infected. If she is, the mother-to-be is given a shot of antibodies that fight the hepatitis B virus (hepatitis B immunoglobulin).

The most common forms of transmission between adults are through sexual contact, blood transfusions or sharing needles. Adults who have been vaccinated against hepatitis B are 80 to 100 percent protected against this illness, but this vaccine can't be given during pregnancy.

Hepatitis C

The incidence of hepatitis C is increasing, notably among people between twenty and forty years old, the same age when most women get pregnant. Hepatitis C is spread in the same manner as hepatitis B, but the risk of infecting the baby is much lower.

Hepatitis D and E

Hepatitis D shows up only when hepatitis B is present, and is spread through contact with the blood of an infected person.

Hepatitis E is transmitted in the same way as hepatitis A, by contact with human feces or contaminated water or food. It's a serious disease for pregnant women, but in the United States it is almost nonexistent. Hepatitis E usually appears in disaster areas where there have been floods and the local water has been contaminated.

HEPATITIS F AND G

Relatively rare, F and G hepatitis have been discovered only recently. They are still being studied.

Acquired Immune Deficiency Syndrome (AIDS)

I remember a few years ago when I did a series of interviews with Latinas who had tested positive for HIV. The story of Gabriela Muñoz really got to me. She was a thirty-four-year-old woman who found out her partner was HIV-positive the same day the big earthquake hit Los Angeles. Gabriela (not her real name, to protect her from *los chismes del barrio*, the neighborhood gossip) not only didn't abandon her partner, but she married him, took care of him and dedicated her life to making sure everyone in her community practiced safe sex, without revealing her personal drama.

That was in 1994. Unfortunately, stories like Gabriela's have been repeated thousands of times. Latinas represent 11 percent of the female population in the United States. But they make up 20 percent of the women with HIV.

❧

The main source of HIV infection for Latinas is unprotected sex with their infected partners.

HIV is transmitted when blood, semen, vaginal fluid or breast milk from an infected person gets inside another person's body.

HIV works in a methodical way to slowly destroy the human immune system. It could be "asleep" from eight to ten years, and although the infected person might not experience any symptoms during that period, he or she could infect other people.

Being HIV-positive is not the same thing as having AIDS. HIV is the virus that causes AIDS; AIDS (acquired immune deficiency syndrome) is a stage of the disease where the immune system does not work anymore and there is no defense left against illnesses. A cure has yet to be found for this infectious disease, but with the appropriate medication and care many women can live a normal life and have a healthy baby.

One of the tests included in the first prenatal visit is an HIV screening, to see if HIV antibodies are in the bloodstream. If they are, it means the virus is present and the immune system is trying to fight it. Given that this virus is transmitted through the blood, a mother can infect her baby at any moment during the pregnancy, the birth or even afterward, while she's breastfeeding. Unless the virus load (the amount of virus present in the blood) is very low, infected mothers almost always give birth by cesarean section.

Before the use of treatments to avoid mother-baby transmission of the virus, around 16 to 25 percent of the babies of HIV-positive women were infected. Today, the use of these drugs combined with extensive prenatal screening for HIV and AIDS has cut down the infection rate from mother to baby to 2 percent. Recent studies have shown that using these medicines does not harm the baby. The most effective medicine against AIDS is zidovudine (also known as ZDV, AZT or Retrovir), which keeps the virus from replicating itself. In the Contact List, you'll find telephone numbers you can call to get your questions about HIV and AIDS answered. The information is available in English or Spanish and it's confidential.

Group B Streptococcus (GBS)

This bacterium is the most common cause of pneumonia and meningitis in newborns. It's transmitted from mother to baby through the vaginal canal during birth.

Group B streptococcus lives inside many healthy people without causing any harm. One of every four women has this type of bacteria in the rectum. But since this illness can be very serious for a newborn, a vaginal sample is taken at the beginning of the pregnancy and between 35 and 37 weeks of pregnancy to determine if the bacterium is present. The test is done so late because the closer delivery is, the more effective antibiotic treatment is.

There is a higher risk of group B streptococcus infection to the baby in premature births, or when eighteen hours go by after the amniotic membranes have broken. For this reason, when no GBS test results are available, it's possible that your obstetrician/gynecologist will want to treat you with antibiotics as a precautionary measure.

Venereal Diseases

Venereal diseases are transmitted sexually. Many of them are considered "silent" because they don't present any symptoms in the men or women who have them. However, venereal diseases can affect the baby, in some cases seriously.

Some of these infections are contagious during birth, as the baby comes in contact with the mother's blood. Others travel through the mother's blood to the baby while it's still in the uterus. At some point during your pregnancy your doctor may take a vaginal swab to see if any type of venereal disease is present, even if you only have one partner.

Many venereal infections can affect your pregnancy, but the most common are the following.

Bacterial Vaginosis

Pregnant women with bacterial vaginosis can give birth to low-birth-weight or premature babies. The Centers for Disease Control recommend that all women who have had a premature birth should be tested to see if the cause was bacterial vaginosis.

Doctors still aren't sure how a woman gets this disease, although studies show that women who have a new sexual partner or who have had several in the past are more likely to suffer it. Nonetheless, bacterial vaginosis also appears among women who haven't had many sexual partners. Surveys done in 2000 show that 16 percent of Latinas have suffered bacterial vaginosis, compared to 9 percent of white women and 23 percent of African-American women.

The infection appears when one of the types of bacteria that live in the vagina starts reproducing madly. The result is an infection that can cause a burning or itching sensation when urinating, and a discharge that is different in color and amount and sometimes malodorous. Typically bacterial vaginosis produces a strong fishy smell, especially after sex. But in other cases there are no symptoms at all.

Chlamydia

As an educational campaign used to say, *la clamidia no es una flor*, chlamydia is not a flower, but one of the most common venereal diseases in the United States. Chlamydia is caused by a bacterium that infects the vagina and can produce a stinging or burning sensation during urination and a heavier-than-normal vaginal discharge. In the majority of cases, no symptoms are present. That's why this infection is so common and becoming more so. The incidence of this disease, which is especially high among women younger than twenty-five, has increased 500 percent in the past fifteen years.

Chlamydia can spread to other areas of the reproductive system and cause pelvic inflammatory disease (PID). The bacterium damages the lining of the fallopian tubes and can cause infertility or ectopic pregnancies. Fortunately, treatment with the proper antibiotics is very effective.

Chlamydia can also infect the baby as it passes through the vaginal canal during birth, and the result is an eye infection or pneumonia. The ointment doctors put on a baby's eyes when it is born is an antibiotic to reduce the risk of an infection in case the mother has undetected chlamydia or gonorrhea.

GONORRHEA

Gonorrhea can cause premature birth and can be transmitted to the baby during birth, causing blindness, blood infections and joint problems. It is treated with an antibiotic, and it usually disappears after one dose.

The majority of the cases appear in people between fifteen and twenty-nine years old, and like chlamydia, it affects Latinos more than other ethnic groups. As with other venereal diseases, the risk is that it could turn into pelvic inflammatory disease. Gonorrhea is commonly seen along with chlamydia.

Men tend to have more symptoms than women, such as burning or stinging while urinating or a yellow discharge from the penis.

GENITAL WARTS

They're caused by a virus known as human papillomavirus. They look like little gray or flesh-colored cauliflowers, and they appear in the genital area. Many infected people do not develop the warts, but still they can transmit the virus through sexual relations. In women the virus can cause cervical cancer.

A baby rarely gets infected with this virus during birth, but if this happens, he/she can get warts in the throat.

SYPHILIS

A disease caused by a bacterium, syphilis develops in stages that can last for years. It's a serious illness for pregnant women, because the virus can cross the placenta and attack the fetus. When this happens, the baby has what's called congenital syphilis syndrome, which is nearly always devastating. It can attack the brain and the liver or cause death.

The latest efforts to treat infected mothers have shown good results, and the number of babies born with congenital syphilis syndrome has gone down. However, that's not the case with the disease among adults. Even though the numbers on a national level have leveled off, there are some cities where the number of cases of syphilis continues to grow.

Genital Herpes

There is no cure for this disease, although the symptoms are treatable. Herpes can appear on the lips or on the genitals. When a person is infected with genital herpes he/she passes through several stages, first seeing the formation of blisters that eventually burst. It's in that stage that the virus is most contagious. On average, an infected person can expect three to five outbreaks a year.

For pregnant women, the danger is if the virus is active during delivery, because the herpes can be transmitted to the baby as it passes through the vagina. The herpes virus can cause serious harm to the baby by damaging its nervous system. The risk of transmission is higher when the mother is first infected during the last trimester of pregnancy, because the first episodes are the most active; the risk is lower if the woman has had genital herpes for several years. But the possible harm to the baby is so severe, many doctors recommend a cesarean section birth if the mother has genital herpes. It's a good idea to avoid oral sex with a person who has herpes lesions on the lips or in the mouth, especially in the last three months of pregnancy.

To treat herpes, doctors use antiviral medicines such as acyclovir, which reduces the severity of the symptoms and shortens the life of the episodes.

Depression

Women get depressed more often than men, and according to one study, depression is a real problem for Latinas: we are among the most depressed women in the United States. Depression is more than just being sad or having *nervios*. It's an official illness, on par with the others described in this chapter, and if it's not treated, it gets worse.

Depression begins with chemical changes in the brain. During pregnancy there are powerful hormonal releases that can affect the brain's chemical balance. Also, the anxiety that some women feel in the face of the big changes that maternity brings can alter the brain chemistry.

It's difficult in our culture to understand how a mother-to-be could be depressed during pregnancy, because this is supposed to be one of the happiest times in a woman's life. Under normal circumstances it's true that pregnancy is a very special and wonderful time for a woman, but there are several situations where this might not be the case:

- *Depression before pregnancy.* In some women, depression gets better during pregnancy, but in some others it gets worse.

- *External circumstances*. Pregnancy is a stage where many women feel vulnerable. If a woman's family is far away or if she is going through economic difficulties, there could be a lot of anxiety that leads ultimately to depression.

- *Hormonal sensitivity*. The monthly hormonal cycles of women apparently play a role in the prevalence of depression among females. Some women are more sensitive than others to hormonal changes.

And for Latinas, there are cultural factors that make us more likely to suffer from this disease. If we feel depressed, we often think, *"Ya pasará,"* "It will pass, I don't need a psychiatrist."

---

§

Depression doesn't pass; it gets worse. You cannot cure it trying to *sentirse alegre*, feel happy, any more than you can cure diabetes by talking your pancreas into producing more insulin. These are chemical processes that you can't control.

If you have depression, you are not alone. Fully 20 percent of women feel depressed during pregnancy, and 10 percent develop serious symptoms.

Depression Symptoms

You may have this disease if you feel depressed during much of the day for two weeks straight and in addition you have:

- Difficulty sleeping or are sleeping too much
- Difficulty concentrating
- Fatigue or lack of energy
- Anxiety or feelings of emptiness
- Lack of interest in recreational activities
- Feelings of guilt
- Thoughts about death or suicide

The difficulty in diagnosing depression during pregnancy is that symptoms such as fatigue, lack of energy, and difficulty sleeping or sleeping too much are the same ones that nondepressed women have during the first three months. Depression is usually easier to diagnose during the second trimester, when the physical discomforts start to disappear.

It's important to diagnose and treat depression during pregnancy, because if it's not, the mother is even more likely to suffer from postpartum depression (see page 341). A depressed mother-to-be may not eat properly or may turn to smoking and drinking, which aren't good for the baby. In addition, this illness will prevent a woman from enjoying her pregnancy.

Treatment for Depression During Pregnancy

The first treatment during pregnancy is usually psychotherapy, which has been proven pretty effective in cases of moderate depression. There are two types of psychotherapy:

- *Personal therapy* focuses on why a woman may be depressed. For example, does she have enough support for her pregnancy? Is she far from her family?
- *Behavioral therapy* focuses on changing situations or external influences.

The effects of therapy are felt more slowly than the effects of drugs, but they are usually longer-lasting. A combination of drugs and therapy is very effective.

The antidepressant drugs prescribed by doctors during recent years have not been shown to have harmful effects on the baby. For ethical reasons, pharmaceutical companies haven't carried out tests on pregnant women, but they are keeping track of all the mothers-to-be who take antidepressants and following the course of their pregnancies and their outcomes. Nothing so far leads doctors to believe they cause problems for the child, but it's still to be seen what the long-term effects are, if any.

The most-used drugs to treat depression during pregnancy are called selective serotonin reuptake inhibitors (SSRIs). In the last few years, scientists have discovered that people who have lower levels of serotonin in the brain are more likely to be depressed. These medicines increase the serotonin level in the brain. The most common brands are Prozac, Zoloft, Paxil and Celexa. Although all of them work in the same way, gynecologists seem to prefer Prozac because it's been used in many pregnancies without problems.

These drugs do have some side effects for the mother, including dry mouth, headaches, insomnia and lack of sexual desire. If they don't work, don't stop taking them without talking to your doctor, because you may get worse by stopping suddenly.

THE LATINA PARADOX

After reading this long list of illnesses, you might be thinking it's a real miracle that even one Latino baby survives from these ailing mothers. But the truth is, despite all our health risks, the fact that many of us don't have health insurance, and the fact that many of us don't have the resources other sectors of the population have, our babies and we turn out better than fine.

So much so, in fact, that the success rate with our babies has some scientists puzzled. Several studies have been done to determine why it is that with all the odds against us, Latino babies are born healthy and at a good weight. One study in particular tried to analyze how Mexican women counted their missed periods to see if they were counting the months wrong and premature babies were not premature.

Well, there are some things that just can't be explained in a laboratory or by statistics. Yes, certain genetic and social factors aren't on our side. But we Latinas hardly smoke and in general don't abuse drugs or alcohol, our diets are much more healthy than the rest of the population, and *sobre todo*, most of all, we've got a strong support network in our families and our communities.

I don't have any doubt the *forma de vivir latina*, the Latino way of living, is what gives us and our babies good health, that is, a mix between strong human connections, healthy habits and good spiritual life. And in fact, statistics show that the further we drift from our roots, the further we separate ourselves from the *buenas costumbres*, our traditional customs, with the passing of each generation, the more vulnerable our health and the health of our children becomes.

So take care of yourself during your pregnancy. Go for your prenatal visits. Watch out for diseases. But more than anything, don't forget to live *la buena vida*, the good life.

6

Pregnancy Medical Tests

It won't be long before parents-to-be carry along photographs of their future babies in their wallets. I'm not talking about those blurry black-and-white sonograms where only a parent is able to clearly see how the baby looks just like *Abuelo* or Grandpa. No, I'm talking about color, three-dimensional images of our babies at four months.

Modern science will also help us confirm once and for all, without having to go through an amniocentesis, which of our co-workers and relatives really master the art of predicting the sex of the baby by the shape of a belly. A simple blood test will determine whether we're going to have a boy or a girl.

Technological advances of the past few decades have included improvements in prenatal care, and doctors can now determine with near certainty if the unborn baby is developing normally. There are even treatments and procedures doctors can perform while the baby is still in the uterus to correct health problems that in the old days wouldn't have allowed the baby to survive.

In this chapter, you'll read about the most common tests doctors perform on pregnant women. Some are routine and are given to nearly all mothers during their nine months but others are used only when the doctor thinks there's a problem that needs to be looked at.

BABY IMAGES

Sonograms are one of the most popular tests among future parents. It's a magical and emotional moment to see for the first time a heart beating inside you, with all the force of life, or the silhouette of a moving hand or, in the case of my daughter Patricia, how an unborn baby can jump as if she were on a trampoline.

Sonograms produce images through sound waves. A small device called a transducer is placed on the abdomen or inserted into the vagina. The unit emits sound waves that bounce off the baby. A computer interprets these waves or "echoes" and sends them to a viewing screen where a doctor or technician analyzes them. That's how the images get their names—sonogram or echography. It's the same principle as radar.

The baby doesn't feel anything during a sonogram, and neither does the mother. Nor have any negative effects after birth been documented for mother or child during the almost forty years that sonograms have been in use.

Generally at least two sonograms are done during pregnancy to make sure everything is fine. The images obtained through the sonogram help the doctor determine several things at different times, including:

- Presence of a heartbeat
- Age and development of the fetus
- Approximate delivery date
- Number of fetuses (surprise!)
- Location and condition of the placenta (important because sometimes the placenta sits at the opening of the uterus, precisely where the baby has to go to be born—it's called placenta previa; see page 165—in which case the baby must be delivered by cesarean section)
- Evaluation for causes of vaginal bleeding
- If there are any physical deformities, either external and internal
- The position of the fetus before it's born
- The amount of amniotic fluid at the end of the pregnancy
- Whether there is an ectopic pregnancy (see page 164)
- To help perform other tests such as amniocentesis or fetal blood tests

There are several types of sonograms. They differ in the way they're given and the techniques used.

Vaginal Sonogram

It's used during the first weeks of pregnancy because it delivers the clearest, most detailed pictures. At the beginning of the pregnancy, it's easier to get to where the baby is through the vagina. With this technology, you can see the baby as early as four and a half weeks. At six weeks, it's possible to detect a heartbeat and more than one amniotic sac. This doesn't necessarily mean that you are having twins because one sac might be absorbed later.

When you get to the doctor's office, a nurse will tell you to take your clothes off below the waist, give you a dressing gown to put on and ask you to get comfortable on the examining table. The sonogram device is about the size of a tampon and is inserted into the vagina. The unit will be covered with a sterile and lubricated condom. Once the transducer is inside the vagina, the doctor or technician will move the device around until a clear picture appears. It doesn't hurt at all, although it can be a little uncomfortable, but I can assure you that the moment you see your baby's little heart beating on the screen, you'll forget about everything else.

If you can't see the screen very well from where you're lying on the table, don't be shy—ask to have the screen moved so you don't miss a single detail. Ask what's what. The images are really better understood if an expert explains them to you, because it's hard to tell what you're looking at most of the time. But remember, if technicians and not doctors, or your doctor, are giving you the sonogram, sometimes they're not authorized to interpret the images for you. That can be frustrating, but ask anyway because they might be able to give you at least a general idea of what you are looking at.

I also recommend you go with your husband or partner to this first appointment. Seeing together for the first time what both of you have created is unforgettable. When you are finished they will give you your first "baby pictures." But don't carry them around for a long time in your wallet, because they're printed on special paper and the ink rubs off. By the time my husband finally handed them over, all that was left was a gray blur. He must have shown the picture more than two hundred times.

Another way to keep these memories is on videotape. In some offices it's possible to record the sonogram on a VHS tape. Ask before you go so you can take your own blank tape. The whole procedure takes between fifteen minutes and an hour, depending on what the doctor is looking for.

Abdominal Sonogram

After the first three months of pregnancy, it's easier to see the baby through the mother's abdomen. This type of sonogram is often repeated at eighteen to twenty weeks.

For this test, all you have to do is leave your abdomen exposed. The

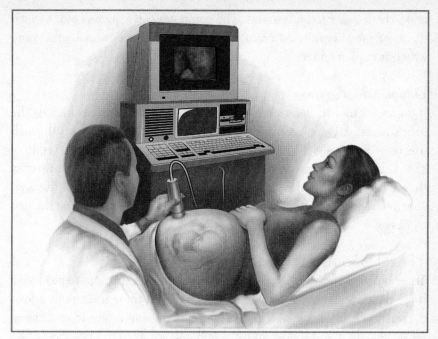

Abdominal sonogram

doctor or technician will apply a gel that allows the transducer (the unit that emits the sound waves) to slide easily. This is the sonogram that in theory can determine the sex of the baby. But it all depends on how he or she is situated and the experience of the technician. I imagine you know a few couples who spend a lot of money on pink clothes or decorations, only to find they should have bought blue, and vice versa.

Level II Sonogram
The technique is the same as the previous sonograms, but the difference is this one is more detailed. It's given between the eighteenth and twentieth weeks to evaluate the possibility the baby has any birth defects. A level II sonogram analyzes each and every organ and structure of the baby. The technician or doctor will look at the four heart chambers, kidneys, lungs, intestines, genitals and extremities and will make sure the brain is normal and does not have fluid accumulated inside. This sonogram offers an abundance of information. Nevertheless, the accuracy of these test results depends on the expertise of the person giving it, as well as the equipment used.

Some doctors are using sonogram machines that print color images to make them easier to understand. The computer can assign a color to each shade of gray. This is different from the three-dimensional sonogram, which is explained later.

Doppler Sonogram

It's a useful tool to determine if there are congenital deformities in the baby's heart. A Doppler sonogram measures how the blood flows through the fetus and assigns different colors to different paths and speeds of blood. These exams are given vaginally or abdominally. The intensity of the waves emitted by the Doppler system is greater than those of the conventional sonograms, which is why they're given with care during the first trimester.

Three-Dimensional Sonogram

Technological advances in computers now permit a sonogram to produce a three-dimensional image. The detail provided in these sonograms allows doctors to clearly see images that were not available before in traditional sonograms. In a 3-D sonogram it's possible to see even the lips. Some factors affect the clarity of the image, such as the amount of amniotic fluid, obesity of the mother, or the expertise of the technician operating the machine, but when quality is good you will be able to count the baby's toes and know who he or she looks like, before you have your baby in your arms.

3D fetus sonogram

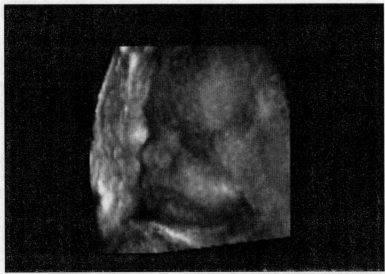

Image: Dr. Fernando X. Marin

Magnetic Resonance Images and Fetoscopy

These are procedures used only in rare circumstances. Magnetic resonance is useful when there is something that needs to be examined in greater detail. The images from these tests are very clear and defined. Fetoscopy is used for certain surgical procedures, such as when there are circulatory problems between twins or to remove placenta tumors. A doctor will make a small incision through the abdomen of the mother and another in the uterus to insert a small camera and the surgical instruments.

GENETIC TESTS

Genetics and its applications have seen some of the most dramatic advances in all of science in recent years. Thanks to a big project, carried out by several countries, scientists are going to be able to identify all the genes in the human body, something only a few years ago thought to be almost science fiction. This project has opened the door to discovering all kinds of hereditary diseases, how to treat them, and in some cases, even how to cure them.

The genetic tests given today during pregnancy allow doctors to see if the baby has certain hereditary diseases or abnormalities in its chromosomes or genes.

There are two types of genetic tests done during pregnancy:

- *Screening tests*. They will *not* tell you if your baby has a birth defect. They only indicate the possibility that your baby has a birth defect. Most of them are done through a blood test of the mother-to-be.

- *Genetic tests*. They *do* determine if your baby has a birth defect because they analyze the fetal chromosomes. The most common one is amniocentesis, where amniotic fluid is obtained from your body through a needle.

Screening tests are performed in a routine way, but genetic tests are done for the following reasons:

- The mother has already had one child with serious genetic defects.
- There is a hereditary disease in the family.
- Other tests done during pregnancy point toward the possibility the baby has a genetic defect.

- The mother is thirty-five years old or older.
- The parents are members of an ethnic group that has a history of suffering from a particular genetic disease.
- The mother or the father is exposed to radiation or chemicals at work.
- The parents are first cousins (although scientists have recently found out the risks of children between first cousins is much lower than previously thought).

The Dilemma

Our grandmothers and most of our mothers only knew if their babies were going to be fine after they were born. Sometimes, it took years to figure out that something just wasn't right. But now genetic science has made it possible to know before birth how our babies are doing. That knowledge carries with it many implications.

On one hand, this information means doctors can treat certain illnesses (unfortunately not many yet), giving some babies a greater chance of surviving and living healthy, happy lives. But on the other hand, it puts us in the terrible situation of having to choose what to do if we discover our baby has a birth defect. Even deciding *whether* you want to know is difficult.

Because these tests are part of modern-day prenatal care, you're going to have to think about them at some point during your pregnancy. Talking about all of this with your husband and your family beforehand will help you make a calmer, more thoughtful decision and will help you keep things clear when you're given the opportunity to take the tests. You'll feel more in control of the situation and less pressured to make a quick decision. Don't forget that each family is a universe of its own, each with different circumstances, ideas, values, and motivations. What's good for one family isn't necessarily good for another. What is good for one pregnancy might not be good for the next one.

Leticia Gomez was given the option of having an amniocentesis done during her second pregnancy, because she was older than thirty-five at the time.

"We brought home all the reading material they'd given us at the doctor's office. After reviewing it, we realized the results wouldn't be 100 percent certain. They never guarantee you and your baby will be 100 percent healthy. And if we can't have that peace of mind *¿para qué?*, why bother with the test? My husband and I decided if something really was wrong with the baby, the sonogram would be enough to detect it. But then I thought: what if they do see something, won't I be an emotional wreck for the entire pregnancy? After all, abortion isn't an option for us. So in the end, *le pedí a Dios,* I asked God for the strength to love my baby, no matter how it was born."

Ana María Caldas chose to do the test:

"When I was pregnant some friends of mine found out that their newborn baby had Down syndrome. I got very nervous. Until then I hadn't even thought about amniocentesis because I was only thirty years old. It's a terrible thing what I am going to say, but I will not bring to this world a child with problems. *No solo por mi,* not just because of me, but for him too. I think it is very unfair to bring to this world a person that is going to suffer. He is going to realize that the rest of the people have a kind of life that he will never be able to have. It doesn't matter. I will take care of him for my whole life, that's not the problem. But *el día que yo muera,* the day I die, who is going to take care of him? How can you leave somebody so helpless alone? They are babies all their lives."

Purpose of the Genetic Tests

One of the reasons for giving a genetic test is to see if the baby has any problems that can be treated before it's born. Treating the baby while it's still in the uterus is still an experimental field of medicine, but in some cases it's proven effective.

Another reason for genetic testing is to evaluate the severity of the abnormalities in order to determine the possibility of putting an end to the pregnancy because chances of survival are minimal, and because there will be suffering for the baby and the family.

Deciding whether to terminate a pregnancy is difficult and painful, and for many Latinas, this is not even an option. Each case is different, and it is important to obtain all the information. The abnormality can produce mild effects that will not interfere with a normal life, or severe malformations. Even in the most common of all genetic problems, Down syndrome, each case is different and disabilities could range from mild to severe.

There are some considerations that might help you in case you are confronted with an abnormal result:

- What kind of life will the child live? What degree of interaction will he/she have with the people around him/her?

- Do you have the means to take care of a disabled child? Can you give him/her the hours of attention that he/she will need?

- Do you have other children to take care of? How will a disabled child affect the rest of the family?

- In case he/she is going to need surgery or specialized medical attention, do you have medical insurance? Will your baby suffer because of the surgical procedures?

- Who will take care of the child when you are not here anymore? Will he/she be institutionalized? Who will pay for this?

Finding out your baby has a genetic defect is heartbreaking. I recommend you learn as much as you can about the problem before making any decisions, since the emotional consequences will be with you for a long time. Talk to your genetic counselor. Talk to another doctor. Look on the Internet. Talk to families who have already made the decision to terminate their pregnancies. Talk to families who have a child with Down syndrome. Don't give up until you're completely satisfied. Ask and ask until you know in your heart you're making the right decision, whatever that may be (see the Contact List for resources to help you).

Although you may not be thinking about ending your pregnancy, some couples prefer to know with certainty about any genetic problems so they can prepare themselves for the road ahead. This allows you to make arrangements for a birth in a hospital equipped with staff and technology to take care of babies with genetic defects.

When the purpose of testing is just gathering information, you'll also have to weigh the risks of the actual test causing a miscarriage. They're small risks, but they do exist.

Finally, genetic tests give precise results. The margin of accuracy is nearly 100 percent in the case of amniocentesis. Nevertheless, the fact that a test has indicated no genetic defects are present is not a guarantee that the baby will be perfectly healthy. Genetic tests only pick up certain abnormalities. Some defects are still undetectable.

Chromosomes and Genes

Genetic abnormalities are produced by genes or chromosomes defects. Genes are microscopic particles of matter that form chromosomes. Chromosomes are found in each of the cells of our bodies, except the red blood cells. Genes determine the physical characteristics of a person, as well as many psychological and emotional traits. The genes will determine if your baby will be male or female, tall or short, thin or fat, have black or green eyes. In other words, chromosomes contain the instruction manual for how to construct a human being.

By some estimates, human beings have between thirty thousand and thirty-five thousand genes, divided among forty-six chromosomes. We inherit half of them from our mother and the other half from our father. The egg and sperm only have twenty-three chromosomes each, and at the moment of conception they combine, so there are forty-six. That's how a new life begins to develop.

The forty-six chromosomes are in pairs; we've got twenty-three pairs. Looked at under a microscope, they resemble pairs of little ribbons. The only ones that are different are the sex chromosomes.

This different pair of chromosomes determines the sex of the baby. They are called X and Y. The mother always passes on the X chromosome, because a mother's egg always contains one X. But the father can pass on either an X or a Y chromosome. His sperm can contain one or the other. He's the one who decides whether the baby will be a boy or a girl. His X with the mother's X makes a girl (XX); his Y with the mother's X makes a boy (XY).

Karyotype

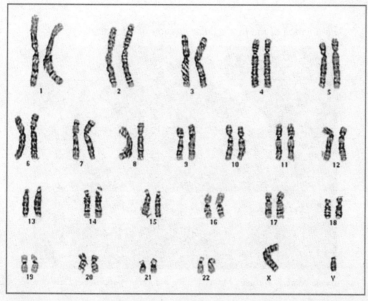

So when your husband says, "Let's see if you can give me a little girl this time," or "Are you going to have a boy?" you can answer with a big smile: "Mi *amor*, honey, that's up to you."

This process of pairing and dividing chromosomes is complicated and delicate and sometimes there are mistakes. Errors can be already present in the chromosomes, passed on from the parents to the baby, which is the case in hereditary diseases, or they can occur because of external forces, such as radiation, medicines that alter them or simply because of a problem in the early division process.

When the sperm enters the egg, that single cell divides into two, and those two into four, four into eight, eight into sixteen, and so on. Each cell has a copy of the chromosomes with the complete instructions on whether to turn into a kidney cell or skin cell or stomach cell or any other. So if there's an error at the beginning of the division, all the successive cells have the same mistake included, because they are copies of the original. That can mean a birth defect, an illness or a problem that causes the fetus to grow incorrectly.

The majority of spontaneous abortions during the first trimester are caused because the initial genetic pairing process didn't go well. Other times these problems don't stop the fetus from developing, despite the fact there are errors in the chromosomes or in a gene. In fact, these genetic mistakes may not have any effect on the baby at all—all of us have a few imperfect genes. In other cases, though, errors could be more serious.

Genetic tests during pregnancy serve to determine or at least rule out

Photograph of the first cellular division of a fertilized egg

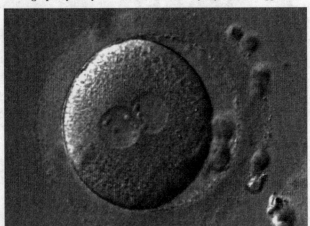

Image: Mark P. Portman, Mt, MHA; Reproductive Associates of Delaware

whether specific problems are present in the baby's chromosomes or genes. These tests obtain, through a variety of methods, samples of the baby's cells. Then a photograph of the chromosomes is made through a microscope to count them and analyze their shape. The photograph of a group of human chromosomes is called a karyotype (see page 119).

Some abnormalities are easy to pick out in the karyotype, such as when there's an extra chromosome; instead of forty-six the baby has forty-seven. The pair where the extra chromosome is present determines what type of abnormality the baby will suffer from. If the extra chromosome is in pair number twenty-one, the baby will have Down syndrome.

Other times, there are forty-five instead of forty-six chromosomes (one too few), and some other times the number of chromosomes is correct but some are missing pieces or they've got extra genetic material attached to them. Certain illnesses are located on a certain gene inside a certain chromosome. For example, cystic fibrosis is a genetic disease that produces dense phlegm in the lungs; it's caused by a malformed gene located in chromosome number seven.

I imagine that as you read all this, your hair is standing on end as you consider the myriad of things that could go wrong. Mothers throughout the ages have suffered the same fears about the health of their babies.

It is true that genetic abnormalities are like a lottery; anybody who plays can get it. But under normal conditions, the probability of your baby suffering some genetic disease are about the same as winning the multimillion-dollar lottery—that is, very low. There are some circumstances in which the chances go up, for example, if your family has a history of hereditary diseases or if you are older than thirty-five. The following table lays out the risks according to age.

Age of Mother	Risk of Down Syndrome	Other Abnormalities
25	1 in 1,250 births	1 in 476 births
30	1 in 952	1 in 384
35	1 in 385	1 in 192
40	1 in 106	1 in 66
45	1 in 30	1 in 21

Genetic Counselors

Before going through a diagnostic genetic test, you and your partner or other members of the family will have an interview with a genetic counselor. These interviews serve to give you more information about the test and its possible results.

First, the counselor will tell you about many of the things you've just read about: what chromosomes are and how genetic defects arise. Afterward, he/she will ask you questions about your family's genetic history in order to create a family tree. This drawing helps the genetic counselor determine whether there's a chance you or your husband are carriers of some type of genetic disease your baby could inherit.

The counselor will also ask you about your ethnic background, because some diseases appear more frequently in certain populations:

- Sickle cell anemia strikes people of African or Latin American descent. This illness causes the red blood cells to take on the shape of a sickle, instead of having their usual appearance, which is similar to a doughnut. The irregular shape means the blood cells don't flow smoothly through the veins and arteries and they get backed up. That causes infections and other problems.
- Anemias such as thalassemia affect people from the Mediterranean and Asia.
- Tay-Sachs disease appears more frequently among Eastern European Jews.

🦢

If certain diseases have reappeared on several occasions in your family's past but you don't remember exactly in whom, talk to relatives who can refresh your memory before going to the genetic interview.

This is important because the genetic tests only detect common abnormalities. To find out if there's a risk of passing on a particular disease, it's necessary to search for a specific gene that might be irregular.

Perhaps you've decided you don't want to have any genetic testing done, but the doctor's office is pushing you to do an interview with the genetic counselor anyway. Other times the doctor's office will require you to sign a form saying you've had the benefits of the test explained to you but you rejected it anyway. Well, you know how it goes in this country when it comes to possible lawsuits. The form serves as a cover for the doctor's office. In case anything goes wrong, you can't complain you didn't have your options explained to you.

SCREENING TESTS

They help determine which women have a higher risk of having babies with problems. However, they are not a diagnosis; the results are only statistical possibilities of certain problems arising. They are not completely accurate. Sometimes they will indicate a possibility of genetic defects being present in your baby when in reality all is well.

The most common genetic abnormality is Down syndrome. Half of the babies born with a genetic defect suffer from this condition. That's why many of the genetic tests focus on this problem.

The American College of Obstetricians and Gynecologists recommends these screening tests be offered to all women, both older and younger than thirty-five.

Alpha-Fetoprotein

The baby produces this substance as it grows; it's found in the amniotic fluid as well as in the mother's blood. Sometimes the baby's spinal column doesn't close up correctly during its development and creates a condition known as spina bifida, which can result in paralysis in the lower body and other problems. Alpha-fetoprotein is found in higher levels in babies who have neural tube defects. The levels can also be high if the baby suffers from kidney and urinary tract problems. On the other hand, if the levels of this protein are too low, the baby could have Down syndrome.

Alpha-fetoprotein is measured through a test of the mother's blood or by taking a sample of the amniotic fluid in which the baby is floating. The test is given between weeks 16 and 18, with the results coming back about a week later.

Triple Marker or Maternal Serum Alpha-Fetoprotein (MSAFP)

This is a blood test that measures not only the level of alpha-fetoprotein but also the levels of two of the mother's hormones (estriol and human chorionic gonadotropin [HCG])—that's why it's called the triple marker. It's given between weeks 15 and 20.

When the levels of alpha-fetoprotein and estriol are low and the HCG is high, it could be because the baby has Down syndrome.

Quadruple Marker

A few years ago, scientists discovered a way to measure yet another protein in the mother's blood. This protein, called inhibine A, allows a more accurate prediction of whether a baby has Down syndrome. Although doctors don't know why, when the levels of this hormone are high, there's a greater chance the baby has a problem.

The test measures the same things as the triple marker, plus the inhibine-A. The triple marker test detects 69 percent of the cases; the quadruple marker test detects 85 percent. Recent studies show this test is also effective in detecting other types of genetic abnormalities.

Nuchal Translucency Test

This strange word refers to the possible accumulation of fluid on the back of the baby's neck, which is common among Down syndrome babies. The test is a sonogram, and it's done between 11 and 13 weeks. If fluid is found on the back of the baby's neck and the blood tests also show abnormal results, doctors can do an analysis of the chorionic villus to confirm the results (see page 129).

The nuchal translucency test isn't widely used yet, but the advantage is that it doesn't present any danger to the baby or the mother and that it's done early in the pregnancy. However, the American College of Obstetrics and Gynecology advises caution when reading the results, because the accuracy depends on the expertise of the screener. Also, given that we're talking about a relatively new test, doctors still haven't determined standard measurements of exactly how much fluid on the back of the neck is considered normal and how much is cause for concern.

PAPP-A and Free Beta-HCG

This blood test measures the level of a hormone and a protein in the mother's blood (PAPP-A stands for "pregnancy associated protein plasma A").

The chance of Down syndrome goes up when the levels of PAPP-A are low and the levels of free beta-HCG are high. When this test is combined early in the pregnancy with the nuchal translucency test, the results are pretty accurate. If both tests have positive results, doctors will recommend the chorionic villus sampling test, which will determine with almost total certainty whether there's a genetic abnormality.

Although the popularity of these new tests is growing, they are relatively new. It's possible that your insurance company will not cover them.

Abnormal Results

When the results of a screening test are not normal, this *could* mean spinal column problems or Down syndrome. But I emphasize *could*, because abnormal values are often found in cases where the baby is perfectly healthy.

Ana Maria Ceballos, now in the seventh month of her second pregnancy, still remembers the scare she suffered waiting for her first baby:

"I remember they took some of my blood and I received a call from my doctor a few days later with the results. According to them—the doctor told me—there was a chance my baby could have Down syndrome, and to be on the safe side, we should do an amniocentesis test. *Me angustié mucho,* the news made me nervous, and when I told my husband, we were both very scared. We didn't even say anything to *la familia,* the rest of the family, because we didn't want to create more anguish. We made an appointment to do the amniocentesis, and when we arrived, the nurse told us we should also talk to the genetic counselor. We asked, 'Is it necessary?' And they said yes, as if we had no other choice.

"During the interview is when I became terrified. She began to explain what the chances were of our baby having genetic abnormalities, and that because of my age, thirty, the probabilities were this, and the chances of birth defects increase with age, and when the results come back as mine did the baby's risks were that. Then she started with the risks of amniocentesis.

"At the end of *todo este rollo,* all this lengthy explanation, I asked why all the pressure, why did we have to do the tests now, immediately. She said, 'It's because you only have until a certain week to decide whether you want to terminate the pregnancy and we're obligated to make sure you understand all the options.' *Jamás en mi vida se me pasó por la cabeza,* never in my life did it even cross my mind that I was going to abort my child. So during the couple of minutes my husband and I had to ourselves before the tests were to begin, I told him: 'Look, Jaime, I think the baby is going to be just fine, and we're going to find out all this was just a big mistake.' I was confident all the warnings were out of proportion and out of line.

"So we went into the diagnostic room and they began with the sonogram. The doctor—who I must say was *de lo más agradable,* most friendly—measured the baby, told me it was a boy and said: 'I think they tested your blood a week early. You decide if you want to go through with the amniocentesis.' I asked, 'What alternatives do I have?' He told me I could do another blood test in a week to see how everything looked then, and if something was out of order, then we could do the amniocentesis. According to my logic, it seemed the greatest risk was losing the baby during the amniocentesis, so I decided to wait. So a week later, we did another blood test, y *todo salió perfecto*, everything turned out fine."

The majority of the cases in which abnormal levels are found are false alarms. The causes of these mistakes can be:

- A miscalculation of the age of the fetus; it's older or younger than the real age
- The presence of more than one baby, so levels are higher
- A mother who smokes, is obese or uses insulin for diabetes; she will have lower than normal levels.

To figure out if a positive result is really false, generally a doctor will do the test again. If it continues to be positive, the next step is ordering a detailed sonogram, or a level II sonogram. If both tests shows no problems, there's no reason to worry. But if some abnormality does show up in the sonogram, then a doctor will continue with a chromosome analysis (chorionic villus sampling, amniocentesis or PUBS).

Despite the false positives, this test will give you peace of mind, and it's done early in the pregnancy. There aren't any risks for the baby or the mother since it's a simple blood test.

DIAGNOSTIC GENETIC TESTS

These tests *can* determine if the baby has a genetic abnormality. We're not just talking about probabilities now. Diagnostic genetic tests actually analyze the chromosomes to make sure everything's in order. However, these test themselves carry some risks, because the doctor must take a sample from inside your uterus, of the amniotic fluid or of the umbilical cord blood to do the analysis.

Amniocentesis
The amniocentesis test is given between weeks 15 and 18. It entails using a needle to extract a small amount of amniotic fluid. Skin cells that have

sloughed off the baby tend to float around in the liquid. These are cultured and the genetic material they provide is analyzed. Also, alpha-fetoprotein levels can be measured with more accuracy through the amniotic liquid obtained in an amniocentesis.

For this test you will lie down on the table and pull up your blouse to expose your abdomen. First the doctor or technician will find the baby inside you through a sonogram and will also search for a place where there's enough fluid to do the test. When the doctor is sure there's an appropriate spot to insert the needle, the area will be disinfected with an antiseptic solution. The needle will never be poked through the mother's belly button. You may be offered a local anesthetic so you don't feel the needle go in, or you can do it without anesthesia.

But the question is: Does the needle hurt when it goes in? And above all, could it poke the baby? As far as the pain, it depends. I have several friends who said they didn't feel a thing or only a little prick. Other women, like myself, did feel some pain. But to tell you the truth, a big part of my problem was how tense I was. If at the moment when they were going to insert the needle they'd tickled me with a feather, I probably would have screamed the same. *Para ser sincera,* to be honest, the only thing

Amniocentesis

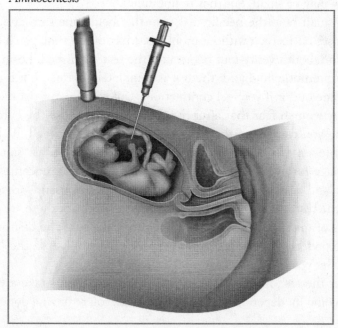

that really hurt was the first prick, which is similar to when the nurse sticks a needle in your arm to draw blood. My doctor didn't use any anesthetic, but if you ask for one, you'll probably get it.

María Cuellar had a better experience than me, but not her husband.

"I told my doctor I didn't want to see the needle, although I was looking at it through the sonogram. It feels a bit uncomfortable, but that's all and it goes away very quickly. My husband was the one *que se puso amarillo*, that turned yellow, and they had to sit him down."

Once the needle makes it into your womb, you won't feel a thing. And if all goes well, it will only take a few seconds for the doctor to draw out the right amount of amniotic fluid. After the needle comes out, that's it! The test is over. You will be able to see in the syringe the fluid your baby is floating in.

The baby isn't really in any danger. It's very rare for a baby to get poked. The doctor is watching through the sonogram where the needle goes after it's inside you, making sure it's away from the baby. According to my doctor's assistant, "babies move away from the needle." Now, I don't know if this has been proven scientifically, but I really could see my daughter move away from the needle in the screen. *Son chiquitos pero listos*, they may be small, but they're not dumb.

The small hole the needle makes in the membrane surrounding the baby closes on its own without problems. Most of the time you'll be told to rest for about twenty-four hours after the test is finished. Losing a few drops of amniotic fluid after the test is completely normal, but if you see more come out or if you feel contractions, call your doctor right away.

Many women fear that after the test they might lose the baby. Plan ahead so you can spend the next twenty-four hours in bed. Risks that the amniocentesis causes a miscarriage or an infection are small: one miscarriage for every two hundred to four hundred amniocentesis procedures and less than one infection for every thousand procedures. When the test is done before week 15 or after week 18, there are greater chances of miscarriage. It's a good idea to make sure the doctor who's going to perform the test has a lot of experience with it. Ask; they're obligated to let you know.

After the test, all you have to do is wait. The results take a week or two to come in, depending on the type of test you're having done.

Chorionic Villus Sampling

Much like amniocentesis, this test detects abnormalities in the chromosomes and genes. The difference is that it can be done earlier, between weeks 10 and 12. Also, the results come back more quickly.

This test works by taking a sample of the chorionic villi, which are similar to fine hairs and which connect the sac surrounding the baby to the uterine wall. The cells of these villi have the same chromosomes as the baby.

There are two ways to do this test. The first is similar to a gynecological exam. The doctor will disinfect the vagina and the cervix and will insert a small, thin tube up to where the villi are. It feels much the same as a Pap smear, but it can be a little more painful.

The other way to do the test is with a needle, much like the amniocentesis. The risk of a spontaneous abortion doing the test this way is higher than the risk during an amniocentesis: one for every one hundred to two hundred tests.

A few years ago, some doctors began to worry that some children of mothers who had this test done were being born with defects in their

Chorionic villus sampling

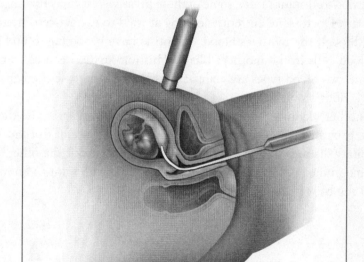

hands, feet and jaw. Scientists have looked into it and found that the risk of this happening is one in every one thousand to three thousand tests. But the risks decrease dramatically when the test is done after the tenth week of pregnancy.

Percutaneous Umbilical Cord Blood Sampling (PUBS)

This test is used when the results of the amniocentesis and CVS aren't clear or when a doctor suspects the baby has an infection such as rubella or toxoplasmosis. It tests the baby's blood taken from the umbilical cord. The advantage of this analysis is that the results come back in twenty-four hours and they can tell a doctor a lot about the baby's health. In addition to genetic problems, it can also show if the baby has anemia or if there are blood clotting problems.

The procedure is the same as in amniocentesis, but it's carried out after week 18 because before this date, the veins in the umbilical cord are too delicate. The doctor guides the needle looking at the sonogram monitor, and extracts a small sample of umbilical cord blood. The baby doesn't feel a thing. The risk of spontaneous abortion and infection are similar to the risks when undergoing amniocentesis.

The Tests of the Future

In the not-so-distant future, some of these invasive tests may no longer be necessary. Doctors are currently looking at ways to extract cells from the fetus through the mother's blood. Scientists have been able to find fetal red blood cells in the mother's blood. This information is used to make sure the two blood types are compatible because otherwise the baby can suffer serious problems.

Another technique doctors are studying is how to determine the sex of the baby by testing the mother's blood. This is a useful test for those hereditary diseases that are only passed on to one sex or the other, such as hemophilia, and of course it's perfect for those who want to know the sex of the baby before he or she is born.

GLUCOSE TESTS

The hormones our bodies produce during the nine months of pregnancy make us do a lot of strange things: sleep seventeen hours a day or cry at every diaper commercial we see on television. They're also responsible for interfering with the normal workings of certain organs during pregnancy.

And no, I'm not talking about the brain. I'm referring to the pancreas. Sometimes these hormones keep the insulin that's secreted by the pancreas from working properly (insulin is in charge of making sure the glucose from the food we eat gets to our cells). When this happens you might develop gestational diabetes. The little cup you're given to urinate in every time you go to the doctor's office helps to determine whether there's sugar in your urine. If there is, it could mean your body is not processing glucose properly.

In addition to the urine test, there are two others commonly used to see if you've developed gestational diabetes.

One-Hour Glucose Tolerance Test

Between weeks 24 and 28, the hormones that interfere with insulin production are raging. The one-hour glucose tolerance test helps to figure out if you're having problems processing the glucose that's derived from the foods we eat (see Chapter 4). In this test you'll be given a glucose drink called "glucola." They may call it a "cola," but don't be fooled by the name—any resemblance to a soda is pure coincidence. It tastes like an orange drink plus a half a pound of sugar—or to be more precise, with 50 grams of glucose added. If you don't like the idea, ask the doctor if you can substitute a few jelly beans for the glucose drink—a study showed that eighteen jelly beans have the same effect as a glucola with 50 grams of glucose. Some doctors even use chocolate bars and other sweets for this test.

One hour after having taken glucose, no matter what form it is, you'll be given a blood test to determine your blood sugar level. That's the amount of glucose in your bloodstream at that time. If the level is lower than 140 mg/dL, that means everything's fine. But if it's higher than 140 mg/dL (this figure might vary depending on the lab or hospital doing the test), that means you could have a problem with your insulin production. To make sure, the doctors will give you another glucose tolerance test that's described in the following paragraphs.

Three-Hour Glucose Tolerance Test or Glucose Curve

This test is similar to the preceding one, but it involves more glucose over a longer period of time. You'll have to go without eating for between eight and twelve hours before the test.

In the hospital or lab, the nurse will take a blood sample to determine what your starting glucose level is. After that, *prepárese*, get ready to learn the true meaning of the word *sweet*. You'll be given a drink with double the amount of glucose compared with the earlier test—100 grams.

During the following three hours after drinking the potion, your blood will be taken once every hour to see how your insulin is handling all that sugar. There are various ways to measure the results, but the most common are the NDDG and the Carpenter scales.

	NDDG Scale	Carpenter Scale
Fasting	105	95
1 hour	190	180
2 hours	165	155
3 hours	145	140

If two of the results are above any of these levels, then you've officially got gestational diabetes. If only one of the results is higher than the levels in the scales, then you don't have diabetes, but you will have to watch what you eat. Chapter 4 is dedicated to gestational diabetes and how to control it.

TESTS FOR THE BABY

These tests make sure the baby's okay, especially if there's a risk during the pregnancy such as diabetes or high blood pressure or if the mother notices the baby isn't moving around enough. It's also done when previous pregnancies had complications and when the baby is late.

Counting the Baby's Movements

This is the oldest and simplest way to see if the baby is doing well. The process involves counting the number of times the baby moves during half an hour. The mother can begin to feel the baby moving between weeks 16 and 20, but the test is best done starting with week 24. It's really easy—all you need is a pencil and paper and a little concentration.

To begin, pick an hour of the day when the baby is usually awake, such as after lunch or dinner. Get comfortable on the couch or lie down on the bed, leaning a little to your left side to improve your circulation, and write down the time you feel the first movement. Count the movements until you get to ten and write down the time again. Movements are whatever sensation you feel from the baby: a kick, a twist, a stretch, whatever. Generally, babies move at least five times in half an hour. If you don't notice anything, it could be because your baby is taking a *siesta* or nap. Try to wake him or her up with a loud noise, by eating something or by changing positions. Keep in mind that the more the baby grows the less space it has to move around in, so the movements you felt during the first weeks of pregnancy will have different intensities, frequencies and durations.

Sometimes you won't feel any movements for a while, and there's still nothing wrong with the baby. But other times the absence of movement is an indication of a problem. Talk to your doctor if more than four hours pass without your noticing a movement, if you notice the movements are coming less frequently as the days pass or if there are periods with frantic movements.

Trust your instincts: a mother-to-be knows how her baby moves. If you think things aren't going well, insist that your doctor or nurse check into how the baby's doing. A false alarm is better than an emergency.

Fetal Nonstress Test

This easy and even enjoyable test doesn't hurt at all. It monitors the baby's heartbeats when it moves. The idea is that if the baby is moving, its heart rate should increase, much as ours does during exercise. But if the baby's heart rate stays the same, it could be a sign of a problem.

The test is usually done in the hospital, with the same machine used to measure your contractions during delivery. After you lie back on the table, the nurses will put a belt around your belly. The belt is lined with electrodes that detect the baby's heartbeat.

External fetal monitor

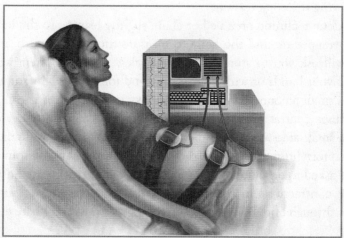

The baby has to be awake to move, so you may be asked to eat something before the test, since eating gets them moving. But if your baby is a heavy sleeper, they might use other methods to wake it up, such as making noise, rubbing your abdomen or having you drink cold water. You may also have to push a button every time you feel the baby move so the machine will monitor the heartbeat at the right time.

Biophysical Profile
This is a combination of the fetal nonstress test and a sonogram. It shows the heart rate acceleration, general movements, breathing movements and amount of amniotic fluid. These results give a pretty clear idea of how the baby is doing.

A variation of this test that measures only the amount of amniotic fluid is called the modified biophysical profile.

Fetal Acoustic Stimulation Test
It's the same as the fetal nonstress test but uses a sound to startle the baby to see how it responds. The advantage of this test is that the baby is awake *de todas todas*, no matter what, so it doesn't last long. The responses of the baby's heart are measured by a belt strapped around the mother's belly.

Contraction Stress Test
This test "stresses" the baby a little. The baby is stimulated by gentle uterine contractions, much weaker than the ones during delivery. The contractions put pressure on the placenta, which is the baby's source of oxygen. The test measures the placenta's ability to supply oxygen to the baby during the compression.

It's done reclining on a bed or chair, slightly leaning to the left, with a belt wrapped around the belly to measure the baby's heartbeats. The nurse will ask you to stimulate your nipples, massaging them with the palm of your hands or with your thumb and forefinger. This stimulation releases small amounts of the hormone oxytocin, which is the chemical that causes contractions during delivery. If this doesn't work, you'll be given a small amount of artificial oxytocin intravenously (pitocin). The test lasts forty minutes. In case the results continue to be abnormal, you may be asked to do more tests, or you may be admitted to the hospital.

The contractions in this test are a little uncomfortable, but you'll make it through fine. Believe me, I'm telling you this, and I hate even the smallest amount of pain. I went through this test during my first pregnancy because of my diabetes.

The tests listed here are the most common. If you don't feel comfortable undergoing any of the tests, relay your fears and concerns to your doctor. Ask questions until you feel better. And don't let a bad or condescending attitude stop you. There is never a stupid question if it's coming from a mother-to-be. Don't refrain from asking *por educación*, to show politeness. Your doctor and the other professionals helping you through your pregnancy could help you better if they know what's causing your concern and why. By law, hospitals that receive federal funds have to provide you with an interpreter.

7

❧

The First Trimester

Congratulations! If you're reading this chapter, it's likely you're pregnant. If that's the case, get prepared for one of the most emotional and thrilling experiences of your life: you will actually be creating another human being inside you. And if this is your first baby, the memories of these next nine months will remain seared in your memory long after your child has gone off to college. You'll recall not only the enormous physical and emotional changes your body is about to experience but also the fact that along with your baby, somebody else will be born: a mother.

And I can guarantee you one thing: from now on your life will take a 180-degree turn. You are about to discover a unique love, one that's profound and fierce, *que le llegará al alma*, that will touch your soul, turn your life upside down and teach you things about yourself that you never knew before—for example, that you can go for weeks on only four hours of sleep a night, and that your hearing will become so acute that you can pick up your baby's cry from half a mile away. Well, maybe *exagero un poco*, I am exaggerating a bit, but not much, believe me.

But let's not get ahead of ourselves. You've got nine great months ahead of you (if you get morning sickness, subtract three) to take care of yourself and to make sure your family takes care of you. Enjoy all of it, because you can only be pregnant for the first time once.

The next chapters will accompany you through this journey, talking you through the physical and emotional changes that come with each month—everything from how your baby is growing inside you to what to expect at your prenatal visits, during delivery and after.

You'll also find a brief monthly guide for dads—don't forget that they're also along for the ride and will be on their own emotional roller coaster. Share this book with your partner; it will give him the chance to learn more about what you're going through. But if he doesn't have time, he can get an idea of what's going to happen with the dad's section in each chapter.

The aches and pains that come with each successive month might not apply to you or not at that time. Look in the index if you don't find what you're looking for in the chapter you're reading.

THE FIRST MONTH
Weeks 1 to 4 (counting from the first day of your last period)

"We went to a place where you swim with dolphins. They were glued to me. There was a female touching my belly with hers. The instructor asked me if I was pregnant; he said they acted like that with pregnant women. I didn't know I was, so I told him, no way! Two days later I did a home test and it came out positive."

—*Ana Cristina Osorio*

First month

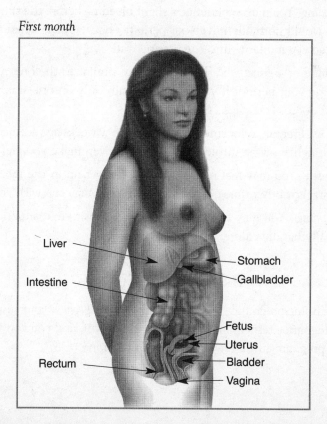

"One night before I knew I was pregnant I started feeling something very strange in my belly. It was not feeling sick, it was like something I have never felt."

—*Ana Miriam La Salle*

"I just wanted to eat banana pancakes with cream and maple syrup. I wanted that to be my dinner. Next day I started to feel sick and I realized: *Estoy embarazada*, I am pregnant."

—*Miriam Gayden*

Along with some pretty strange feelings and cravings for certain foods, there are other physical signs that may show up during the first weeks of your pregnancy, even before you miss your first period.

Pregnancy Symptoms

- *Breasts*. They will feel sore and be very sensitive to touch.
- *Frequent urination*. You'll go to the bathroom a lot, during the day and at night.
- *Bleeding*. You may experience a slight bleeding before the time when you would normally have your period. That happens when the fertilized egg implants into the uterine wall.
- *Cramps or uterine pain*. These pains are similar to the ones you feel during your period. If you feel sharp pain only on one side, talk to your doctor (see page 164).
- *Odors*. Fragrances or smells that up to a few weeks ago seemed pleasant might now be intolerable and could even make you feel sick.
- *Nausea*. You may feel nauseous when you get up in the morning or during any other time of the day. This nausea may end with vomiting.
- *Emotions*. You may feel more irritable or sensitive in situations you usually handle calmly.

Pregnancy Tests

A simple home pregnancy test can confirm *sus sospechas*, your suspicions. Home pregnancy tests are more accurate than ever, and you can find out if you're pregnant just a few days after conception.

When the fertilized egg has implanted into the uterine wall, your body secretes a hormone called beta-HCG. This hormone is the one pregnancy tests detect. It appears after the egg is implanted, not before. Implantation usually takes place between eight and ten days after conception. So suppose you got pregnant halfway through your menstrual cycle—in theory you could do a home pregnancy test three days before the date you expected your period to start.

Not all pregnancy tests have the same ability to detect the small amounts of this hormone that are present in the urine in the first days of pregnancy. For that reason, if you do the test too early you may get a negative result but still be pregnant. Test yourself again a few days later after your period was supposed to have started; at that point there will be a greater amount of hormone in your urine.

Pharmacies and supermarkets sell these home tests. They can detect between 25 and 250 mIU/ml of beta-HCG. That's a broad range. Although each woman is different, generally a pregnant woman will have around 100 mIU/ml of beta-HCG in her urine on the date she expected her period to start.

The following table lists some of the most well-known and sensitive brands of home pregnancy tests. The lower the mIU number (milli–international units), the more sensitive the test is. If the test you buy doesn't list the amount of beta-HCG it detects, you can find out by calling the toll-free telephone number in the instructions.

Answer Early Result	25 mIU/ml
First Response Early Result	25 mIU/ml
One Step Be Sure	25 mIU/ml
EPT	40 mIU/ml
Fact Plus One Step	40 mIU/ml
ClearBlue Easy Earliest Result	50 mIU/ml

The reliability of these tests is pretty good: a positive result means an actual pregnancy in 99 percent of cases. If you like to shop on the Internet, you will find tests with a sensitivity of 20 mIU/ml that also are usually cheaper than the ones sold in pharmacies and supermarkets.

If you take these home tests and you still aren't sure if you're pregnant, your doctor can confirm it through a blood test and an internal exam.

The Calendar

This simple calendar shows you what date you can hold your newborn in your arms for the first time. Look for the day when your last period began in the columns in bold. The number that appears below is the approximate birth date.

More than one husband has had a shock in the first prenatal visit after hearing that his wife was already one month pregnant, when a month ago he was out of town or not even in the country. Pregnancy is not counted from the date of conception but from the first day of the last menstrual period.

The table is based on a forty-week pregnancy or 280 days, counting from the first day of your last period. However, these dates aren't exact and there could be a difference of as much as two weeks before or after the date you pick out on the table.

A woman with twenty-eight-day menstrual cycles tends to ovulate and therefore get pregnant two weeks after the beginning of her period. If her cycles are shorter or longer, then the pregnancy may happen a week earlier or later. That's why women are told to use the date of the beginning of their last period as a starting point. Under that system, at the date on which you were supposed to get your next period you are considered a month pregnant, when actually the fetus may be only two weeks old.

The date of your last period is important in order to calculate the age of the fetus and to know if it's developing properly. If you don't remember exactly or you're confused about when you got pregnant, don't worry. The first sonogram will allow the doctor to figure out exactly how many weeks old the fetus is.

Actually, if you count four weeks per month, a pregnancy isn't nine months but ten. Counting by months is a bit confusing—that's why they talk about weeks of pregnancy instead of months: at six or eight weeks is when the first sonogram is done, at twelve weeks morning sickness is usually over and at sixteen weeks you can begin to feel the baby moving. To make things easier, in this book the first five months of pregnancy are counted as four-week months. After the sixth one we add one week per month. That way you have exactly nine months of pregnancy (five four-week months and four five-week months).

🦋

	1	2	3	4	5	6	7	8	9	10	11	12	13	14	15	16	17	18	19	20	21	22	23	24	25	26	27	28	29	30	31
January	1	2	3	4	5	6	7	8	9	10	11	12	13	14	15	16	17	18	19	20	21	22	23	24	25	26	27	28	29	30	31
Oct/Nov	8	9	10	11	12	13	14	15	16	17	18	19	20	21	22	23	24	25	26	27	28	29	30	31	1	2	3	4	5	6	7
February	1	2	3	4	5	6	7	8	9	10	11	12	13	14	15	16	17	18	19	20	21	22	23	24	25	26	27	28			
Nov/Dec	8	9	10	11	12	13	14	15	16	17	18	19	20	21	22	23	24	25	26	27	28	29	30	1	2	3	4	5			
March	1	2	3	4	5	6	7	8	9	10	11	12	13	14	15	16	17	18	19	20	21	22	23	24	25	26	27	28	29	30	31
Dec/Jan	6	7	8	9	10	11	12	13	14	15	16	17	18	19	20	21	22	23	24	25	26	27	28	29	30	31	1	2	3	4	5
April	1	2	3	4	5	6	7	8	9	10	11	12	13	14	15	16	17	18	19	20	21	22	23	24	25	26	27	28	29	30	
Jan/Feb	6	7	8	9	10	11	12	13	14	15	16	17	18	19	20	21	22	23	24	25	26	27	28	29	30	31	1	2	3	4	
May	1	2	3	4	5	6	7	8	9	10	11	12	13	14	15	16	17	18	19	20	21	22	23	24	25	26	27	28	29	30	31
Feb/Mar	5	6	7	8	9	10	11	12	13	14	15	16	17	18	19	20	21	22	23	24	25	26	27	28	1	2	3	4	5	6	7
June	1	2	3	4	5	6	7	8	9	10	11	12	13	14	15	16	17	18	19	20	21	22	23	24	25	26	27	28	29	30	
Mar/Apr	8	9	10	11	12	13	14	15	16	17	18	19	20	21	22	23	24	25	26	27	28	29	30	31	1	2	3	4	5	6	
July	1	2	3	4	5	6	7	8	9	10	11	12	13	14	15	16	17	18	19	20	21	22	23	24	25	26	27	28	29	30	31
Apr/May	7	8	9	10	11	12	13	14	15	16	17	18	19	20	21	22	23	24	25	26	27	28	29	30	1	2	3	4	5	6	7
August	1	2	3	4	5	6	7	8	9	10	11	12	13	14	15	16	17	18	19	20	21	22	23	24	25	26	27	28	29	30	31
May/June	8	9	10	11	12	13	14	15	16	17	18	19	20	21	22	23	24	25	26	27	28	29	30	31	1	2	3	4	5	6	7
September	1	2	3	4	5	6	7	8	9	10	11	12	13	14	15	16	17	18	19	20	21	22	23	24	25	26	27	28	29	30	
June/July	8	9	10	11	12	13	14	15	16	17	18	19	20	21	22	23	24	25	26	27	28	29	30	1	2	3	4	5	6	7	
October	1	2	3	4	5	6	7	8	9	10	11	12	13	14	15	16	17	18	19	20	21	22	23	24	25	26	27	28	29	30	31
July/Aug	8	9	10	11	12	13	14	15	16	17	18	19	20	21	22	23	24	25	26	27	28	29	30	31	1	2	3	4	5	6	7
November	1	2	3	4	5	6	7	8	9	10	11	12	13	14	15	16	17	18	19	20	21	22	23	24	25	26	27	28	29	30	
Aug/Sept	8	9	10	11	12	13	14	15	16	17	18	19	20	21	22	23	24	25	26	27	28	29	30	31	1	2	3	4	5	6	
December	1	2	3	4	5	6	7	8	9	10	11	12	13	14	15	16	17	18	19	20	21	22	23	24	25	26	27	28	29	30	31
Sept/Oct	7	8	9	10	11	12	13	14	15	16	17	18	19	20	21	22	23	24	25	26	27	28	29	30	1	2	3	4	5	6	7

Pregnancy calendar

ALCOHOL, DRUGS, HERBS AND OTHER PRODUCTS NOT RECOMMENDED DURING PREGNANCY

The first weeks of the baby's development are important because that's when the basic structures of the nervous system are being formed, including the brain and spinal column. In these first weeks, the baby is most vulnerable to toxic substances such as alcohol, drugs, certain prescription medications, vaccines and some foods. These are the same substances that you should stay away from when you are trying to conceive. You can read more about them on page 6, but the most important to avoid are:

- Alcohol, tobacco and drugs
- Medicines not prescribed by your doctor
- Paints and food contaminated with lead
- Cosmetics that contain mercury
- Cat litter
- Some raw foods, soft cheeses and certain fishes
- Coffee and herbs
- Certain cleaning products
- Vaccinations with active viruses
- Saunas or very hot baths

ALCOHOLIC DRINKS, CIGARETTES AND DRUGS BEFORE GETTING PREGNANT

Perhaps you're a little worried because you had a few drinks or took drugs or smoked cigarettes before you found out you were pregnant. A couple of drinks or even recreational use of some drugs before you take the pregnancy test doesn't usually have major consequences for the baby because the exchange of blood between mother-to-be and child isn't that great. Nevertheless, drugs and alcohol are very dangerous for the fetus during pregnancy, and continued use can result in birth defects or even a miscarriage.

As far as cigarettes go, fortunately we Latinas aren't heavy smokers. But if you do smoke, think about quitting now. When you smoke, you're depriving your baby of the oxygen it needs to develop normally. It's tough to quit but not impossible. Talk to your doctor about which strategies are best for you to quit smoking.

X Rays Without Knowing You're Pregnant

X rays and other tests involving radiation are something you want to avoid during your pregnancy because they can cause birth defects. Still, if you've been to the hospital and were given an X ray before you found out you were pregnant, don't fret, because the risks are much lower than you think. There are many different tests using X rays or radiation. Their intensity varies a lot and so does the risk to the baby.

Radiation levels are measured in rads. Radiation greater than five rads can harm the fetus. The most common tests that use radiation and their corresponding rads are in the table that follows:

- Dental X ray—0.00001 rads
- Lung or breast X ray—0.06 rads
- Barium enema (to see the inside of the intestines)—0.8 rads

These levels are way below the dosage of 5 rads needed to harm the baby. One way to reduce those risks even more is to use a lead apron during the X ray to protect the womb if you're of childbearing age.

Medical Attention During Pregnancy: Whom to Choose

A positive pregnancy test tells you two things: the first is that you're pregnant, and the second is that you should make an appointment with your doctor as soon as possible for a prenatal checkup.

¿Cuál es la prisa?, what's the hurry? After all, our mothers and grandmothers waited for a couple of months after missing a period before going to the doctor. True, but in those days, our mothers and grandmothers couldn't count on modern science to determine whether they were really pregnant so soon after conception. Now, doctors can see the baby's heart beating only weeks into the pregnancy. But there are also other reasons to go as soon as possible.

Latinas suffer more than other women from certain illnesses that can have consequences for the baby. The tests that are done during the prenatal visit help determine whether there are any illnesses the mother may be suffering from, such as diabetes, high blood pressure, infectious diseases or sexually transmitted diseases. With the proper treatment, none of them will have consequences for the baby. That's why it's important to get to the doctor right away. In general, mothers-to-be who don't get proper prenatal care during the first trimester have more complications later compared to women who do go to the doctor early in their pregnancies. So the next question is: with whom?

You've got several options. You can choose among an obstetrician/ gynecologist, a certified or licensed midwife, a family doctor or a perinatologist (for high-risk pregnancies).

Obstetrician/Gynecologist

This is the most common option. Obstetricians/gynecologists (or OB/GYNs) are specialists in taking care of women during pregnancy, labor and birth and after the baby is born. These doctors are qualified to do a cesarean section or other surgical procedures if they're necessary. The key word here is *obstetrician*, because there are some gynecologists who don't specialize in attending pregnant women.

There are several things you should keep in mind when choosing an obstetrician/gynecologist:

- *Latino or not?* Spanish-speaking or not? If it's important to you to have a person who shares your culture treating you, who possibly speaks Spanish, then you'll feel more comfortable with a Latino doctor. On page 34 you'll find a few tips on how to find a Latino obstetrician/gynecologist.

- *Male or female?* Some women feel more comfortable being treated by a woman during their pregnancies. Medical insurance plans and clinics have several doctors to choose from.

- *Individual office?* Here the doctors work by themselves and attend their patients individually. One important question to ask is who substitutes for him/her when he/she is not there. If for some reason he/she can't attend your birth, you may end up with a doctor you've never met during your delivery.

- *Group office?* In this case, two or more doctors work together out of the same office. You'll receive more of your prenatal care from only one doctor, but the delivery will be overseen by whomever is on duty that day. It could be your obstetrician/gynecologist or any of the other doctors working in the office. Generally, during your pregnancy you'll be introduced to all the doctors so you will know the one that will be attending your delivery, in case it is not yours.

- *Obstetrician/gynecologist or midwife?* Some doctors offer the option of being taken care of by a certified midwife in the very same office or hospital, although the doctor will oversee the delivery.

How to Tell if This Obstetrician/Gynecologist Is Right for You

Trusting and feeling comfortable with the obstetrician/gynecologist who will deliver your baby is very important. This is the person who is going to be in charge of your health during one of the most important times of your life. Birth is also one of the moments when you might feel most vulnerable. You should spend some time choosing the right doctor. Don't assume that just because a person carries the title obstetrician/gynecologist, he or she will be right for you.

One of the best ways to choose a doctor is to ask the advice of other mothers. Ask your friends or the women you work with how they felt with their doctors. Were they warm and caring? Were they serious or did they have a sense of humor? How did the deliveries go?

It's also possible your health insurance plan or your clinic will only allow you to choose among two or three doctors. Generally, you're allowed to change doctors at least once if you don't feel comfortable.

The best way to find out more about a particular obstetrician/gynecologist is by talking to him or her. Sometimes it can be a little embarrassing to ask so many questions, because it seems as though *usted no confía*, you're doubting the professionalism of the doctor. But if you explain you're only asking because you want to make the right choice of doctor to take care of you during the delivery of your baby, they'll usually understand. Remember, you're the client who is looking for a service, just the same as when you go to buy a car or anything else.

Before going to the doctor, make a list of the questions that are most important to you. You will not be asking him or her, "Are you agreeable and friendly and patient?" Still, the way the doctor answers your other questions may give you an idea of what kind of personality you're dealing with. And try to bring your partner to these interviews. Make sure he likes the doctor, too. If he doesn't, it will be a tense relationship.

Here are some examples of questions you can ask:

- *Are you board-certified by the American College of Obstetricians and Gynecologists?* In order to be board-certified, an obstetrician/gynecologist has to pass a test by the American College of Obstetricians and Gynecologists. They must repeat this exam every ten years. A board certification is a professional warranty.

- *Do you deliver babies yourself? How many babies do you deliver every month?* If he or she works alone, ask who is his/her substitute and how many deliveries he/she attends every month. Ten is a normal figure, but more than twenty means that you are not going to see much of him/her, since it's not possible to be in the office and at the hospital at the same time. Even when they have an individual office, obstetricians/gynecologists often use substitutes. It's important to know who will take care of you if your doctor is not there.

- *How much time will you spend with me during my delivery?* Sometimes obstetricians/gynecologists will arrive just before the baby is born. Up to that point, the nurses in the hospital will be taking care of you. However, there should always be a doctor there for emergency situations.

- *Which hospitals do you deliver babies in?* Make sure your health insurance covers the hospital your doctor works in.

- *What percentage of your deliveries are by cesarean?* You may not like the idea of a cesarean delivery (as long as there is no emergency), so asking this question gives you an idea of what to expect. If the answer is higher than 20 percent, that doctor does cesarean deliveries frequently.

- *What's your policy regarding amniocentesis and other genetic prenatal tests?* Some doctors really like them and put some pressure on expectant mothers to do them. Other doctors refuse to interrupt any pregnancy and don't see much need for genetic testing.

- *How many people will be with me during my delivery?* In part, this depends on the policies of the hospital you're in, but some doctors don't feel comfortable with a lot of family members in the delivery room.

- *When would you recommend an epidural?* Some might recommend it from three centimeters or less but others like to wait as long as possible.

- *If everything looks as though it's going well, may I use the hospital's birthing center (if there is one)?* This option allows you to have a delivery without a lot of typical help from a doctor, but still within the hospital where there's assistance if there's an emergency.

- *Do I have to have an intravenous line?* This is the needle they stick into the back of your hand to give you medicines in case there's an emergency. The norm is to insert one as soon as you arrive at the hospital, so it will be ready in case of emergency. That means you'll be connected to a hanging bag during the delivery. Some doctors allow their patients to go without the intravenous treatment or they give an anticoagulant (heparin lock) that will allow you to move around freely.

These are only a few examples of the kind of questions you could ask your doctor. Talk with other mothers about their experiences. Ask them what they liked and what they would have liked to know about their doctors beforehand.

Midwife

Prenatal care can also be provided by a midwife. In the United States, there are several types of midwives, classified according to their level of education and licenses they've earned.

- *Certified nurse midwives.* These professionals have been to college and graduated as nurses. Later, they earned a master's degree in midwifery. They are authorized to give prenatal care and gynecological exams and to attend to women during delivery and afterward, as long as the pregnancy progresses according to plan. Most of them work with doctors in hospitals, but they can't do surgery. Health insurance plans almost always pay for the services of a certified nurse midwife.
- *Licensed midwives.* These professionals have to pass an exam to earn a license to practice in the state where they live. Although they've got some of the knowledge a nurse has, they haven't been through university training. Instead, their studies are focused on midwifery. They offer the same help as certified midwives, but they don't usually work in hospitals. Instead, licensed midwives set up shop in natural birthing centers or in the homes of the mothers. Licensed and certified midwives can work under the supervision of a doctor but can't take charge of a pregnancy or delivery that's likely to be problematic. Generally but not always, health insurance plans cover the costs of licensed midwives.
- *Direct entry midwives.* Direct entry midwives do not have a state license to practice. They aren't covered by health insurance plans and doctors do not supervise their work.

- *Lay midwives.* These women learn the trade through apprenticeships. They don't have formal midwifery education. Health insurance plans don't cover their services and a doctor doesn't oversee their work.

Many women choose midwives because they give a much more personalized treatment with more natural options for dealing with discomfort and pain before and during delivery. Also, unlike your obstetrician/gynecologist, who will probably only be with you in the moment the baby is born, a midwife will be with you during the entire delivery, from beginning to end.

Family Doctor

This is a common choice in places where you may not have easy access to a specialist. A family doctor is a general doctor or primary care physician who has received a varying number of years of training on how to treat a mother-to-be and deliver her baby. As the name implies, this doctor may be able to treat the entire family, just as in the good old days. If you've established a good relationship with your family doctor, this could be your best option for prenatal care. However, you should ask if he/she is working closely with an obstetrician/gynecologist, and who is his/her backup if there are complications during pregnancy or birth.

EMOTIONS

A positive pregnancy test can set off a landslide of contradictory emotions, even if you were already trying to get pregnant. Sometimes you'll feel joy and anticipation, and other times you'll feel apprehensive and scared and uncertain. Sometimes you'll feel all of that at once.

"It was a surprise. I felt very happy but also a bit scared of the new situation. *Un poco de todo,* a little bit of everything."
—*María Teresa Díaz-Blanco*

"I was not married yet and I was concerned about my boyfriend's reaction, but I was very happy."
—*Lorena Asbell*

"It was the happiest day of my life. The second happiest day of my life was when I realized I was pregnant with my second son. It was something I had been looking for my whole life."
—*Ana Cristina Osorio*

The arrival of a new human being represents a complete change in who you are, how you live, how much free time you'll have and how you work. And if your pregnancy is a surprise, you'll feel even more confused about how to adapt to these changes.

One of the reasons your emotions change so much during pregnancy is because after conception your hormones begin to increase their levels dramatically. To give you an idea: during the first month of pregnancy you've got thirty times the amount of estrogen in your body than you do when you're about to get your period. You know those days shortly before your period is due when your emotions go haywire? Imagine thirty times that.

It is normal to feel as if you are on an emotional roller coaster. But if you feel as though your anxiety is really spinning out of control, talk to your doctor. Sometimes these hormonal changes can spark depression during pregnancy, which can be treated.

THE *BEBÉ*

How can two people make another? The process that's going on inside you right now is truly one of the miracles of nature. The moment sperm fertilizes your egg, an exquisite biological chain of events begins whose ending is *nada menos*, nothing less than the creation of another human being. Although pregnancies are said to begin on the first day of your last period, the moment of conception is two weeks later. That's why the description of what's happening to your baby begins with week three.

Fertilization and implantation of the egg

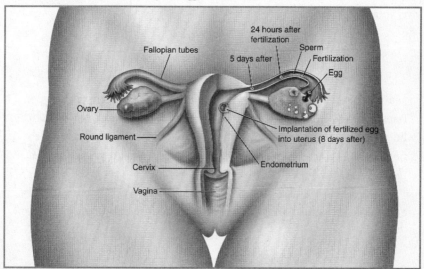

Week 3

The lucky sperm that beat out the other five hundred million fighting for the right to fertilize ran into your egg in one of your fallopian tubes. Those are the tubes that connect the ovaries with the uterus. The egg had just recently left one of the ovaries to begin its travel down the tube. When the sperm and egg met, they fused together and the sperm lost the tail that had propelled it up to this point. This happens twenty-four to seventy-two hours after making love. Once fertilized, the egg begins to roll like a little ball down the fallopian tube until it arrives at the uterus. That long trip usually takes more than a week. The future baby is at this point a mass of cells that divide every twelve to fifteen hours.

Week 4

Once at the uterus the fertilized egg literally implants itself into the uterine wall, which is ready to receive it.

The tissue that covers the inner uterine wall is called the endometrium. It grows after ovulation in preparation to nurture a possible fertilized egg. If there is no pregnancy, this tissue is destroyed and flushed out, which is what happens every month during the menstrual cycle. Sometimes the implantation causes a small hemorrhage that's known as implantation bleeding. Once attached to the uterine wall, the embryo begins to grow rapidly.

This week the cells are already organized: some will form the baby, others the placenta and another group the amniotic sac. At this point your period should have started, but it won't. Your baby is now two weeks old, but according to the pregnancy calendar, you're already four weeks into your pregnancy.

FOR DAD

Maybe the news you're going to be a father is a total surprise, or perhaps you had a feeling something was up by the way your wife has been acting. But what you probably haven't anticipated are all the new feelings you're going through as you contemplate becoming a father.

Upon hearing the news, many dads-to-be feel contradictory emotions. On one hand, they're very proud because, among other things, they've proven that all their equipment works well. You're a man in every sense of the word, and you've fulfilled what nature intended for you.

On the other hand, you might be worried and fearful about what kind of father you'll be or whether you'll be able to support your growing family. You might even ponder strange thoughts such as "Am I really the father?" even when you know so.

All this is normal, and many men, even though they don't talk about it, go through exactly what you're feeling as they wait for their child to be born. The problem in our Latino culture is that there isn't much room for a man to express his doubts, fears and worries. After all, you're supposed to be the rock of the family, the one everyone can depend on, especially now that you're going to be providing for an additional person. It's true that the ideal Latino man is supposed to be *el proveedor de la familia*, the family provider, but talking about your feelings and recognizing what you're going through is very healthy. It will help you deal with the changes in your relationship with your partner and the rest of your family.

Happily, the modern father doesn't have to play the role of spectator during pregnancy and especially during delivery. Most doctors will count on your participation, which will allow you to better understand what the mother of your child is going through.

Remember that when your wife's home pregnancy test gives a positive result, a huge amount of hormones have already begun flowing through her body so the baby can grow. It's as if you were given a massive shot every day of some strong medicine that would be good for the baby but would make you feel nauseous, moody and tired. A good dose of *paciencia y comprensión*, patience and understanding, is one of the best ways you can help your wife through this difficult time.

THE SECOND MONTH
Weeks 5 to 8

Your baby is still small and your abdomen won't show any signs of all that's going on inside you. But you still could be feeling other symptoms

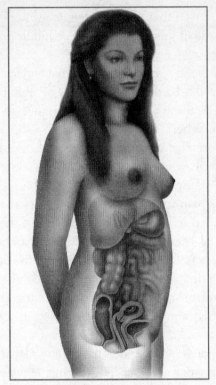

Second month

of pregnancy, such as nausea, the need to urinate frequently, or emotional ups and downs, all due to the hormones running through your veins. You'll likely discover you're pregnant in this month, because your period won't have arrived on time. The second month is a time of physical and emotional adjustment.

MORNING SICKNESS

Nausea is one of the most unpleasant sensations our bodies are able to muster. If you find yourself among the unlucky 89 percent of women who feel nauseous during pregnancy, you'll probably agree with me that it's simply no fun. If you're also one of the many women whose sense of smell suddenly becomes so acute it would put a hunting dog to shame, many smells will trigger a bout of nausea. And of course, the more nauseous you feel, the worse things smell.

Morning sickness may only be a feeling of dizziness or queasiness, or it may also be accompanied by vomiting. It can happen in the morning or in the afternoon, but for many women it doesn't have a schedule. Moms-to-be who are expecting twins or triplets are more likely to feel nauseous.

No one knows for sure why so many women suffer morning sickness during the first weeks of their pregnancies. Nor is there an explanation why 1 to 2 percent of pregnant women suffer severe nausea and vomiting for the whole nine months, a condition called hyperemesis gravidarum.

Commonly, it is believed that hormones cause morning sickness. Scientists have discovered that the most frequent feelings of sickness coincide with the highest levels of hormones. This time is usually between weeks two and eight.

A new theory posits that nausea came about millions of years ago to protect the fetus from the toxic plants its mother was eating. The first three months of pregnancy are when nausea is most common, and that's also precisely when the fetus is most vulnerable to outside toxins that could affect its development.

If you're going through nausea or vomiting right now, all these theories *no le servirán de mucho*, won't make you feel any better. Perhaps the most uplifting news is that, according to some studies, women who suffer from nausea during the first trimester have fewer miscarriages. The higher the level of the pregnancy hormone beta-HCG, the better the fertilized egg has implanted, but the sicker you'll feel.

There are some things you can do to help you survive this second month, which is usually the most difficult.

- If you feel sick in the morning, try to eat light, easily digested dinners the night before.

- Keep crackers next to your bed and eat a few before getting up in the morning.

- Take many small meals during the day, and don't let two hours go by without eating something.

- Some women don't seem affected by chiles, hot sauces or spicy foods, but try going without them for a few days to see if you feel better.

- Get as far away as you can from things that smell bad to you. You might keep something that smells good to you in your purse, perhaps a lemon. Take a whiff of that when you are surrounded by a smell you can't escape.

- Don't force yourself to eat healthy foods if they make you sick. Only eat what you can keep down.
- Acupressure bands worn on the wrist (advertised for seasickness and carsickness) help some women. You can find them in supermarkets and pharmacies, and they're not too expensive.

If your nausea is severe, ask your doctor if you can try either of the following:

- *Natural ginger pills*. This works well for women who get seasick easily and also some pregnant women. Take it in moderation.
- *Vitamin B$_6$.* In some cases this vitamin helps to reduce bouts with nausea, but a doctor should watch how much you're taking. More than 200 units a day of vitamin B$_6$ can affect the development of the fetus.

There are some drugs that your doctor may prescribe if you have severe nausea. Even though it's difficult if you're feeling really sick, try to drink as much water and other liquids as you can. If you're vomiting a lot, you'll get dehydrated.

Nausea, Nutrition and Vitamins

Even though you feel terrible, the baby is doing just fine. Maybe you're not eating as healthily as you should, or you may even be losing weight, but your baby is still very, very small and doesn't need much to nourish itself. Eat as many healthy foods as you can, but ones that are easy to digest, such as soups, yogurt or roasted potatoes. Don't forget to drink a lot of liquids and rest as much as you can. Fatigue and nausea aren't a good combination.

Prenatal vitamins will help you during this period, but you may not be able to swallow an entire pill because you feel so ill. Ask your doctor about liquid vitamins.

Excessive Saliva

Sometimes nausea is accompanied by an excess of saliva. It's not clear why this happens, but one-third of women who go through this say when they eat or drink dairy products they produce more saliva. Fruits appear to be one of the foods that have the least chance of causing this problem, which doesn't result in any difficulties in the pregnancy and usually disappears in a few weeks. There is no cure for excessive saliva, but eating something every two hours will help a little. You can also try using a mouthwash frequently.

APPETITE

Fifteen percent of pregnant women don't suffer from nausea, and some of those even see their appetites increase. If you're among those women who feel more hungry, you'll likely eat several times a day because your stomach will feel full quickly. Listen to what your stomach is telling you. Taking small meals every two to three hours helps to maintain a stable sugar level in the bloodstream and avoids difficult periods of indigestion. Easily digestible foods are recommended during this time, but for some women there are exceptions, such as those who still find chiles tasty.

CONSTIPATION AND GAS

There are several other things you can blame your hormone levels for, and constipation and gas are among them. Foods now spend more time in your intestines because digestion is slower. During that extended stay in your colon, more water is taken out of the food. The result: the stools get harder, you get constipated and the digested food produces more gas.

Constipation is something you might deal with in private, but flatulence is a different story. Green leafy vegetables, grains, legumes and fruit will come to your rescue because they will absorb a lot of water and counteract much of the loss of liquid that occurs during periods of slow digestion. Drinking a lot of water helps too.

As far as the gas goes, if you can avoid constipation, you'll feel a lot better. Stay away from foods that made you gassy in the past, and don't get too stressed out about it—the flatulence usually goes away after the first three months.

FREQUENT URINATION

As your hormone levels increase, so does your need to pee. The amount of blood passing through the kidneys during the first trimester is 70 percent greater than normal. The greater the amount of blood in the kidneys, the greater the amount of fluid that's filtered out. So it's no wonder you feel as though *se pasa la vida en el baño*, you're spending half your life in the bathroom. Plus, as your baby grows so does your uterus, and that puts pressure on the bladder, making you feel—that's right—as if you need to go to the bathroom again.

Beginning with the fourth month, the uterus starts to grow upward and the pressure disappears. But later the baby's head will once again produce that same sensation of having to urinate at all hours, even though when you go, it's only a few drops. To avoid having to get up so many times in the night to go to the bathroom, you might drink your eight daily glasses of water earlier in the day and stop at midafternoon. But don't limit your fluid intake—your kidneys need it.

Sometimes a frequent urge to urinate indicates that there is a urinary tract infection. Talk to your doctor about it, especially if you feel a burning or itching sensation when you go to the bathroom.

LACTOSE INTOLERANCE

Half of all Latinos are lactose-intolerant. People with lactose intolerance lack an enzyme that helps to break down lactose in the stomach. Lactose is a type of sugar that's found in milk and milk products. Without this enzyme, lactose can't be digested into small particles to be absorbed into the bloodstream. Instead those sugars ferment in the intestine, which causes stomach pains, gas, diarrhea and nausea—which already appear during pregnancy without any help.

Milk is one of the most recommended foods during pregnancy because it contains so much calcium. But even if you're lactose-intolerant, it's still possible to provide your baby with calcium.

- Take calcium supplement pills. During pregnancy you need 1,200 mg of calcium a day.

- Try yogurt made with lactobacillus bacteria. These bacteria predigest much of the lactose, making yogurt more digestible.

- Low-fat cheeses are a good source of calcium and contain less lactose than milk. You can also find low-lactose cheeses and yogurt in many supermarkets.

- Increase your intake of other foods rich in calcium, such as green leafy vegetables, sardines, and breads fortified with calcium. Another source is calcium-fortified soy milk.

- The enzyme needed to digest lactose is available in pill form. Take one at the same time you eat foods containing lactose.

- Sometimes you can drink small amounts of milk without problems.

HEADACHES

If you had migraines before your pregnancy, you may have hit the lottery. Pregnancy improves cases of migraines in seven of every ten women. But in the other third, it makes them worse. Why? You guessed it: changes in hormone levels.

Even if you've never had migraines, it's possible you'll still suffer from some headaches during the first weeks of pregnancy. Tension and fatigue, along with hormones, cause them. At the end of the first trimester, these headaches tend to disappear, but while you've got them, try to battle them with natural remedies, because taking migraine medication is a risky proposition during the first months of pregnancy. A Tylenol or two might help you during a crisis, but talk to your doctor before taking any. And don't use aspirin because it can cause bleeding and other problems. Some of the natural approaches you might try are:

- Resting with your eyes closed and with a cold damp cloth on your forehead

- Doing relaxation exercises

- Keeping a diary of when the headaches come and what sets them off (what you ate, when were you tense or tired, etc.)—you may notice that sometimes the pain appears because of changes in your routine

- Exercising regularly

I was one of the unlucky 30 percent who suffered more painful migraines during the first three months of my pregnancies. Mine usually started at the back of my neck. I treated them by lying down in a darkened room with my eyes closed and placing a bag of ice wrapped in a towel under my neck. When the migraines spread from my neck to the rest of my head, a cold towel over my eyes helped.

However, severe head pains during the second trimester could indicate another type of problem, such as a sudden rise in blood pressure. Contact your doctor if you suffer a severe headache, especially after the fifth month.

HAIR COLORING AND PERMANENTS

Even though there's no direct evidence that hair coloring or permanents cause birth defects, the consensus is that it's better to avoid them during the first months of pregnancy because the fetus is so vulnerable to toxic substances.

Some hair products are absorbed into the body in small amounts through the scalp. The type of coloring or permanent and the time it's in contact with your hair determine how much gets into your system. Temporary colorings, the ones that disappear after just a few washings, are absorbed less than the semipermanent or permanent colorings. Another option during pregnancy is to use temporary vegetable-based color.

Always keep an eye on how much lead is in the coloring, because in different countries there are different rules governing the allowable amount. Use only well-known brands. Lead and other metals such as mercury can harm the fetus.

IMMIGRATION AND TRAVEL VACCINES

Vaccines may contain weakened or inactive forms of the virus. Your body uses these debilitated viruses to create antibodies in case the real virus tries to attack your body later. But because of the possible effects even these weakened viruses may have on the fetus during the first stages of development, some vaccines aren't given during pregnancy or the three months preceding conception.

The following vaccines are required to earn residency status in the United States:

- Diphtheria
- Tetanus
- Mumps
- Measles
- Rubella
- Hepatitis B

If you're pregnant, you will not be given these vaccines. But there is no exception for women planning on getting pregnant, so if you're going to go through the immigration process, you should avoid getting pregnant for the next three months. Also, if you prove through a blood test you've already developed antibodies for some of those vaccines, you don't have to get that vaccine.

Another situation that may require you to get a vaccine is if you're planning to travel to countries where they are recommended. The Contact List has telephone numbers you can call to get information about which vaccines are required in which countries. After you find out, talk to your doctor.

The vaccines that contain living but debilitated viruses and which are therefore not recommended during pregnancy are:

- Rubella
- Measles
- Mumps
- Chicken pox
- Tuberculosis (BCG)
- Vaccinia

The following vaccines contain inactive viruses that pose less of a risk to the fetus, and are therefore used in some cases:

- Hepatitis A
- Hepatitis B
- Influenza
- Tetanus and diphtheria
- Meningococcal meningitis
- Rabies

If you have been vaccinated just before getting pregnant or you didn't know you were pregnant, there are tests to determine if the baby has been infected.

INSOMNIA

With all the changes your body is going through and all the emotions involved with having a baby, you may have trouble sleeping. The famous or infamous hormones of pregnancy are working full speed day and night and they can affect your ability to sleep, even if you feel exhausted. Some simple things you can do to help you sleep include:

- Taking a relaxing bath before going to bed
- Drinking a glass of warm milk or chamomile tea
- Eating a light dinner and not drinking a lot of water before going to bed, so you don't have to go to the bathroom in the middle of the night
- Listening to a relaxation tape or soft music while in bed
- Counting sheep (it does work)

Try not to get worked up about how many hours you lie awake in bed or how much longer you've got until it's time to get up. The secret is in relaxing.

Later on you may find other things can make it difficult for you to sleep. The baby might decide its favorite hour to practice *zapateado*, a traditional Latino dance, is at three in the morning. That's what my daughter Adriana did. Take it with calm and some humor if this happens, because it's just a preview of what's to come. The heavy, deep sleep you enjoyed before becoming a mom will soon be permanently a thing of the past. But in a few weeks your hormones will relax and you will too. You'll get accustomed to being pregnant and eventually return to sleeping at night.

FATIGUE

You might go through periods where you fall down exhausted on the sofa at seven in the evening and don't wake up until seven the next morning. Fatigue is one of the most obvious symptoms of pregnancy. It's a type of fatigue that makes your body feel heavy, as if screaming for a *siesta* or nap. It's normal during these months to sleep anywhere, anytime—even at work. And it's no wonder. Your body is working day and night to create millions of new cells that will form the placenta, increase the volume of your blood, and perform other complex tasks to protect and nourish your baby. Listen to what your body is saying during these months and rest as much as you can. You'll have time during the second trimester to buy baby clothes and get the baby's room ready.

THE FIRST PRENATAL VISIT

It's likely your first prenatal visit will be during your second month of pregnancy, because it takes a couple of weeks before you notice you've missed a period, decide to take a home pregnancy test and then make an appointment to see your doctor. This will be the longest visit of all because your doctor or midwife needs to get a lot of information from you.

Urine
When you arrive at the doctor's office you'll be given a small plastic cup which you have to write your name on and then urinate into, in this order. (Sometimes I forgot to write my name first, and believe me, *se hace*

complicado, it gets complicated!) This urine, which you'll have to provide every single visit, helps to measure a variety of things:

- *Urinary tract infections*. It's important to keep urinary tract infections in line during pregnancy because they can cause premature birth.
- *Sugar*. When glucose appears in the urine, it could be a sign of diabetes.
- *Albumin*. If this protein is present in the urine, there's a chance of preeclampsia. However, this illness only appears after the twentieth week of pregnancy.

Blood Pressure

The normal levels for a pregnant woman are between 110/60 and 120/80, but yours can be higher or lower and still be fine. Remember that during pregnancy, the volume of your blood increases and the veins and arteries relax to allow more liquid to flow through them. That's why your results will change.

Weight

Office scales *no perdonan*, are really unforgiving, even when you take off your shoes, your watch and your hairpins. During the first months you won't gain much weight, especially if you're nauseous or vomiting. But in the second trimester you'll begin to see the scales tip, and it only goes more quickly from there.

Blood Test

The first blood tests are thorough. Your obstetrician/gynecologist will use them to confirm your pregnancy and see if there are any illnesses that need to be treated to avoid complications. For more information on these diseases see Chapter 5. The blood work will test for:

- *Hepatitis B*. This is an inflammation of the liver produced by a virus that can infect your baby (see page 101).
- *Rubella*. This is also known as German measles. The blood test will show if you've got antibodies to this virus. If you do, that means you were vaccinated in the past and there's nothing to do. If you don't have the antibodies, you should be careful to avoid contagious children and adults because the virus can cause birth defects (see page 95).

- *HIV (human immunodeficiency virus)*. This is the virus that causes AIDS. If HIV is detected soon enough, the mother can be treated and the risk the baby will be infected is reduced. The sooner the mother's infection is known, the greater the chance of avoiding the baby's infection.

- *Syphilis*. It's a sexually transmitted disease. Just like HIV, if it's treated soon enough, the chances of the baby being infected are reduced.

- *Hemoglobin*. Figuring out how many red blood cells the mother has in her bloodstream helps to determine if she's anemic. It's common to have anemia during pregnancy because the volume of blood increases so dramatically, but the red blood cells don't increase in the same proportion. Medication corrects this problem.

- *Rh Factor and blood type*. If your Rh is negative and your baby's is positive, you might react to your fetus's blood. There are treatments for this problem. The analysis will also show what your blood type is: O, A, B, AB. Then the doctors know which blood to give you in an emergency.

- *Glucose*. This is the sugar level in your blood. This test is more precise than the urine test and also helps to figure out if you've got diabetes. The glucose test isn't done routinely, only when doctors suspect something might be wrong. Another test will be done later with a sugary drink (see page 138). But since diabetes is so common among Latinas, you might ask your doctor to include the glucose test in your blood analysis, especially if you have a family history of diabetes.

- *Toxoplasmosis*. This test is also done only when the doctor thinks there might be a problem. If you've got a cat in the house that spends a lot of time on the street, your doctor may want to know if you're immune to the disease, since it can harm the baby (see page 12).

- *Chicken pox and cytomegalovirus*. The tests for these diseases are not routine. But if you're a teacher or spend a lot of time with children and don't know if you've had chicken pox or cytomegalovirus already, tell your doctor. The test will determine if you've developed antibodies to these diseases (see pages 97–98).

Vaginal Exam

The doctor will likely do a vaginal exam to make sure the cervix is well closed. The uterus or womb is where your baby is growing. The cervix will dilate during delivery, but during pregnancy it's closed to protect the baby.

This test will also include the use of the speculum, that small device to open the vagina so the doctor can clearly see the opening of the cervix. The doctor will take a few samples of the cells of the cervix and of vaginal secretions with a cotton swab, a spatula or a brush. It's the same test you get during your annual pelvic exam and it doesn't affect the baby at all. The samples of your cervical cells and secretions will be sent to a laboratory to be analyzed.

- *Pap smear.* The cervical cells are looked at under a microscope to see if they're normal. This is the way doctors check for cervical cancer. If the results show some abnormal cells, it is necessary to do more tests and a follow-up as well as any appropriate treatment.

- *Chlamydia and gonorrhea.* These are sexually transmitted diseases. When they are present, it's necessary to treat the mother so the baby's eyes aren't infected during birth and so it doesn't get pneumonia.

- *Genital herpes.* Doctors don't usually look for genital herpes in this test because it has to be active for it to be detected. However, if you think you may have herpes, it's important to tell your doctor about it. Why? Because if the herpes is active during delivery, it can infect the newborn as it passes through the birth canal and cause serious nervous system damage. But if your doctor knows about your condition ahead of time, the risks are much lower.

- *Group B streptococcus.* This bacterium can live in the mother's vagina and can cause pneumonia and meningitis in newborns. This test is repeated in the last weeks of pregnancy (see page 103).

The First Sonogram

Sometimes doctors will do sonograms in their offices and may give you one during this first visit, depending on how far along you are. Try to bring your partner. Seeing your baby's heart beat for the first time is an emotional experience. It's still too early to know whether you're going to have a boy or a girl—that usually can be detected at 18 to 20 weeks.

The first thing the doctor or technician will look for is if there's an amniotic sac (or more than one), if there is a heartbeat and where the placenta has implanted. Normally it should be in the upper half of the uterus. But sometimes it could be in other places and cause problems:

- *Ectopic pregnancy.* Sometimes the fertilized egg begins its journey from the fallopian tube toward the uterus but doesn't make it. It gets stuck along the way and begins to grow inside the tube. That's dangerous. The fallopian tubes stretch from the ovaries to the uterus (see illustration on page 149), and if you've ever had an infection, surgery or endometriosis, it's possible the tissues have scarred over and don't allow the fertilized egg to pass through. In endometriosis the tissue that covers the inside of the uterus grows in other places, such as in the tubes, creating obstructions. Other times this happens for reasons doctors still don't understand.

  When the embryo begins to grow, it literally bursts the tube, producing internal bleeding that can be grave or even fatal for the mother. An ectopic pregnancy can also occur inside an ovary, in the cervix or even in the abdomen.

  Ectopic pregnancies are usually discovered as a result of the amount of pain they produce in the lower part of the abdomen. It's a sharp, throbbing pain on the right or the left side of your lower abdomen, similar to menstrual cramps. The pain comes and goes as the tube tries to expel the embryo. Sometimes the pain is also felt in the shoulder corresponding to the side the pregnancy is on. It can also be felt as pressure in the rectum or intestinal cramps. In addition to the pain, other symptoms of ectopic pregnancies include bleeding, low blood pressure and a rapid pulse.

  Fortunately, this type of pregnancy isn't common (about one in every thirty pregnancies). Still, there are some conditions that make it more likely to occur:

  - Venereal diseases (chlamydia, gonorrhea, pelvic inflammatory disease)
  - Infections caused by an intrauterine device (IUD)
  - Surgery
  - Endometriosis
  - Extrauterine pregnancies in the past

  Along with a sonogram, a blood test will show if hormone levels correspond to a pregnancy. When an ectopic pregnancy is detected, doctors can do a laparoscopic surgery to repair the broken fallopian tube. The doctor will make a few small cuts in your abdomen to introduce a small instrument with a camera on the end of it. That allows the doctor to see where the damage has been done and to repair it.

- *Placenta previa.* One of the things the first sonogram will tell you is where the placenta is situated. Placenta previa happens when the placenta is located too low in the uterus, partially or totally obstructing the cervix. No one knows why this happens, but it's most frequent in women who have had cesarean sections, several pregnancies, or twins or triplets or who are older than thirty-five. It's a serious condition that requires a close follow-up. It's very possible that you'll have to stay in bed. The good news is that in 90 percent of cases, if placenta previa is detected early enough, it will resolve itself before birth. If the situation doesn't improve and the placenta is completely covering the entrance to the uterus, there is a risk that it will rupture during contractions, so close monitoring and a C-section will be required.

- *Fibroids.* During or after your first sonogram they might tell you that one or several fibroids are in the uterus. A fibroid is nothing more than a benign tumor. The only problem that might appear is if the placenta is implanted on top of it because the baby might not get the proper nourishment. Also, if they're very large, they may obstruct the passage of the baby through the birth canal, but usually fibroids don't present any problem. Fibroids grow with estrogen, so they're likely to get larger during pregnancy as estrogen production and blood volume go up. Sometimes they can be painful or show up as a bump underneath the skin during the last weeks of pregnancy, but they usually return to their original size after birth.

- *Molar pregnancy.* This is a benign and relatively rare tumor produced in the placenta. It's a pregnancy that doesn't get organized. The lining of the uterus looks like grapes. Sometimes these tumors cause lots of nausea because they elevate the levels of the hormone beta-HCG. They're detected through an ultrasound test and are removed via suction.

- *Corpus luteum cyst.* This type of cyst appears frequently in the ovaries during pregnancy and usually doesn't have any effect at all. The corpus luteum is the wrapping that surrounds the egg before it's released from the ovary.

FEELINGS

During this month, you'll have the chance to experience just how varied and disparate your range of emotions is, a phenomenon that will surely get your partner's attention. In other words, in less than thirty seconds you may go from laughing to sobbing, getting furious along the way—all this because your husband commented on the weather during breakfast.

But you're not losing your mind. These are just the mood swings of pregnancy. It's an interesting mix of the increase in your hormonal levels and the feelings that pregnancy brings up. The result is something like premenstrual syndrome multiplied by a hundred.

You may feel happy and radiant one minute and the next feel that *todo le molesta*, everything annoys you, while at the same time the least little bit of care or affection shown toward you makes you cry. And if in addition you're nauseous or can't sleep, the feeling can be one of complete loss of control, particularly if it's your first pregnancy. It will all pass. By the end of the third month, most women who have suffered morning sickness begin to feel a lot better and their mood swings lessen.

Another symptom of the first months is *despiste*, forgetfulness. You might forget where things are, commit obvious mistakes in your work or not remember a conversation you had just five minutes before. Who wouldn't pay less attention to the outside world when she's going through all these emotional and physical changes?

There's no cure for all these emotions and feelings, but being tired aggravates them. Remember that all this will pass soon.

THE *BEBÉ*

Week 5
The cells of the embryo, which is what the baby is called at this stage, have begun to take shape. The future baby looks like a little *frijol* or bean with thousands of cells organizing themselves in three layers. From the outside layer will come the spinal column, brain and nerves. Bones and muscles will grow from the middle layer. And the innermost layer will give rise to the lungs, intestines and other internal organs.

Week 6
During week 6, millions of cells now make up the embryo. Even though it only measures a quarter of an inch (6 millimeters), it really does have a small heart the size of a pencil tip, which is pumping blood. The head

is beginning to form, and there is the start of a rudimentary spinal column. The eyes and the umbilical cord are already present.

Week 7

During the seventh week some of the facial features begin to appear, such as a nose and mouth. The eyes are even more well defined. The embryo now has arms and legs and it's starting to form fingers and toes and some internal organs, such as the intestines and lungs.

Week 8

At this time, the vertebrae, ribs and teeth have appeared, as well as the abdominal muscles and the skin, including pores and hairs. The intestines are still located inside the umbilical cord. The heart beats quickly, between 190 and 200 times a minute. The embryo now measures half an inch (a little more than a centimeter) and it moves nearly constantly.

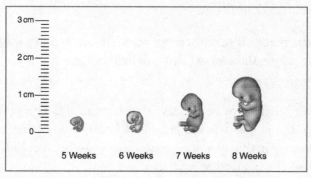

Fetus at 5, 6, 7 and 8 weeks of pregnancy (real size)

FOR DAD

Even when you know for sure that your partner is indeed pregnant, the fact that you are going to have a child might still be an abstract idea for you, not something as real as it seems for your wife. You also may be confused and worried about how quickly her moods change, or you might feel left out and abandoned because she's so tired and she can't take care of you as she once did. She'll probably not want to make love with you as much because she feels sick half the time, and you might feel frustrated because you can't help her feel better.

The second month of pregnancy might be a little difficult for her because of how bad she's feeling emotionally and physically, and it might be challenging for you as you learn to live with a person who's changing. Some of the things you should keep in mind are:

- The nausea, fatigue and mood swings your wife is feeling aren't psychological, but real. They're caused by the huge influx of hormones her body is producing during these first weeks. She can't do anything about it.

- What's happening to your wife *no es su culpa*, isn't your fault and there's nothing you can do about it either. Sometimes men feel the need to fix what's wrong when their loved ones are suffering. In this case, the only tools you've got at your disposal are being understanding, caring and patient as you wait for nature to take its course.

On the practical side, there are some strategies for dealing with your wife during these weeks that will help her get through morning sickness.

- Your partner may be sensitive to certain smells. The aftershave lotion you use that she once loved now makes her vomit. If you smoke, the odor of cigarettes will make her feel bad. Try to avoid the smells that make her nauseous.

- Your wife's body is now making a great effort to create the placenta and other basic structures to support and nourish the baby. This takes a lot of energy; that's why she's so tired all the time. Help her to rest. Cook meals yourself or order food in. Encourage her to drink a lot of liquids and to take her prenatal vitamins.

- Your wife might not want to make love with you because she feels bad physically or just because she doesn't want to. A pregnant woman's desire to have sex can change from month to month as her hormone levels fluctuate. Be patient, because her levels of desire might switch in a few weeks to heights you've never seen before!

- Be understanding with the mood swings and don't take them personally. She's in a temporary state of hormonal imbalance. Remember at the end, you'll have a baby.

- Don't be alarmed if you find you're also getting nauseous and dizzy along with your wife or if you start to gain weight. No, you're not pregnant, but it's such a common phenomenon it's got a name: couvade. Psychologists think it's a way for husbands to unconsciously try to share some of the struggles and discomforts their pregnant wives are going through.

- If you've got a cat, please take charge of changing the litter box. An infection called toxoplasmosis is spread through cat feces. This illness is harmful to the baby.

During this month, you'll make your first prenatal visit. Two important things to keep in mind:

- Try to accompany your wife to the prenatal visits, even though other family members are going. She'll appreciate it and it will give you a chance to participate more closely in the pregnancy by asking questions and helping to make decisions.

- Make sure you like the doctor, too. If you don't get along with the physician, you are going to feel tense during prenatal visits, labor and delivery.

And more than anything, be calm during this month. In a few weeks, when the hormonal crisis has passed, you'll see things in a different light.

THE THIRD MONTH
Weeks 9 to 12

At the end of this month, the pregnancy hormones have begun to calm down a little bit. That means the nausea and dizziness are much less frequent, and in the next few weeks you'll begin to feel a whole lot better. Also, at the end of this month, doing up your pants will start to become difficult. Your baby is completing critical stages in its development, and soon you'll begin to gain weight.

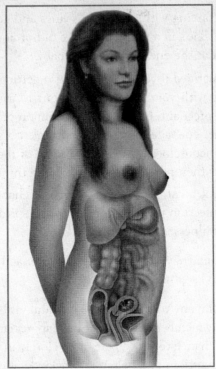

Third month

SWELLING

Your belly isn't growing, but the rest of you is. The sensation of being swollen is common during these weeks. This is because of the effect of hormones on your intestines. On one hand, the intestines are more relaxed, and on the other, they're working more slowly than normal, which allows things to back up, making you feel bloated. On page 155 you'll find some ideas to fight constipation and gas.

But the only real cure for this feeling is time. As the days go by and your belly begins to grow, the sensation of feeling full will go away. Looser-fitting clothes will make you more comfortable.

WEIGHT GAIN/LOSS

The American College of Obstetrics and Gynecology recommends gaining between three and four pounds during the first trimester. But that doesn't happen to everyone. If you're really suffering from serious nausea and vomiting you may even lose weight. Don't worry about that for the moment. The baby has more than enough reserves to survive.

It's also possible your appetite has increased and your weight is going up quickly. Try to gain weight gradually. During the first months, the fetus doesn't weigh much, which means the extra pounds you put on are in the form of fat, not the weight of the growing baby.

HEARTBURN

The feeling of having a match lit inside the top of your stomach is also common during this time. What else but the hormones? During pregnancy, hormones relax the valve that separates the esophagus and the stomach. As a result, the acids that help you to digest food, which are pretty strong, escape from the stomach up to the esophagus and cause a burning sensation.

During the final months of pregnancy, the acids are pushed up into the esophagus because the baby's growth doesn't leave them anywhere else to go. Some simple things you may try include not eating spicy or heavy meals, sleeping with your torso raised slightly and not bending from your waist down. There are also some medicines your doctor may prescribe for you during pregnancy.

BLEEDING

You might have a little bleeding or red-colored staining during the first weeks. Even though it's scary, there's no reason to worry. This light bleeding can happen for the following reasons:

- *Implantation*. Eight or ten days after fertilization, the egg implants in the uterus wall.
- *After a medical exam*. The blood flow has increased at the cervix, and it's possible the doctor broke a few capillaries.
- *After sex*. Just as with the medical exam, sometimes the penis will reach the cervix and cause bleeding.

Even though this is completely normal and not cause for concern, talk to your doctor anyway about slight bleeding. However, other types of heavier bleeding are dangerous. If you see any of the following symptoms, call your doctor immediately or go to a hospital.

- *Copious amounts of blood or blood *. Call immediately if you use more than one pad per hour or if the light bleeding lasts for an entire day.

- *Bleeding accompanied by abdominal cramps or persistent pain on either side of your abdomen or in a shoulder.* It could be an ectopic pregnancy (see page 164).

- *The appearance of gray or pink material.* Keep a sample of it in a plastic bag so your obstetrician/gynecologist can analyze it to see if it's a spontaneous abortion.

URINARY TRACT INFECTIONS

Urinary tract infections are common during pregnancy. A urinary tract infection is caused when bacteria that live on the skin outside where you pee make their way back up into the bladder or even the kidneys. The bacteria have an easier time getting into the urinary system during pregnancy because hormones make the sphincter tissues (the muscles that help you hold your urine) relax and because the growing baby pushes the tubes where urine flows out of their normal positions.

Urinary tract infections during pregnancy need to be treated immediately because they can cause uterine contractions that result in premature birth.

Sometimes urinary tract infections don't have any symptoms, but most of the time they do. The most common are:

- Burning or pain during urination in the bladder or the tube where the urine exits (urethra)
- The constant need to urinate, even though there's nothing there
- Urine that's cloudy, milky, bloody or smells bad
- Fever, vomiting or kidney pain

Urinary tract infections during pregnancy are treated with antibiotics that don't affect the fetus. Once you've had an infection, there's a good chance you'll get another during the pregnancy. That's why doctors will continue to test you for them, to make sure the bacteria haven't reappeared.

One way to prevent these infections is to drink cranberry juice. A recent study showed drinking this type of juice helped women avoid urinary tract infections. Water helps as well.

SEX

All the changes your body is going through might be reflected in your sexual relations with your partner. But the changes might surprise you. During pregnancy, some women feel a greater desire to have sex than normal, and they enjoy it for the entire nine months.

However, at the beginning of the pregnancy, the opposite is usually true. If you've gone through morning sickness and you're really tired, the last thing on your mind might be *una noche de pasión*, a night of passion with your partner.

Sometimes it's the husband who has a tough time having sex, because he worries about harming the baby. This is one of the most common fears of dads-to-be. But if the pregnancy is going according to plan, there is no reason to deprive yourselves of this experience, except under certain circumstances:

- Prior miscarriages
- Placenta previa
- History of premature deliveries
- Pregnancy with more than one fetus
- Genital infections

Although you might not be able to have sexual relations with penetration, you can still feel romantic, caress each other and practice other forms of sexuality. Your doctor will tell you whether you should avoid orgasms to prevent the uterus from contracting.

MAKING THE ANNOUNCEMENT

Perhaps there are no more family members left who don't know you're pregnant. Or maybe you and your partner are waiting a little while before telling everyone, especially if you've been through a miscarriage in the past. By the end of this month, the pregnancy will be well on its way, and it's a good time to make the announcement.

Think about how you're going to feel emotionally when you decide to tell everyone. If you're still sensitive or irritable, you might decide to tell just a few people at a time. Another option is during a *gran comida familiar*, a large family reunion.

If you've got other small children, they'll surely have noticed that "Mom's different." Explain to them in words they can understand that the family is going to have another baby and mommy is going to feel a little tired for a while and that she needs help. But remember, a child's concept of time is different from an adult's. To a child, six to nine months doesn't mean much. One suggestion is to tell them the next time it snows or the next time they go to the beach, the baby will have arrived. Pick a big event that coincides with your due date.

Telling the good news to your boss may be a little more complicated. Perhaps the weeks are going by and you just can't find the right moment to speak up. Nevertheless, there are several reasons to tell your boss before your pregnancy becomes obvious:

- It's much better if your supervisor hears it from you than from a third person.

- If you tell your boss several months ahead of time, it will show you're dealing in good faith because you're allowing the boss time to make plans to find your substitute.

- If you want to return to work after your baby is delivered, you should show you're interested in the well-being of the company. You may even help search for your own substitute.

By law, you can't be fired simply for getting pregnant. And if you have difficulty doing certain tasks, you should be treated as any other worker with a temporary illness. Also, depending on the requirements of your job, your company and the state where you live, you may not have the right to take time off for pregnancy (see page 27).

MATERNITY CLOTHES

At the end of this month your body is going through some obvious changes and you may not fit into many of your old clothes. Perhaps you can get by with leaving the top button of your pants undone or borrowing something from your partner. But soon you will have to buy something new to accommodate your new and changing shape. I have some friends who loved to go shopping at maternity stores, while others preferred to buy regular styles a few sizes bigger until there was no way to hide their bellies.

You don't have to spend money if you don't want to, unless you're going to have twins, in which case there's not many options other than to buy maternity clothes to accommodate your growing belly. However, some tricks for the first few months are:

- If your pants are not closing, you can use a rubber band. Tie one side around the button and thread the other through the buttonhole and back to the button. You will have to use a long shirt to cover this quick fix.
- Borrow some shirts or even pants from your husband.
- Use elastic-waist pants. They are cheap and they grow with you.
- Borrow some clothes from relatives or friends who have already been pregnant.

If you'd rather go shopping, fortunately maternity clothes have evolved a lot in the last years and you will find lots of styles to choose from. Almost all large clothing chains now carry a maternity section.

Undergarments
One of the things that receives more than a dozen different names in Spanish, depending on the country, is panties. Panties are known as *calzones, chones, pantaletas, trusas, bombachas y bragas*, among other things. But no matter what you call them, you will have to agree with me on one thing: tight panties are very uncomfortable, especially during pregnancy. The belly and the breasts are the first parts of your body to grow, so the first thing you might notice is that your underwear and bras don't fit well anymore. As far as panties go, the ones our grandmothers wore are likely to be the most comfortable because they cover the entire belly. But if this is too retro for you, perhaps you can use a bikini style that leaves your belly bared.

Your breasts will continue growing throughout your pregnancy, especially at the end. Maternity bras have several hooks that make them expandable as the months go by. They're not very sexy, but they do provide good support. If your breasts are sensitive, you may consider wearing a bra while you sleep to keep you in place.

Shoes

Comfortable shoes are a necessity during pregnancy. Your feet may swell as the months go by, and your shoe size may actually go up a little. Shoes that don't have laces or buckles are a blessing during the last months of pregnancy because reaching your feet is a real undertaking. Shoes with short or no heels are also welcome because as your belly grows, your center of gravity keeps changing, making walking with heels a challenge.

PRENATAL VISIT

Just like in your first visit, you'll be given the urine cup and they'll take your blood pressure and your weight. Your urine will be tested using several special strips of paper that detect protein and sugar.

They might also try to listen to the baby's heartbeat with an instrument that's placed on your belly to amplify the sound of the baby's heart (it beats much faster than yours). Another thing they'll do is measure your belly with a small metric tape measure, to follow the growth. You'll see how the centimeters go up more as the months pass.

During this visit you'll be given the chance to do a genetic test that's called chorionic villus sampling (see page 129). This test is done between weeks 10 and 12 for the following reasons:

- A sonogram detected something abnormal.
- You've had other babies with genetic problems.
- You've got a genetic hereditary disease in your family.
- You're older than thirty-five.

Although they are not very common yet, it's also possible to do two screening tests (nuchal translucency test and PAPP-A and free beta-HCG, see page 124) before the chorionic villus sampling. When the results of these two tests are combined, the accuracy is high. But these tests only determine the likelihood of your baby having Down syndrome— they don't confirm that your baby has that genetic defect. Confirmation is available only through a genetic test, such as chorionic villus sampling or amniocentesis.

Before going to your prenatal visit this month, I recommend you write down all your questions to take with you. Ask until you're satisfied. Remember, you're paying; you're the customer.

FEELINGS

Your hormones may have begun to give you a little break from the roller coaster they've had you on for the last weeks. The mood swings and irritability tend to disappear at the end of this month. On the other hand, they might not. Continuing morning sickness during these weeks and your varying emotional states may make you wonder *cómo va a sobrevivir,* how you can survive six months more.

Some women take several weeks more before they begin to feel better, and for an unfortunate few, they never do—it lasts the entire pregnancy. You may be among the fortunate ones who haven't felt nauseous or irritable at all, and you feel *mejor que nunca,* better than ever. Or perhaps you're among the women who felt sick, and you are now feeling better, just in time to start worrying about other things.

Now that the pregnancy is more established, you've entered the stage of actually feeling pregnant. You don't appear pregnant to those around you, because your belly isn't sticking out yet. But still, you feel a baby is really inside you. That's why it's normal to begin focusing at this stage on the baby's well-being and how the pregnancy will progress.

One of the most common worries during this trimester is the risk of having a miscarriage, especially if this has happened before. As the days pass, the possibility becomes more remote, because the majority of spontaneous abortions happen during the first weeks of pregnancy.

You may also be worried about how something you eat or drink or touch is affecting the baby. Don't be intimidated by *esos cuentos,* those myths that are so common in our culture. In the past, there wasn't any other way to explain problems during pregnancy or birth defects other than to make up stories. Today, we know why birthmarks appear and how cleft palates form (see Chapter 12 regarding myths of pregnancy).

During this time you may also find yourself less outgoing. Instead you're focusing on who's inside you, and you may even begin to converse with your baby. It's all part of the process of becoming a mother-to-be.

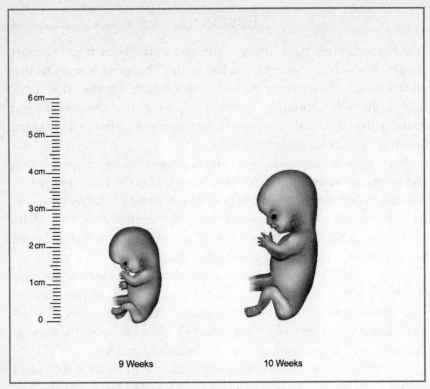

Fetus at 9 and 10 weeks of pregnancy (real size)

THE *BEBÉ*

Week 9

The nerve cells of the brain are beginning to make their first connections as they multiply hundreds of times over. The ears are two little buttons on the side of the head. The structure of the eyes is more advanced now, and there's even a tongue. The embryo will be moving side to side, and it measures 1 inch from head to buttocks (2.5 centimeters).

Week 10

In this week, the embryo has graduated into a fetus. The most critical stage of development has passed. By now all the major organs have been formed and all that's left is growing in size and refining the functions of each one. The fetus definitely has a human shape, with shoul-

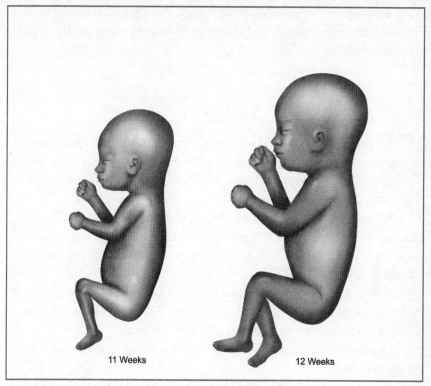

Embryo at 11 and 12 weeks of pregnancy (real size)

ders, ankles, elbows, fingers and toes. It measures about 1½ inches (4 centimeters).

Week 11

The fingers and toes are fully formed now, and the fingernails and toenails are soon to come. The head is one-third of the length of the entire fetus and it's starting to get upright. The eyelids are present, and even though they remain closed, beneath them the iris that gives color to the eyes is forming. This is the beginning of a rapid growth stage. The fetus measures 2½ inches (about 6 centimeters).

Week 12

The amount of amniotic fluid in your belly surrounding the baby begins to increase. The baby can now urinate and its intestines are moving.

Urine ends up in the amniotic fluid, which the baby swallows. The fingers and toes are separated, and the genitals begin to take on their male or female form.

FOR DAD

If the previous weeks have been difficult for your partner, then surely they have been for you as well. Morning sickness, nausea, mood swings and other maladies may have left you wondering how you are going to make it through the rest of the pregnancy.

Fortunately, by the end of this month there's a good chance things will be better. The hormones flowing through your partner's veins are beginning to level off and the mood swings and nausea are becoming less severe.

Along with your partner, you may also be worried about a miscarriage, especially if she's had one before. As the weeks go by, you can become more confident that this won't happen.

During this month, you'll notice your wife becoming more distant and more thoughtful, or maybe she's becoming closer to her mother or another woman in her family. And if she doesn't feel like making love, you may feel distanced from all that's going on, or even resentful.

Her attitude doesn't mean *que ya no le ama*, she's stopped loving you. It means that after the initial surprise, the pregnancy is now a reality for her—in her body and in her mind—and she's thinking about it a lot. Maybe she's beginning to have conversations with the baby. Also, it's normal for her to try to get closer to her mother now that she's becoming a mother herself. If your relationship with your mother-in-law isn't the best, have a little patience. This is only a stage, and soon your wife will need you more than ever. Whatever happens, remember:

- The self-involvement your wife is going through is normal, and you shouldn't react by distancing yourself from her even further. That will only make things worse.

- Don't scold her for not paying attention to you. She's not doing it on purpose. It's a healthy and normal stage of pregnancy.

- Let her know in a calm and friendly way how you feel. Perhaps she hasn't noticed how she's focusing so much of her attention on the baby.

- Talk with other fathers who have already been through the same thing. It helps a lot to know you're not the only one.

MISCARRIAGE

The majority of miscarriages happen during the first trimester. Of those, half are caused by chromosomal abnormalities. That means the cells didn't organize themselves properly to form a fetus, or there were serious errors that impeded normal development.

The most common signs a spontaneous abortion has occurred are:

- Abdominal pain and contractions
- Heavy bleeding (one pad per hour) or bleeding for an entire day
- Appearance of gray or pink matter

When you experience pain and bleeding but the cervix hasn't dilated and the doctor confirms through an ultrasound that there's still a heartbeat, sometimes there are ways to stop the miscarriage from happening. Among them are bed rest, limiting sexual relations, or even medication. Nevertheless, this depends on the condition of the fetus, because if it does have a serious birth defect, it's possible these measures won't help and nature will take its course anyway.

Once the symptoms of a miscarriage have appeared, your obstetrician/gynecologist will determine if there has been a complete expulsion. If this has occurred, nothing is done. If it hasn't, there's a chance that what remains inside the uterus will cause an infection. That's why the doctor will order a cleaning or D&C (dilation and curettage) to get rid of the remains. After a miscarriage, the expelled material is usually analyzed to see if there are any genetic defects.

If after a miscarriage (whether you had a D&C or not) you continue to experience severe bleeding, pain or fever, call your doctor.

Your doctor will tell you when to begin trying to have another baby, though if you've just had a miscarriage you might not want to think about it for now.

Another possibility in case there is no infection or bleeding is to allow the fetus to be reabsorbed by itself. It's a slower process, you will need close follow-up and it depends also on how many months you were pregnant. But if your doctor approves and you don't want to go through a D&C, this is a less traumatic option to consider.

Two important things to remember after going through a miscarriage:

1. *It wasn't your fault.* The majority of miscarriages during the first trimester are caused by cells that couldn't organize themselves properly to develop into a fetus. This is a lot more common than you think. Ask among your relatives and friends and you'll find that maybe your aunt or cousin or neighbor or even your mother has been through it. Having a miscarriage doesn't necessarily mean there are genetic problems in your family, nor that you'll have more in the future. It's just how nature works. Creating a human being is complicated.

2. *You didn't do anything to cause it.* Don't spend many sleepless nights trying to figure out how this happened: "Maybe if I hadn't picked up those boxes," or "Maybe if I hadn't eaten that food," etc. If you live a normal life and don't take drugs or drink (and I'm not talking about just a couple of sips to celebrate a birthday) but you have a miscarriage anyway, it's because of complications or problems way beyond your control.

That doesn't mean you won't feel a great disappointment and pain for the loss of your pregnancy. Although your belly wasn't swelling yet, the baby was something as real to you as the sun rising and setting every day. However, others might have a difficult time understanding what your relationship with the baby was, and they might feel that two weeks is enough recovery time and you should start thinking about trying to have another baby.

Nhora Estella Saxon, mother of two girls, went through this during her second pregnancy. She was bleeding for several days, but the sonogram showed everything was fine. One night, she began to feel severe pains and went to the hospital with her husband, where they confirmed she'd had a miscarriage.

"They gave me a strong painkiller and I spent the entire weekend bleeding *con una pena y un dolor muy grande*, with a big sadness and pain in my heart. It was just like my period. On Monday we went to the doctor and they suggested we come back Tuesday to clean out the remains of the baby. If they hadn't known me so well, they surely would have committed me to an insane asylum. *Yo no entendía*, I couldn't understand how they could make me wait—I wanted this nightmare to be over.

"On Tuesday I woke up and went to the hospital. I was overcome by sadness. When they sent me back home, I saw all the things we'd bought for the baby and I began to cry again. I took a week off from work and that was tough, because a lot of people don't know what's happened, they ask you about the baby and then they don't know what to say. Some tell you it was for the best because the baby wasn't developing properly, and others tell you it's God's will. *A mi se me hizo todo una pelota*, everything got very confusing for me. I couldn't even talk to my husband about it because he was so upset.

"Finally I went to a psychologist. There I learned to accept that what happened was important and not a nightmare. I have the sonograms and all the test results. You shouldn't deny what happened but accept it. I returned home and told everyone: 'I need to talk about this baby. I need to talk about what would have happened had it been born. I don't need you to go running out of the room when I begin to broach the subject.' *Fue duro*, it was tough.

"We waited six months before deciding to try again. Then I couldn't get pregnant. I felt I was a failure, I was frustrated, I thought I had done something wrong, I thought I was broken. But the psychologist told me about many women who have gone through the same problem. I really think in the majority of cases, most people aren't given enough support to overcome the loss of a baby."

The loss of a baby, even in the first weeks, is a real hardship. And because it's real, you should mourn it. Take the time you need. Talk about the pain you're feeling with your husband, your family, your friends. Tell them it's the same as losing a loved one: there is a mourning process. And if you need to, do what Nhora Estella did—seek out professional help if you feel overwhelmed by your emotions and you don't know what to do with all your feelings.

And for Dad, your pain is real, too. Keeping all your feelings bottled up inside doesn't do anyone any good. They'll end up coming out in one way or another, in the form of rage, anger or distancing yourself from your wife through your work or with your friends.

Talk about it with your wife and share what you're going through with the husband of another woman who's also lost a baby. For people who haven't been through it, it's difficult to understand just how painful it is and how profound those feelings are. Just like any other injury, they need attention and time to heal.

8

The Second Trimester

After the storm, calm sets in. If you've had or continue to have morning sickness, if you feel completely exhausted and your emotions are fluctuating between euphoria and despair every five seconds, you may have felt shipwrecked at times. But this stage of your pregnancy may soon be over and you will start feeling much better. The pregnancy hormones—responsible for all this turmoil during the past three months—will now begin to level off. On the other hand, if you're one of the lucky women who had a pretty good time during the past three months, you're likely to feel even better during the second trimester.

This stage of pregnancy is an enjoyable time for most women. It's when you will feel the baby move for the first time, the glow of pregnancy starts to appear, your energy will go up, fatigue diminishes, your belly isn't so big yet that it gets in the way and the trips to the bathroom are cut way down.

So, enjoy the next few weeks and celebrate with your husband. You're one-third of the way through your pregnancy!

THE FOURTH MONTH
Weeks 13 to 16

ANTOJOS, CRAVINGS AND WHIMS

"I craved chocolate. Before getting pregnant I didn't want anything to do with chocolate."

—*Miriam Gayden*

"I just craved *cosas saladas*, salty things like salami or olives. Nothing sweet."

—*Laura Loustau*

"I craved crushed ice. I thought I was lacking some vitamin. I wanted the crunchiness. I was constantly asking my husband to stop in places I knew you can serve yourself crushed ice."

—*Leticia Gutierrez*

Women can crave just about anything during pregnancy. No one knows for sure where these desires come from, but many people have tried to explain them:

- They make up for lack of nutrients during pregnancy.
- They're psychological, only a way to get attention.
- They're a way to avoid the baby being born with birthmarks.

Fourth month

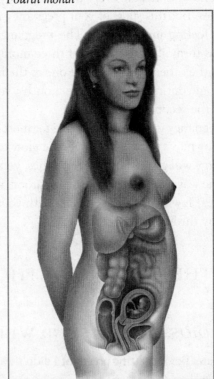

The sudden need to eat a fresh salad or a grilled steak could justify the first reason. Waking up your husband at three in the morning to ask him to go buy you a candy bar from the corner store could be an example of the second reason. And the third reason can only be used nowadays with relatives from past generations, since it's proven that cravings have nothing to do with birthmarks.

Still, if you've got someone who can help you fulfill these whims and cravings, *¿por qué no?*, why not do it? The only thing you have to be careful about is your weight, because satisfying your frequent cravings for sweets or fatty foods can make your weight go up quickly. Sometimes it's possible to substitute another, healthier food for the one you're craving. Instead of an ice cream, try a frozen yogurt that has fewer calories and less sugar. Or if you are craving something crunchy, like some *churros*, try some low-fat cookies instead.

There's another type of craving that strikes some pregnant women, called pica. Women with pica have a strong desire to eat dirt, ashes, ice, soap, plaster or coffee grinds. Some of these substances are toxic and can harm the baby. Talk to your doctor if you feel these cravings, because it could be an indication of a physical or psychological problem that could be treated.

While you may feel cravings for foods you've never tried before, you may also suddenly find your favorite things to eat are now disgusting. All this is normal, and in the next weeks or after the birth of the baby, you'll get back to your normal likes and dislikes.

SKIN DARK SPOTS

One of the hormones that increases its presence in the bloodstream during pregnancy is the melanocyte-stimulating hormone (MSH). Melanocytes are cells that live in the skin. Depending on how concentrated they are, your skin can have a lighter or darker color. Some of the changes you'll notice during pregnancy are attributed to this hormone. The most common are:

- Chloasma or pregnancy mask, light brown patches that appear on the mother's face, usually on the cheeks and forehead
- Darkening of existing moles

- Linea nigra (black line), a dark-colored line that runs from the pubis up to the belly button and sometimes even higher
- Darkening of the nipples

Other changes in the skin are due to the increase in estrogen production:

- Varicose veins in the legs
- Veins visible through the skin
- Red or purple capillaries that spread out at the skin's surface (spiderweb veins)

And sometimes little skin tags can show up on the neck, eyelids and other places on the body. Although no one knows for sure why they appear, they're nothing to worry about.

STRETCH MARKS

These marks come in pink, purple and white and appear on the abdomen because the skin stretches too much. The marks usually show up on the sides of the abdomen and underneath it. I was happy after my first pregnancy, thinking *que me libre de ellas*, I'd avoided them altogether. That was until it occurred to me to grab a mirror and look at the underside of my belly.

In theory, if you use some type of cream on your skin during pregnancy, you can help to increase the elasticity of the skin and reduce the chances of getting stretch marks. But the reality is there's no miracle way to avoid them. You might improve your look a little, but stretch marks are usually a permanent reminder of your pregnancy.

ACNE

The skin goes through many changes during pregnancy. Hormones make the skin more oily, and pores get clogged. It's the same reason you get acne as a teenager. Nevertheless, you must be careful with acne treatments such as Retin-A and Accutane because they can cause birth defects.

Also look out for the contents in beauty creams (see page 8).

CHANGES IN HAIR AND NAILS

"My hair was much more manageable and it looked *hermoso*, beautiful. Without the big belly it would be perfect!"

—*Gloria Villalobos*

One of the good things about pregnancy hormones is they make your hair grow more quickly, keep it from falling out and help strengthen your nails. But that hormonal stimulation also makes body hair begin to appear in places it didn't before. One thing for the other.

Be careful about chemical products for beauty treatments during pregnancy. It is unknown whether products to remove hair or to dye it have any negative effects on the baby. A small amount of hair coloring products is absorbed through the scalp, and this could be a problem, especially if they contain lead (see page 6).

The hormones help fingernails and toenails to grow more quickly and become stronger. Manicures and pedicures are fine during pregnancy. Just make sure the salon you go to is well ventilated, because breathing the fumes of the chemical products used isn't a good idea. As far as acrylic nails go, there haven't been any studies done to see if they harm the fetus, but it's better to be cautious, since strong chemicals are used in the process.

BLEEDING GUMS

The volume of your blood has increased dramatically in the last few weeks, and those hormones have made tissues all over the body softer and more sensitive. That can cause the capillaries in your gums to bleed when you brush your teeth. Also, you may be eating many small meals but not brushing as often. Gum irritation at this time is called pregnancy gingivitis. It's not all that serious and it gets better the more you brush. Don't forget to floss your teeth and use a mouthwash after each meal.

A few purple blisters may appear on your gums that also bleed easily. Even though they look scary, don't worry about them. They're common among pregnant women. They won't harm the baby and they'll go away after delivery.

Periodontal Disease

Another problem that shows up during pregnancy that's more serious is called periodontitis (or periodontal disease or pyorrhea). This disease is caused by pieces of food that stick to the teeth below the gum line and turn into plaque. This plaque is full of bacteria that irritate the gums and cause them to bleed. If periodontitis isn't treated, the gum begins to recede and the tooth can become loose and finally fall out.

The danger with periodontal disease during pregnancy is that it can affect the fetus. A recent study showed that pregnant women who suffered this disease had a higher incidence of premature births. Scientists have discovered that bacteria in the mother's gums actually pass through to the baby.

If you've had gum problems before getting pregnant, it's likely they'll get worse during pregnancy. You should make an appointment with the dentist during this trimester.

Nosebleeds and Nasal Congestion

Your nose may bleed during pregnancy for the same reason the gums do: an increase in the volume of blood and the tissues becoming more sensitive. In dry or cold climates, the changes in temperature or the lack of humidity can cause minor nosebleeds. Use your finger to apply a little olive oil or Vaseline, or use saline drops to moisten the tissues on the inside of your nose. But if your nosebleeds are frequent and abundant, talk to your doctor, because it could be a sign you've got high blood pressure.

To stop a nosebleed, lean forward and pinch your nose with your thumb and forefinger for about fifteen minutes, the same as if you were going to jump into a swimming pool. If you feel as though you're swallowing a lot of blood and the bleeding doesn't stop, call your doctor or go to a hospital.

Vaginal Discharge

An increase in vaginal discharge during pregnancy is normal. It's usually white or a little yellowish, and it can be thick and dense or nearly liquid. It's known as leucorrhea, and it's caused by changes in hormone levels.

Soaps, douches and other similar products don't work during this time, because the flow will continue no matter what. Be careful with strong soaps that can be irritating. Ask your obstetrician/gynecologist about douches during pregnancy. Not all are in agreement about their effectiveness and safety. Wearing cotton underwear and changing it frequently helps, or you can use panty liners.

If the fluid is white and doesn't smell bad, everything should be fine. But if it does have a bad odor or looks a little greenish and yellowish or like cottage cheese, talk to your doctor, because you may have developed an infection. Yeast infections during pregnancy are common and are easily treated (see page 258).

DIZZY SPELLS

The most common causes of dizziness are insufficient blood flowing to the brain and a low blood sugar level. One of the most common times to suffer a dizzy spell is right when you stand up after being seated or lying down. Gravity literally pulls the blood down to your feet as you get up, and because your veins and arteries are relaxed during pregnancy, the body takes a while to reestablish the proper blood flow to the brain. Also, as the months go by, the uterus begins to put pressure on one of the mother's principal arteries, and that can restrict blood flow and oxygen to the brain. Get on your feet slowly to give your circulatory system time to adjust to what you're doing and make sure enough blood is getting to the brain. If you get really dizzy, try lying down with your feet elevated higher than your head.

The other cause of dizzy spells is a low blood sugar level. Eating several small meals a day can help to maintain blood sugar levels. Take cookies, crackers, nuts or dried fruit with you in your purse to eat when you feel dizzy. If you're diabetic and you often feel dizzy, talk to your doctor.

SLEEPING POSITIONS

During this month you might find it's a little difficult to find a comfortable position to sleep in. Sleeping facedown might become a challenge and soon it will be impossible. The recommended sleeping position during pregnancy is lying on your left side. Sleeping on your back puts all the weight of the growing uterus on the aorta and the vena cava, two important blood vessels. The weight on these blood vessels can restrict the blood flow that you and your baby are getting.

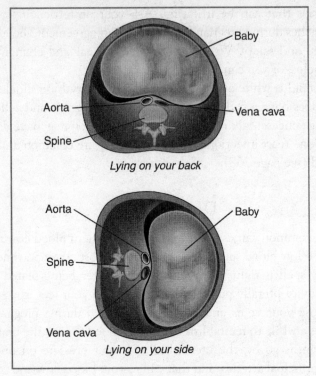

Vena cava compression during sleep

But *que no le quite el sueño*, don't lose sleep over this piece of information. Remember, before scientists figured this out, millions of women slept on their backs during pregnancy and had healthy, happy babies. In other words, doctors recommend you sleep on your left side, but don't worry if you're really uncomfortable that way, and don't feel bad every

Sleeping position

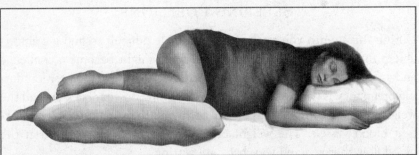

time you wake up and realize that you are sleeping on your back. Sleep the best way you can. Your body knows what it needs and will alert you when it's time for a change. However, if you've got high blood pressure, the baby is developing behind schedule or you've got kidney problems, you really should try to avoid sleeping on your back.

Many pregnant women learn to sleep on their left side by putting a pillow between their legs and supporting their right arm with another pillow. Maternity stores sell all kinds of sleeping pillows. You can also find them on the Internet. And if you get used to sleeping this way, you may never change. That's what happened to me.

THE NAUSEA CONTINUES

It's possible that after reaching the promised land—12 weeks—you may continue to feel nauseous. Sometimes relief doesn't come at exactly week 13. Unfortunately, some women never feel better, and some get worse. If you're of Mexican descent, your doctor might want to look at your gallbladder, because it might be contributing to your queasiness (see page 92). Being pregnant with more than one child could also be the cause, because your hormones will be in an even more elevated state.

If the nausea keeps you from living normally, your doctor can prescribe you some medicine to get over it. It's stressful and at times overwhelming to have to feel ill day after day. But no matter how bad it gets, there are women who have felt nauseous during their entire pregnancies, and they have survived.

"I had nausea during my first pregnancy but I thought, okay, I am ready to do this but this is *la última vez*, the last time. I thought I should be able to handle it. But in the second pregnancy, after the first few months the nausea came again and it was worse than the first time. On top of that I had a little one. I couldn't hold anything down, not even water, *nada, nada*, nothing. I got dehydrated like three times. Finally, around the eighth month it started to get better."

—*Leticia Gutierrez*

If you vomit every day and can't keep even liquids down, you ought to talk to your doctor. An illness called hyperemesis gravidarum can sometimes strike during pregnancy, and it can require hospitalization.

Hyperemesis Gravidarum

It's a rare disease and its cause is unknown. Instead of getting better, morning sickness and nausea gets worse. As a consequence of the constant vomiting, the mother can become dehydrated and lose minerals and weight. When the body doesn't have food, it takes energy from the fat stores. The fat-burning process produces a by-product called ketones that could harm the baby. Generally, when a pregnant woman is vomiting more than three times a day and is not able to retain any liquids, she may need to be checked in a hospital so she can get fluids intravenously. Sometimes the symptoms get better after this treatment, but later on they reappear and she might have to be hospitalized again.

Each case of hyperemesis gravidarum is different. Some women respond to a B-vitamin treatment, and some others might have thyroid or hormonal problems that are causing the constant sickness. Women expecting more than one baby, who are overweight, who are in their first pregnancies or who have suffered extreme nausea and vomiting before have a greater chance of developing this illness.

Domestic Violence

Physical and verbal abuse against women is a problem in all social classes and cultures and at all ages. It's a plague that affects millions of women around the globe. There are some circumstances when a woman is more likely to suffer abuse: Being pregnant or being between the ages of nineteen and twenty-nine are two scenarios common when there's a first appearance or worsening of abuse in a relationship.

In the United States, experts believe that two of every ten pregnant women suffer physical or verbal abuse at the hands of their partners or husbands. The statistics are likely even much higher, because many of the cases of abuse are never reported. An unwanted pregnancy or the abuse of alcohol or drugs increases the chances that the mother-to-be will be a victim of domestic violence.

The risks for the woman who suffers physical abuse during her pregnancy include spontaneous abortion, premature birth, babies born dead or at a low birth weight or with injuries, including broken bones. Punches can separate the placenta from the uterus or damage the mother's internal organs. Other effects of physical or verbal abuse include anemia, infections and bleeding.

A pregnant woman often feels vulnerable and dependent on her companion. She may try to justify the abuse or even get herself to believe it's not really abuse. But domestic violence isn't limited to punches, kicks and rape. It's also shouts, insults, criticism, exaggerated jealousy, obsessive control, isolation or any other attitude that make the mother-to-be feel afraid of her partner or husband.

Remember, there is no justification for domestic violence. You don't deserve it. You haven't caused it. It's not your fault.

Pregnancy is a time of great change and requires a lot of adjustment for all couples. Some men feel jealous of the baby that's on the way. They may feel angry about the decreased sexual desire their partners are showing during pregnancy. Or they may detest the shape of a pregnant woman's body. None of these reasons, or any other reason for that matter, is justification for physical or verbal abuse. Problems are resolved by talking and taking measures, not by punching.

Abusive men don't limit themselves to their wives. Newborns or other children in the family can suffer similar consequences, sometimes for years to come.

The vulnerability a pregnant woman feels may make her think the only option she has is to put up with the abuse because she's got no place else to go. She may think she's got to *aguantar*, to put up with it and *callar*, don't tell anybody because she does not have anywhere to go and *por el qué dirán*, for fear others might think badly of her.

But the truth is there are options for pregnant women who are suffering abuse. The National Domestic Violence Hotline (1-800-799-SAFE) has operators who speak both Spanish and English and accepts confidential calls twenty-four hours a day (see Contact List). There you can find out which organizations will help you free of charge. No one will ask you your immigration status. You'll learn about shelters that protect pregnant women who need to escape from their abusive partners right away and about support groups made up of women who have gone through the same thing.

Feelings

If your hormones have begun to stabilize, you'll feel a great relief (and so will your husband). Your mood swings will be milder, and you'll begin to react to situations as you did before you got pregnant.

Nevertheless, the changes your body is going through may begin to provoke new feelings. Your belly is beginning to grow. But you may be in that stage where it is not clear whether you've just put on a few pounds or you're expecting. Maternity clothes are still too big for you, but your regular clothes are now too small, and people don't dare ask about a possible pregnancy in case you really are just gaining weight from eating too much.

> "I was in a stage where pregnancy clothes were too big but my clothes were too small. I felt depressed about gaining weight, even when I knew it was only for a while. I didn't like pregnancy clothes and I didn't use them until I had no other option. I was always looking for clothes for *flacas*, thin women."
>
> —Ana Miriam La Salle

This won't last long because in a few weeks there won't be any doubt in anyone's mind as to why you can't do up the top button on your pants.

In this stage you're going to say goodbye to your body as you've known it up to now. That experience can provoke some contradictory feelings. On one hand, you might really like the idea of being pregnant, of having your belly expand. But on the other hand, you might begin to have doubts about how attractive you will be as a woman or whether your partner will like your new, expanded silhouette. Maybe just thinking about all this may put you in a bad mood. Be patient, because in a few weeks you will have a new perspective on things.

Prenatal Visit

During this visit, the routine will be repeated: blood pressure, weight, urinate into the cup, measure the size of the uterus, check water retention and the best of all, listen to the baby's heartbeat.

Your doctor will also offer you a genetic screening test (see page 123) to see what the chances are the baby could be born with Down syndrome or neural tube defects.

THE *BEBÉ*

Week 13
The third trimester is one of the periods of most rapid growth for the baby. At this moment it is 3 inches long (around 7.5 centimeters) and weighs about ½ ounce (15 grams). The placenta provides all its nutrition. The ears and eyes are in their appropriate places and vocal cords are forming. The intestines are in the process of moving out of the umbilical cord and into the abdomen.

Week 14
The placenta is now the principal source of nutrition for the baby. The liver and pancreas are working on their own. The head will now grow more slowly and will stop resting in the chest as the neck grows longer. The baby can make a fist and has begun practicing breathing. It measures 3½ inches (almost 9 centimeters).

Week 15
The baby's bones are still getting stiffer and stronger. That's why at this stage it absorbs a lot of calcium. The little bones in the ear are forming, and it's possible your baby can hear noises from outside. The skin is still thin and appears covered with a fine layer of hair called lanugo. An ultrasound done during this week may show the baby sucking its thumb. That's its way of practicing suckling, which is how it will feed itself later. The baby measures 4½ inches now (more than 11 centimeters) and weighs nearly 2 ounces (about 57 grams).

Week 16
If you want to know whether you'll have a boy or a girl, this is the week to find out. An ultrasound will tell you—if the baby positions itself so that the doctor can see. The sexual organs are now sufficiently formed to tell what's what. The baby now measures 5½ inches (almost 14 centimeters) and weighs nearly 3 ounces (more than 85 grams). Beginning in this week, some mothers can feel the baby begin to move.

FOR DAD

Your Wife's Figure

Dear dads, let me tell you a little secret so you can maintain harmony in your household during this month: don't even think about telling your wife that she looks fatter. Don't even joke about it. You know it's true and so does she. But this is the stage where it is difficult for others to know if she is pregnant or just fatter. The fact that her normal clothes are fitting tighter may put her in a bad mood. Just tell her she looks *más bella que nunca*, more beautiful than ever. Caress her belly and be affectionate.

Cravings

After the self-centered stage of the past few weeks, now begins the time when the mother of your child will need you more than ever. Your wife could be wondering if you'll still want her as she gains pound after pound after pound. This is the time, or maybe even before, when all those *antojos* or cravings for strange food combinations begin to appear.

There are different theories to explain why pregnant women ask for weird foods. Some say it has to do with getting the right nutrients for the baby. Others say it's a way for the pregnant woman to see if her husband really loves her. No matter what the cause, if I were you, I'd make a list of the nearest grocery or convenience stores that are open all night. She's more sensitive to what you do at this stage, and she'll appreciate every little effort you make to please her. So in addition to your 2 A.M. expeditions to find *dulce de guayava*, try giving her a bouquet of flowers, a romantic greeting card or maybe even prepare dinner or vacuum one day without her having to ask. All this will win you lots of points in her eyes.

Money Worries

The idea that you're going to have a baby might bring out the provider and protector in you. You may be worried about how much it costs to take care of a baby, how secure your job is or if your wife will continue to work after the baby arrives. A normal reaction among men to all these worries is to distance themselves from the family and the home. That might mean you look for a second job to earn more money, or you might hang out with your friends more frequently or you may just be colder with your wife. Although this is a normal reaction for men who are suddenly realizing there's a lot more pressure on them, remember your wife is sensitive to what you do and she may feel abandoned. So talk about your worries and plan together what you can do to improve your economic situation. Some things you should talk about are:

- Will your wife stop working? Calculate how much it will cost to have someone else take care of the baby. Sometimes paying the nanny or day care costs as much as what your wife is earning. But even if there's no financial gain from her working, your wife may not want to abandon her profession.

- Will you stop working? Among Latino families, this isn't really a common consideration. How many Latino fathers do you know who iron and do the laundry and cook dinner and take care of the baby? But if your wife is making more money than you, *¿por qué no?*, why not?

- Who will take care of the baby? *Abuelos*, grandparents are a blessing when it comes to child care. If they live nearby, you'll have to establish where the child will be cared for: In your house or in their house. If it's the grandparents' home, go check it out to make sure it's safe for babies. But if they live far away, you may consider having *Abuela* and/or *Abuelo*, Grandma and/or Grandpa, live with you for a while.

THE FIFTH MONTH
Weeks 17 to 20

FACIAL CHANGES

The famous glow that many pregnant women get appears in these months. Pregnant women glow not only because they're happy about expecting a baby, but also because the volume of their blood has increased so much that they have a natural rosy color in their cheeks. While you may not have noticed anything, friends and family might begin to tell you how pretty you look.

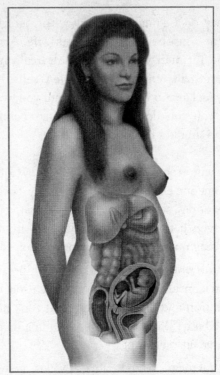

Fifth month

Another change to the face isn't so common. One of my cousins suffered a curious transformation when she got pregnant: her nose got wider and she looked like a completely different person. It also happened to her mother, my aunt, during her pregnancies. These changes occur because of the effect pregnancy hormones have on the tissues. After birth, everything returns to normal.

But don't confuse these normal changes with fluid retention in the face, which can be a symptom of preeclampsia (see page 88).

ABDOMINAL ITCHING

Your abdomen's skin is working overtime to make room for the baby. As it stretches it gets drier, and you may notice itching. Applying some olive oil or a nourishing cream might help. However, the only cure for the itching is delivering the baby. You skin will keep stretching for as long as the baby grows inside you.

However, if the itching begins to spread to other parts of your body, call your doctor. It could be due to other reasons (see page 227).

FETAL MOVEMENT

It's during this month mothers-to-be begin to feel their babies move inside them for the first time. The baby is still floating in the amniotic fluid, and it's got plenty of space to move around. But now it's just big enough to brush the walls of the uterus. If you've never felt it before, you may not know what's going on, because it's often more subtle than a direct kick. What you may feel is:

- *Fluttering*. It's a sensation like butterflies in your stomach. Imagine something very soft brushing up against your insides for only a few moments.
- *Bubbles*. Similar to a little cascade of bubbles rushing across your abdomen, or maybe like a bubble bursting.
- *Little punches*. Like someone knocking very lightly on the door. They're rhythmic punches, different from a movement in your intestines.
- *Involuntary movements*. What you feel when a muscle twitches involuntarily for a few seconds.

These are only a few examples. There are many other sensations you may feel.

"I was in bed. It was like a fish swimming in the water. Like he was moving his fins."

—*Laura Loustau*

"It's a strange movement. Like when somebody is very hungry and the intestines move. Like some gas inside."

—*María Teresa Díaz-Blanco*

These movements can be felt from around week 16, or even earlier if this isn't your first pregnancy. After week 22, the movements are clearly felt. If you haven't felt anything by this time, talk to your doctor.

As the weeks go by, you will continue to feel your baby more and more. The first movements don't have any type of schedule. They happen day or night. But later on, the baby will establish a sleeping pattern. For example, it's normal to feel the baby begin to move more vigorously as you try to go to sleep. That's because while you're awake, your movements "rock" the baby as if it were in a cradle. Sometimes, half an hour or so after you eat, the baby will begin to move a lot because he/she will get a boost from the glucose that arrives through your blood.

During the final months of pregnancy, there's not much room left for the baby to move around in, and that's why you'll feel fewer movements. A good way to know that everything is fine is counting fetal movements (see page 132). Don't get worried if you notice an absence of movements for a few minutes. Remember, babies can go to sleep themselves, or even get lazy. However, if you feel something strange, you should call your doctor right away.

Nasal Congestion

Your nose is one of the body parts that receives more blood during pregnancy. This increase in blood flow, along with an elevated hormone level, makes the inside of the nose become softer and more easily irritated. That can make it bleed (see page 190) and produce more mucus. Just as with many of pregnancy's discomforts, there isn't a surefire remedy for this problem. Still, you may feel a little more comfortable using saline nose drops. Also, try using a humidifier if you live in a dry climate or use central heating in your house. A few drops of essence of eucalyptus in the humidifier may help, too.

Advice from Family and Strangers During Pregnancy

In Latino culture, a pregnancy is a family affair. There's almost always an army of aunts, cousins and other relatives ready to take care of the mother-to-be. They help with household chores or watch the other kids. But the help doesn't come without advice. The family army of helpers wants to tell you what you should and shouldn't do during pregnancy. Sometimes it's difficult to deal with all these comments about what you should do, especially if you're more connected to U.S. culture than your relatives are. How are you supposed to convince Aunt Lupita your eating meat won't make the baby have a big head, or raising your hands over your head won't cause the baby's neck to get caught up in the umbilical cord? Latino folklore is rich with pregnancy myths. You will find some of them in Chapter 12.

One way to look at all these pieces of advice is to consider them a sign of how much people want to help. Don't let them make you nervous (even though that's sometimes difficult). Ask your aunt, mother or grandmother about their pregnancies and what their beliefs were. Telling the stories will give your relatives the acknowledgment they want. Afterward, explain *con cariño*, in a caring way, that you and your husband have talked to your doctor and decided to do things another way.

You'll also notice that it isn't just your relatives who have something to say about your pregnancy. Complete strangers will come up to you in the elevator, in the supermarket, at the movies. Your popularity will grow as your belly does. There really isn't a way to avoid having these strangers tell you what they think, but at the same time you don't have to stand there listening for hours on end to unpleasant stories just to be polite. Thank your storyteller for the advice and walk away.

Above all, don't get scared by what conventional wisdom and old wives' tales, Latino or not, say will happen to your baby if you do this or don't do that. Your hormones are enough to deal with, and you don't need to add more stress to your nervous system. Most pregnancy myths were only a way to explain the unexplainable.

DEPRESSION DURING PREGNANCY

It's hard to recognize depression during the first trimester because the symptoms are so similar to being pregnant (see page 106). But if during this month you feel emotionally overwhelmed, without any joy about having a baby, anxious or panicked, then you have to do something about it. Don't let your friends and family tell you that *es parte del embarazo*, it's all part of being pregnant. Talk to your doctor about the possibility you might be suffering from depression, especially if you've been through it before. Depression is a very common illness among Latinas and it usually gets worse during pregnancy, but it has a cure.

Don't feel ashamed if you don't experience the happiness a pregnant woman is supposed to feel. The huge hormonal changes your body is going through can affect the chemical balance in your brain and cause depression.

It's important to treat this illness during pregnancy because if you let it go, it will very likely get worse after delivery, when the hormone levels change again. Your baby is going to need all your attention and energy when it's born.

INCOMPETENT CERVIX

The cervix is the opening of the uterus into the vagina. It's the part of the uterus that dilates during pregnancy to let the baby out. Sometimes this tissue is weakened and can't bear the weight of the baby. In those cases, the cervix opens during the third trimester and the amniotic sac sticks out. That can cause a miscarriage. An incompetent cervix doesn't cause contractions.

The causes of this condition can be severe tearing in prior pregnancies, improperly done surgeries or abortions, genetic problems or unknown causes.

The way doctors usually correct this problem is called cerclage. It consists of sewing the cervix closed until the pregnancy is over. Doctors recommend bed rest for these women and no sex. The good news is that the procedure works.

WHERE TO GIVE BIRTH

If you still haven't decided how you want to deliver your baby, this is a good time to begin making your final choices. Here are a few of the options you can choose from. (To get an idea of how much the different options cost and whether insurance covers them, read Chapter 2.)

Delivery in a Hospital

Of the more than ten thousand women who give birth every day in the United States, 99 percent of them do it in a hospital. The hospital is the place to have your baby in the following cases:

- You've had complications during your pregnancy.
- Your pregnancy is going according to plan but you don't want to take any risks in case your baby or you need urgent medical attention.
- You want to use medication or epidural anesthesia to deal with delivery pain.

The majority of hospitals have a series of procedures and the basic equipment needed to take care of a woman who's about to have a baby.

But some have more sophisticated options you can take advantage of. Depending on what your insurance will pay for, what you can afford or what area you live in, you may be able to choose some of them.

Hospitals invite mothers- and fathers-to-be to come in for a visit beforehand so they can get an idea of what the process is like and what services are offered. This list will give you an idea of what you can ask about when you go for this visit.

PERSONAL ATTENTION

- *Is there an obstetrician/gynecologist at the hospital at all times?* In case your doctor cannot make it on time or there is any complication when you arrive at the hospital, it's important to know who is going to be taking care of you.

- *What role will the nurses play during delivery?* An obstetrician/gynecologist should be available at all times; however, you will spend the major part of your delivery with the nurses and midwives who work at the hospital you've chosen. Ask if they will help with breathing and relaxation techniques, and inquire about how many patients each nurse will be taking care of at once. If you're there on a day when many women are giving birth, you might not see much of your nurse. See if you like the attitudes of the nurses at the hospital and how they treat you. Find out if they answer your questions in a friendly manner. Ask if anyone speaks Spanish (very useful to talk to waiting relatives).

- *Will I be in the same room during the entire delivery? How many delivery rooms are available?* In the olden days, labor was in one room, delivery in another and recovery yet in another. Today, everything can happen in just one place. They are known as LDR rooms (labor, delivery and recovery). These new delivery rooms are decorated in a more friendly manner, so they feel more like a home instead of an antiseptic hospital. The beds have several modules that can be positioned in a variety of ways to make you more comfortable while you push. However, some hospitals only have a limited number of these modern, comfortable rooms. Ask what happens when there are more women than rooms.

- *Will I have access to an interpreter?* Hospitals that receive federal funds must have interpreters. If you live in a Latino area, it's possible that they have them anyway. Ask if there can be an interpreter during labor and at what times.

Baby Care

- *How soon will I be able to hold my baby and begin breastfeeding? Will the baby stay in my room?* The norm today is to leave the baby in a cradle in the same room as the mother, but some hospitals don't allow it. Ask what exactly will happen to the baby once it's born. Do they hand the baby to you right away so you can hug him/her? Will they take him/her for a checkup? Will he/she have to sleep in a separate room?

- *Does the hospital have a neonatal unit? What level?* Neonatal units are the areas where hospitals take care of newborns. They come in three levels, depending on the services they provide. Level 3 units have the most sophisticated equipment available to take care of your baby.

- *Is a pediatrician available at all times in the hospital?* Some hospitals have a neonatal pediatrician (specializing in taking care of babies) on duty permanently. Other hospitals only have one on call for emergencies.

- *Does the hospital have a breastfeeding consultant?* There are professionals who will help you begin to breastfeed your baby and will answer all your questions.

- *Will the hospital respect your wish to exclusively breastfeed?* Some hospitals will give the baby a bottle shortly after birth.

Anesthesia

- *Is an anesthesiologist on duty at the hospital at all hours?* Some hospitals don't have anesthesiologists on duty twenty-four hours a day. They're only called in when necessary. This means you'll have to wait until they arrive if you need one.

Mobility

- *What type of intravenous catheter will the hospital use?* A catheter is a very fine tube that's inserted into a vein. It allows doctors to put drugs or anesthesia directly into your bloodstream, if necessary. Some hospitals use a traditional catheter that's connected to a dripping bag hanging over the bed. If you need to walk, you have to take the dripping bag with you, dragging it on wheels. Other hospitals have a catheter system called a heparin lock, which includes an anticoagulant. This option lets you leave the catheter in your hand but disconnected from the tube so you can walk around freely.

- *Does the hospital have fetal telemetry systems?* The fetal monitor is a machine that measures your contractions and the baby's heartbeat. The traditional monitoring system is a belt with two bands that are strapped around your abdomen and connected to a computer that measures the contractions (see page 133). This means when the belt is in place, you've got to be lying in bed. The telemetry system measures the contractions and heartbeats from a distance so you don't have to be confined to your bed. It's similar to a television remote control—the signals are sent through the air. This system is not very common yet. If the hospital you're in doesn't have a telemetry system, ask how often they need to measure your contractions. Sometimes they monitor your contractions and the baby's heart at intervals and you can get up and walk around in between.

FRIENDS AND FAMILY

- *Can your husband be with you at all times, including during a cesarean delivery?* Nearly all hospitals allow your partner to be with you, even in the operating room. Still, it doesn't hurt to ask.

- *How many family members are allowed to be with me during delivery? Can my other children be there?* Some hospitals put restrictions on the number of visitors who can attend the delivery, and some don't allow children.

- *Can my partner spend the night with me in my room?* There are hospitals that even include a bed for your husband or another family member who may stay the night with you. In others, the guest will have to make do with a couch or chair but is allowed to stay anyway.

- *Can I have the delivery videotaped?* Some places don't allow this.

Birthing Center

In most states, choosing to deliver in a birthing center first requires a determination by an obstetrician/gynecologist that the pregnancy is risk-free. The midwives of these centers should be certified or licensed and work under the supervision of a doctor. The physician intervenes if there's a problem. If you or your baby needs urgent care during birth, you will be transported to a hospital.

There are no epidurals or any other medical help at a natural birthing center. The midwives there use massages, warm baths and change of positions to ease the pain. There aren't any restrictions as far as your walking around because you're not attached to any machines.

The services offered in natural birthing centers vary depending on the state where you live and the center you've chosen. In most, you'll find:

- A *delivery bathtub*. It may be a big Jacuzzi, a small whirlpool or a small collapsible pool used for this purpose alone. The idea is tepid water will help to ease the pain of the contractions and will make the change from inside the mother to the outside world less traumatic for the baby.

- *Stethoscope or Doppler*. These devices help to hear the baby's heartbeat. The midwife will put the unit on your abdomen to make sure the baby's heart is working properly.

- *Oxygen*. Some centers have oxygen masks that help you breathe during delivery.

- *Family room*. Your relatives can bring their own food to eat and get comfortable to accompany you through delivery.

Some of the questions you should ask are:

- *Are the midwives licensed or certified?* A certified or licensed midwife has to go to school to get a degree and works with a doctor. Lay midwifes don't have the backup of a doctor (see page 147).

- *What will you do to control the pain? What happens if I can't take it?* In some pregnancies the baby isn't in quite the right position to be delivered and the pain can be excruciating. If you find yourself in this situation, you can ask to be taken to a hospital. If your medical insurance is covering the birthing center delivery, make sure it will also cover a last-minute trip to the hospital. Sometimes the pain of delivery isn't considered an emergency and some insurance policies don't cover it. You'll find more information about pain on page 273.

- *What's the procedure if there's an emergency? Who will take me to the hospital?* You may have to go to the hospital in your own vehicle, an ambulance may pick you up or the firefighters may come.

- *How far away is the hospital in case of an emergency? How long does it take to get there?* Make sure to include traffic in your planning.

- *Who will take care of me at the hospital?* You may have your midwife accompany you from your birthing center, but she won't give you medical attention.

Birthing Center in a Hospital

This possibility has become available in the past few years as hospitals begin to accommodate the wishes of those women who want more natural deliveries. These centers are generally on the maternity floor of the hospital. They may include a tub for delivery, or you may be able to rent it and have the delivery overseen by a midwife or doctors. Because they're inside the hospital itself, these rooms provide you with immediate medical care if an urgent need arises.

Home Delivery

It's likely your grandmother or maybe even your mother was born at home, helped by a midwife. In those days, there weren't many options for pregnant women, and the mortality rates for the infant and the mother were high. Most of today's deliveries at home are done under the watch of a licensed or certified midwife with a doctor's approval. In the case of a home delivery, the circumstances are similar to a birthing center delivery: the licensed or certified midwives can help only pregnant women who have low-risk pregnancies, or they will lose their licenses. The advantage of giving birth at home is you're in your own house, with all its comforts. But the disadvantage is it can take a while to get to the hospital if there are unexpected problems. Giving birth at home is a risky proposition. A very recent study has shown that it presents more risks for the child and the mother even in uncomplicated pregnancies. Severe hemorrhage and death can occur in a matter of minutes.

Choosing where to have your baby is very personal. Some women feel safer in a hospital; others believe medical interventions aren't necessary and actually cause cesareans and other problems. Some other women prefer the cesarean option because it eliminates certain risks as well as the pain of the delivery itself.

I recommend you first analyze the status of your pregnancy and your priorities. If you've got a medical problem such as diabetes or high blood pressure or anything else that could cause problems down the road, a hospital is the only place where you will get the medical attention needed to make sure you and your baby will come through all of it *sano y feliz*, healthy and happy.

Sometimes, even when everything should be fine, problems arise no matter where you have the baby: in the hospital, in a birthing center or at home. The difference, of course, is that when the problem arises, the hospital has the resources to deal with it. For example, if the baby isn't getting enough oxygen through the placenta, the doctor at a hospital can perform an immediate cesarean section and help the baby to breathe artificially. If the same delivery takes place in a birthing center or at home, at least fifteen minutes will have passed before you get to the hospital. Just so you know, brain damage occurs after seven minutes of oxygen deprivation.

On the other hand, when everything goes well, women who had their babies in birthing centers or at home are very satisfied with their experiences. Sandra Hernandez had her two babies at home:

"I really enjoyed both my labors. The midwives gave me massages during every contraction. I was walking around the whole house while the babies came. Not one time did I lie down on my back. My mom was with me along with my brother and my husband. I hate telling people about my experience *porque nadie me cree,* because no one believes me, they think I'm making it up. But honestly, I didn't scream even once. The contractions at most felt like a lower back pain that went up and down a little. I didn't rip or need any stitches. As soon as my babies were born they were handed to me and I breastfed them. Really, I enjoyed my deliveries. There's no other way to say it."

Fortunately, more and more hospitals offer birthing centers with no or very few medical interventions, but at the same time with a full medical staff nearby if they're needed. You can have the best of both worlds.

Another option if your pregnancy is going according to plan is to choose to have a certified midwife oversee your delivery. Midwives have a more natural approach to giving birth. The use of certified midwives in hospitals has increased 95 percent in the past few years.

Also, before giving birth you can discuss with your doctor the possibility of not having an intravenous catheter that obligates you to stay in bed and to have your contractions and baby's heart rate monitored at intervals so you can move around. You can also choose not to have an epidural and instead use the services of a doula, who will help you manage the pain (see page 235).

PRENATAL VISIT

You already know the routine: urinate in the plastic cup to see if there's any protein or sugar there, take your blood pressure, check to see there's no abnormal swelling, get weighed, measure the uterus and listen to the baby's heart.

Now your weight will begin to increase rapidly. The American College of Obstetricians and Gynecologists recommends a gain of three to four pounds per month in this trimester and the final one. But still, this depends on your doctor's advice and your personal circumstances.

During this visit your doctor may talk to you about doing an amniocentesis (see page 126). If you don't want to go through an amniocentesis, another way to see how the baby is doing is through a level II sonogram (see page 113), although this test isn't as accurate as a genetic test such as amniocentesis.

In case you don't have any of these tests, your doctor will likely order a normal sonogram between weeks 18 and 22 to make sure everything's going well. This is the test where, if you want, you can find out if you're having a boy or a girl. If you don't want to know the sex of your baby, tell the doctor ahead of time so the news doesn't slip out.

Another genetic test that is sometimes done during this trimester, PUBS, checks for certain fetal illnesses (see page 130).

FEELINGS

The mood swings begin to disappear during this month, although you may still feel irritable on occasion or you may begin to cry without any particular reason. But besides a couple of infrequent episodes, in general your humor and moods will be stabilizing.

This is also the month when you may feel the baby move inside you for the first time. This sensation confirms once and for all that you are really going to have a baby. Feeling the presence of another human being inside you will give you a lot of joy and connect you to the baby in a way you haven't yet felt up to this point. But it could also bring new worries about all the incoming changes.

During this month and the next one, you may feel a newfound energy and a desire *de hacer cosas*, to get things done. Many couples decide to move during these months, or renovate their existing house in preparation for the baby's arrival. It's great to prepare for the changes in your growing family, but don't overexert yourself. Even though you're feeling a lot better, remember your body is still working overtime to develop and grow your baby. It doesn't really need any extra work to do.

THE *BEBÉ*

Week 17
Your baby is accumulating fat for the first time. It moves its extremities constantly and even makes faces. The body is covered in fine hair called lanugo. It measures around 6 inches (15 centimeters).

Week 18
The baby's digestive system begins to work and stores meconium (baby feces) in the intestine. Bones continue to solidify. Legs now have bone but in most of the rest of the body there's only cartilage. There's still a lot of extra space in your uterus, so the baby can move side to side and kick.

Week 19
Fingernails and toenails are fully formed now, and the hair on the head begins to grow. The baby will continue to move freely inside you, and it's possible during this week or the next one you'll feel the movements for the first time. The baby now weighs 8 ounces (227 grams) and measures 6½ inches (more than 16 centimeters).

Week 20
The baby's skin is covered with a white waxy substance called the vernix caseosa. It's a mixture of fat that comes from the pores in the skin and dead skin cells that have been shed. This substance works to protect the baby's delicate skin as it floats in the amniotic fluid. The fetus weighs about 10 ounces now (283 grams) and measures around 7 inches (17.5 centimeters).

FOR DAD

"My Baby Is There!"

If you've been lucky enough to feel the baby kicking inside your partner's abdomen, then the pregnancy may have become something different for you, something more real. The baby isn't just an idea anymore. This discovery, which your wife made a few weeks ago, can provoke a series of contradictory emotions for you. You may feel extremely happy and at the same time have *dudas*, doubts about what kind of father you'll be, or worries about whether you're actually ready to take care of a baby. And just as your wife was, you may be immersed in your own thoughts. Talk to your partner about what's on your mind, because she more than anyone will be able to understand what you are going through.

Connection

One way to stay connected to your baby and your wife is to do certain activities together. For example, if you like the water, swim with your wife or play in the pool. It's a great form of exercise for pregnant women, and it's fun too. Also, you might work on creating a photo album to document the memories and stages of pregnancy. A video can do the same thing. Take weekly recordings to see how her belly grows!

The Birth

This is the appropriate month to begin discussing with your partner where the delivery will take place, if you haven't made up your minds already. It's important that you think about where you are going to feel more comfortable. Also, work out who will make sure you get medical attention if you need it in an emergency, or perhaps think about a natural birth (see page 204). Think where you'll feel the best and how much you want to participate in the delivery process. Tell your wife.

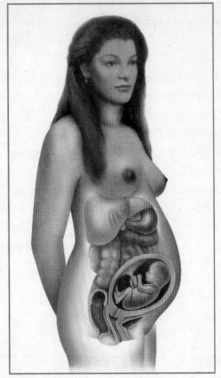

Sixth month

THE SIXTH MONTH
Weeks 21 to 25

BACK PAIN

The increasing size and weight of your abdomen means you'll start to lean backward as you move, in order to balance yourself. This forces your spinal column to curve in an unnatural way and tenses the muscles in your back. Maintaining this unusual posture for weeks on end results in lower back pain. Pregnancy hormones also have an effect on muscles because they make them relax and they don't support your spine as well as usual.

Back pain is one of the most common complaints among women during the second half of pregnancy. There are some things you can do to alleviate your pain:

- Sleep lying on your left side with a pillow between your legs.

- Put a firm mattress on your bed or a piece of plywood under the mattress you're currently using.

- Use shoes that support the arch of your foot and have low heels.

- Don't bend at the waist to pick up another child or anything heavy. Bend at the knees instead, using your leg muscles to stand up, not the ones in your back.

- Don't spend a lot of time sitting down. Get up and walk every twenty minutes. When you are sitting down, use a pillow to support the lower part of your back.

- If you're in the kitchen or doing an activity that requires you to spend a lot of time on your feet, find a small box or piece of wood that's about 15 inches tall (around 25 centimeters). Rest one foot on top of it so your other leg supports most of your weight, and then switch after a few minutes.

Swimming is one of the best exercises you can do to help with lower back pain. And there are other exercises you'll want to try to help with your back pain and to reduce tension and stress (see pages 58–59).

Be careful if you go to a chiropractor or *huesero* because sometimes the adjustments can actually make your condition worse. Your muscles and your spinal column are in an abnormal position compared to before you got pregnant. But even though they may be causing you pain, they're in the proper position for carrying a baby. Also, because the pregnancy hormones have relaxed your muscles, they may not react normally to the adjustments a chiropractor makes.

If you believe a massage may help your pain, there are masseurs who specialize in treating pregnant women. They even have special tables for you to lie on, with space for your abdomen. Make sure the masseur is qualified and has taken the proper courses.

ROUND LIGAMENT PAIN

The round ligaments on each side of the uterus maintain it suspended above the abdominal cavity. They're like two cords that stretch from above the uterus to the lips of the vagina. As the uterus grows, these ligaments stretch and stretch and can cause a lot of discomfort. The pain is

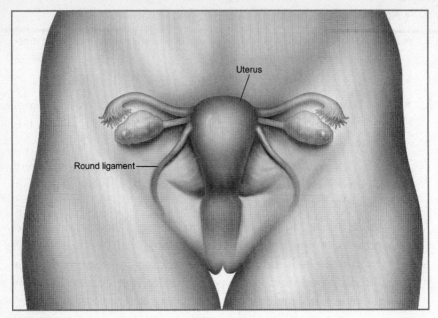

Round ligaments

sharp and sudden in any part of the vagina, groin or abdomen. It can happen while you're walking, standing or sitting or even when you roll over in your sleep. It usually affects the right side more than the left.

Baths or warm towels applied to the painful area can help. Also, a recent study done with women suffering this problem revealed that tilting the pelvis in a special way (see page 59) helps to reduce the pain when the exercise is done at least six times a day.

Sometimes the pain these ligaments cause is severe and can be confused with other gynecological problems. Talk to your obstetrician/gynecologist if the pain is accompanied by a fever, bleeding and pain during urination or if it gets progressively worse.

LEG CRAMPS

One of the discomforts of pregnancy that made my husband's heart race during my second trimester were leg cramps. Not because of their severity, but because they always happened in the middle of the night and were accompanied by a scream—just to make them a little more *dramáticos*, dramatic.

Cramps in the calf muscle are relatively common during the second and third trimesters. The muscle contracts suddenly and produces a sharp leg pain. There are many theories as to why these spasms happen: changes in blood circulation in the legs that make the nerves react, excessive phosphorous combined with a lack of calcium, or a lack of magnesium. But before taking more or less vitamins, talk to your doctor—studies where women took calcium supplements to alleviate leg cramps showed it didn't work.

There is one exercise that can alleviate some of the pain when a cramp hits: Stick the heel of the leg that is hurting on the floor. Without bending your knee, point your toes toward your head as hard as you can. Lean all your weight on this leg and bend forward. Maintain this position till the pain goes away.

You can also walk, apply heat, or make your husband give you a leg massage, because he's probably not sleeping anymore anyway!

SCIATICA

Relaxin is one of the hormones your body produces during pregnancy. It makes your ligaments relax to allow the uterus to grow and makes your cervix and vagina more flexible at delivery. But a secondary effect of this hormone is that your joints and back will be less supported by the ligaments and muscles surrounding them. When you combine that with the extra weight of the baby and the change in the spinal column arch, it sometimes results in the cartilage between the vertebrae slipping out a little and putting pressure on one of the sciatic nerves. We have two sciatic nerves that begin at the lower back, run through the buttocks and then down each leg. When these nerves are inflamed, they can cause pain and discomfort in any of these areas.

"Around the fifth month I started feeling a very acute pain in the lower part of my back, *hacia un ladito*, to one side. It's a pain that goes down to your heel. The nerve hurts. When I stood up I could barely walk. I couldn't use high heels anymore."

—*Ana Cristina Osorio*

Sciatica, the name of this condition, can happen at any time during the pregnancy, but it's most common during the second trimester. The pain changes depending on how you're moving or sitting, and it can range from a slight lack of feeling or a burning sensation to a paralyzing pain. You can feel sciatica as pain in the lower back or as a painful line in the buttocks or down the back of the leg. It usually happens only on one side.

If the problem isn't too severe, the pain can be alleviated by applying ice to the affected area and keeping the back as straight as possible. But if the pain gets worse, your obstetrician/gynecologist may prescribe an anti-inflammatory drug or recommend you use a special girdle for pregnant women that helps to take some of the pressure of the abdomen's weight off the back. Talk to your doctor about this discomfort if you feel you are losing sensitivity in any area, because you might need to see a specialist.

SWOLLEN FEET

From this month on you might feel as though your feet belong to someone else. This swelling, that can also happen in the hands, is usually due to three things:

- Increased blood volume. Now you've got 40 percent more than before you got pregnant (see page 86).

- Pressure from the uterus on the pelvic arteries. Blood doesn't circulate in your legs as easily.

- The law of gravity. Some of the liquid flowing through your body is pulled down to your hands and feet.

Swelling usually happens at the end of the day, or after you have been sitting or standing for a long time. Still, if you notice a sudden swelling in your hands, feet or face, talk to your doctor, because this could be a sign of preeclampsia.

Here are some ways you can reduce swelling:

- Elevate your feet at the end of the day for at least 30 minutes.

- If you work sitting down, get up often to walk around and elevate your feet for fifteen minutes every two hours. Avoid staying in the same position for long periods of time.

- Lie down on your left side to improve circulation (see page 192).

Special socks put pressure on your legs to improve circulation, but ask your doctor before using them.

DISCOMFORT AND NUMBNESS IN THE HANDS

All the fluid that accumulates in your body during pregnancy can cause discomfort besides swelling. During their last months of pregnancy some women feel tingling, needles or even pain in some of their fingers. The discomfort can spread up to the forearm. This is because of pressure put on the median nerve, which passes along various tendons from the forearm toward the arm. This nerve controls the feeling in the thumb, index and middle fingers. The nerve pathway, which is called the carpal tunnel, is very narrow. Fluid retention makes the tendon put pressure on the nerve, which causes the weird sensations in the hands, fingers and forearm. And if you work a lot with your hands, the nerve can be even more irritated. The pain is usually worst at night, because that's when the most fluid has accumulated.

This problem is called carpal tunnel syndrome and can become quite painful. You should try to rest the affected arm and hand as much as possible. Pharmacies sell hard plastic braces to immobilize the affected wrist; this may help you, especially at night.

TRAVELING

If this is your first baby, it'll be a while before you get another chance to go on a vacation alone with your husband. So take the opportunity now if you can. Still, if you plan on traveling, whether for business or pleasure, keep a few things in mind.

Traveling by Plane

You can fly without worry up to the eighth month, as long as your doctor agrees. After week 36, most airlines require a letter from your doctor explaining you've been given permission to fly. That letter must be signed by your doctor forty-eight to seventy-two hours before your flight. Even though the airlines say they require the letter, you'll probably be able to get on the plane without one, unless you appear as though you're about to deliver in the next few minutes. Other airlines ask you to sign a paper saying that you accept the risks of flying and promise not to sue the airline if anything goes wrong. Just call the airline you're using ahead of time to find out exactly what its policy is.

The trip itself isn't what's risky; traveling by air is perfectly safe for the pregnant woman. The problem comes if you go into labor at thirty thousand feet without a doctor on board. So if there's any chance whatsoever you may go into labor during your travels, postpone the trip. In any case, take these precautions, especially if you're going on a long trip:

- Call ahead of time to reserve a comfortable seat. Some rows don't have any seats in front of them, which means you can stretch your legs out and maybe even elevate them. If you tell the reservation agent you're pregnant, you may get one.

- Walk around the plane. Get up from your seat often and walk through the aisle. This will help to avoid leg swelling.

- Drink a lot of water. The air inside the plane is dry. Saline drops may keep your nose from drying out.

- Take crackers, juice or other snacks with you in case the dinner served on the plane is late in arriving.

Certain short flights in small planes don't have pressurized cabins. You should avoid them because changes in pressure can affect the baby.

Traveling by Car

Many couples find themselves changing jobs and houses during pregnancy. That's what happened to my husband and me as we were expecting our first child. Our move was about as far as you can go in the United States: From California to Florida. I was seven months pregnant and we drove. The only thing my gynecologist told me was to take things easy. So my idea of making it from Los Angeles to Miami in one and a half days went out the window. We changed plans, deciding to visit some friends along the way and stopping to do some sightseeing. In the end the trip was much more enjoyable that way. I didn't have any problems taking my turn behind the wheel. I barely noticed the seat belt. In fact, *me fue tan bien*, I was having such a good time in charge of the car, my husband finally told me to stop because he was afraid our daughter would be born with a steering wheel imprint on her forehead. My little car didn't have an adjustable steering column.

Jokes aside, your baby is protected inside you. The important thing is to stay well supported and strapped in yourself. Always wear your seat belt, even if the trip is just five minutes to the store. Run the lower part of the belt below your abdomen, as low as it will go. The shoulder harness should be worn normally, but make sure it stays to one side of your abdomen and not right over the middle of it.

Traveling by Ship or Train

On short trips by boat, watch out for seasickness and for your balance. Even though you may have not suffered from seasickness before your pregnancy, you may now find your stomach can't handle it because of your pregnancy hormones. Also, your center of gravity has changed, so hang on to the railings tightly. On cruises and longer trips keep the same things in mind. The danger of spending an extended period of time on the high seas is an unexpected delivery. Most cruise ships have doctors on board, but their infirmaries aren't equipped to deal with a premature baby.

Train trips have the advantage that there's more space for your legs and you can get off at any station to get to a nearby hospital.

On trips and any other activity you may do during your pregnancy, listen to what your body is telling you. Rest, sleep a sufficient number of hours, eat right and drink plenty of water. All of that will help you overcome the fatigue one usually feels when traveling.

VISION

If you're thinking about getting new glasses or contact lenses because you can't see well, wait until you've given birth. Your pregnancy is changing your sight. Some things hormones can do to the eyes include:

- Relax the normal tension of the eyeball. That is great for women who have glaucoma (excessive pressure inside the eyeball). But for the ones who don't suffer from this disease, it can change their eyesight.

- Affect the cornea through fluid retention. The cornea is the transparent outer layer of the eye. It acts as a lens that allows us to see. When the shape of the cornea changes, so does our sight.

- Dry out the eyes, which may make them red or irritated. This can be easily fixed with a few eyedrops. But ask your doctor which ones you should use because some drops, such as the ones used to treat glaucoma, can cause premature births.

If you suddenly experience blurry vision or flashes, talk to your doctor, because this could be a sign of high blood pressure.

If you've had diabetes before pregnancy, it's a good idea to get an eye exam now. Chronic diabetes can affect vision and the changes in hormone levels during pregnancy usually make the situation worse. The good news is that once you've given birth, your vision, along with most of your other bodily functions, will return to normal.

CLUMSINESS

Some mothers-to-be feel as though they've lost control of their bodies, not only because they're getting bigger, but also because they feel clumsy. They drop things and they bump into corners and doorways, like Gloria Villalobos.

> "I had to be careful when I stood up. *Se me caía todo*, things would fall out of my hands, I bumped into things. I couldn't move my feet as fast as before. It bothered me a lot, although I knew it was normal."
> —*Gloria Villalobos*

If you consider for a moment all the real changes your body has gone through, it won't seem so strange for you to get suddenly clumsy. The pregnancy hormones have relaxed your tendons, and your center of gravity has changed, too. You've got a belly that now sticks out several inches, your hands and feet are accumulating fluid, and a mental fog is pretty common during pregnancy. Fortunately, all this will pass. Soon you'll be walking around as you did before you got pregnant.

THE NAME

In Latino families, sometimes the name of the baby is determined even before the baby is conceived. It can honor a grandfather or grandmother or beloved aunt. But what are you supposed to do when your husband wants to name the new daughter after his mother and you don't exactly like that name? In the United States, there can be as many names as will fit on the birth certificate. So your baby might have your mother-in-law's name and your mother's and yours and another two or three for good measure. You can even combine names or make one up. For example, if you've got one grandmother whose name is Salvadora and another named Isabel, you could call your daughter Dorabel.

But make sure the first name goes with the last name. If your husband's last name is Fuertes, don't call your daughter Dolores ("heavy pains" in Spanish). And if the last names is Casas, forget naming your son Armando ("putting houses together"), unless of course you plan on him working in the construction business.

If you're looking for a little inspiration, many libraries have books with thousands of ideas. So does the Internet. But here are some less common Latino names:

FOR GIRLS

Alegra	Camelia	Jazmín	Naila
Alvera	Candelaria	Lavinia	Nereida
Amira	Casandra	Leila	Regina
Arabela	Delia	Liria	Sabina
Begonia	Dina	Maya	Yasmina
Berenice	Edita	Miren	Zenaida

FOR BOYS

Adalberto	Efraín	Hipólito	Severiano
Aldo	Erasmo	Homero	Urbano
Arquímedes	Ferdinando	Ladislao	Valeriano
Baldomero	Fortunio	Laureano	Venturio
Borja	Guido	Lisandro	Vidal
Cornelio	Heriberto	Reinaldo	Virgilio

These Aztec names are beautiful and uncommon:

FOR GIRLS

Amalinalli (water from a flower)	Huitzillin (hummingbird)
Atlanxochitl (ocean water)	Quiahuitl (rain)
Auachtli (dew)	Tepeyolohtli (heart of the mountains)
Epyoloti (hidden pearl)	Yaocihuatl (warrior woman)

FOR BOYS

Atzin (venerable water)   Ilhuicoatl (celestial snake)
Auexoti (willow)   Iztacoyotl (white coyote)
Cuauhtzin (venerable eagle)   Tonalcozcati (sun necklace)
Ehecatl (wind)   Topiltzin (our little boy)

Prenatal Visit

You are now between weeks 21 and 25, and the routine is the same as in previous months: blood pressure, weight, urinate in the cup, measure uterus, listen to baby's heartbeat and check to see if there's swelling in the hands and feet. The urine sample on this visit is an important one, because after week 20, the symptoms of preeclampsia can begin to appear (see page 88).

Remember to write down ahead of time all the questions you want to ask your doctor.

Feelings

The fact you're feeling heavier and there are still three months to go might not be a pleasant thought. You may find the extra weight is cumbersome and uncomfortable and leaves you unable to do much at all.

On the other hand, you can clearly feel your baby kicking now, and you can imagine having him or her in your arms soon. If you don't have much family nearby to depend on, this might be a good time to start thinking about who is going to come and where you are going to accommodate them. It's a good idea to have a plan already drawn up if the baby comes early. Talk to your husband about those plans, because what seems perfectly normal to you (like having your mother live with you for six months) he might not like, and vice versa.

The *Bebé*

Week 21

The rapid growth of the past few weeks has slowed down a little. Now the baby is getting used to the functions of its growing organs and is storing fat. The limbs are growing and the baby can brush the uterine walls. This is the fluttering sensation that you feel sometimes.

Week 22

The brain is in a period of rapid development, with millions of nerve cells growing all at once. The eyelids are fully formed, and you can make out the eyebrows through the lanugo, the hair the baby has all over its body. Ovaries and testicles are fully formed. The baby weighs nearly 1 pound (a little less than half a kilogram) and measures 8 inches (20 centimeters).

Week 23

The baby now looks like a real newborn, although it's not as chubby as it will be. The eyes move beneath the eyelids, and the lungs are developing small sacs called the alveoli. They will allow the baby to breathe after being born.

Week 24

The baby's hearing is getting better, and he/she will react to exterior sounds such as loud bangs or even music. Internal organs are sufficiently developed to allow the baby to survive if it were born now, though it would need help breathing. It weighs 1 pound 10 ounces (almost 700 grams) and measures about 9 inches (22.5 centimeters).

Week 25

During these weeks you will feel some rhythmic jumps in your belly. The baby sometimes hiccups. The nasal passages are slowly opening and the lungs will soon have blood flowing through them, which is necessary for breathing. The baby measures 9½ inches (almost 24 centimeters) and weighs about 1½ pounds (around 800 grams).

FOR DAD

What type of father would you like to be? Strict? Playful? Disciplined? Involved? Do you plan on changing diapers and giving the baby a bath? Or is that the mother's job? The picture you have in your head of what kind of father you'll be has a lot to do with what kind of father you had. You might now be thinking a lot about what kind of relationship you had with him.

If your father was a role model, you might want to pass on the same values to your children. But if you had a lot of fights with your dad, you might want to raise your child in a completely different way. It's normal now to dream a lot about your father.

If you don't have any family who live nearby, another thing to think about is who will come by to help during the first few days after delivery. Where will they stay? For how long? How will you get along? The first weeks after delivery are a time when you'll appreciate all the help you can get.

Your wife's belly is growing and growing, and she may begin to feel uncomfortable. One of the most obvious places where you'll notice that is in your sex life. From now on you will have to try new positions because the traditional missionary one just doesn't work. Some men find this new shape attractive; others think it's a little weird, and the majority are afraid of harming the baby by having sex. Now you can feel for yourself the kicks and movements—the baby is very real. But *no se preocupe*, don't worry. Unless your doctor says to avoid sex, making love presents no danger to the baby.

There is no rule that determines what the correct amount of sex during pregnancy is. This depends on you and your partner. But if you are not having as much sex as before, talk about it, lest she think you're rejecting her. For example, if you are rejecting sex and you don't tell your wife why, she's likely to think you don't find her attractive anymore, when in reality you are just afraid of harming the baby. Talk to your obstetrician/gynecologist if you need to confirm that having sex is fine.

9

The Third Trimester

Beginning with the seventh month, the discomforts caused by your ever-growing abdomen increase slowly but surely. You're now on the final lap of pregnancy and your baby is gaining weight daily. This constant increase in weight is felt in your back and joints, and it affects your blood flow and your mood. Moving around might start feeling a bit difficult, and soon you'll walk with that distinct "pregnancy waddle." Even though you never thought it possible, you'll actually have to go to the bathroom even more frequently, because the growing baby is putting pressure on your bladder.

Despite all these bothersome side effects, the third trimester is very special for the mother-to-be. There will be times when you can see a hand or foot pushing against the inside of your belly. There will also be times when you will feel the baby is actually responding to your voice, to a change in your posture or to a noise outside. The baby becomes more and more real every day, not only for you but also for your husband. And if you haven't already done it, now is the time to go shopping to begin setting up the baby's room and getting his or her clothes ready.

THE SEVENTH MONTH
Weeks 26 to 30

SKIN ITCHING

Itchy skin during pregnancy is caused by the increase in blood flow. It's normal to go through this during the first trimester. When the itch is in

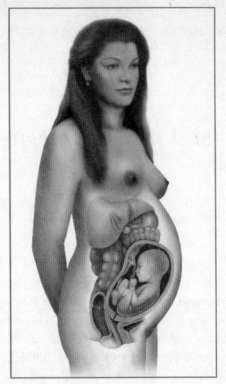

Seventh month

the abdomen it's also caused by the stretching your skin is doing. This type of itching can be helped with a moisturizing lotion and by wearing loose-fitting cotton clothes that don't make you sweat.

However, if the itching during the third trimester is more than just bothersome and you find it difficult to put up with (with or without skin redness and eczema), you should talk to your obstetrician/gynecologist. Certain changes in the skin during pregnancy are symptoms of other illnesses. One of them is a condition called intrahepatic cholestasis of pregnancy or ICP. It is more common among women of Chilean ancestry. The liver doesn't correctly process bile, and the salts this substance carries accumulate in the skin. The resulting itching is very uncomfortable. This is a serious disease that needs immediate medical attention.

Another condition that's relatively common after week 34 of pregnancy involves little red bumps or pimples that itch like mad. This is called PUPPP, or pruritic urticarial papules and plaques of pregnancy.

These bumps appear on the abdomen and run down to the thighs. They're not a danger for you or the baby, but the itching can be the worst. Cold compresses help, but you may need to see your doctor for a prescription for a steroid cream or pills. The itching disappears after delivery.

ANEMIA

Anemia means you have an insufficient number of red blood cells. This is a common problem during pregnancy, especially during the third trimester.

Red blood cells are in charge of transporting oxygen throughout the body. Red cells do this with hemoglobin, a substance they carry inside them. One essential component of hemoglobin is iron. Without a sufficient amount of iron, the body cannot produce a sufficient amount of red blood cells. Even though our body recycles iron from dead red blood cells (each one lives about 120 days), during pregnancy the volume of blood has increased so much, the need for iron increases too. The recycling process just can't keep up (see illustration on page 87). The iron you get through the food you eat usually isn't enough to supply the amount needed during the rapid blood cell production of the third trimester. And if there aren't a sufficient number of red blood cells, there's no good way for the oxygen to get to the rest of your body. Some of the most common symptoms of anemia are fatigue, weakness and shortness of breath.

During pregnancy, 95 percent of anemia cases are caused by a lack of iron; iron tablets remedy the problem. Doctors often prescribe iron along with prenatal vitamins to prevent anemia.

A small percentage of pregnant women suffer anemia because they don't have enough folate or folic acid. This type of anemia is also easily treated, by taking folic acid supplements.

LARGER FEET

Some women discover a surprising side effect of pregnancy: Their feet grow by half a size to a size. Your pregnancy hormones have relaxed the ligaments in your feet and allowed them to expand. If you add to this the twenty pounds you've gained during the past months, you end up with feet like Donald Duck.

Perhaps you won't need to add as much as a full size to your shoes. Instead, you could find comfort in wearing shoes that are wider; that's the direction many pregnant women's feet go. There really isn't much you can do about this. But think on the positive side: You can buy a whole new shoe wardrobe without having to make up excuses.

LOSS OF BALANCE AND FALLING

As your abdomen grows, your walking posture changes. You find yourself trying not to fall forward. Your center of gravity has changed. Also, the pregnancy hormones have softened your tissues and your balance isn't quite as good as it used to be. You may feel uncomfortable or precarious walking up and down stairs.

But even if you do fall down, remember that your baby is well protected inside you. It's rare for any real damage to occur to a baby when its pregnant mother falls. Still, if you notice bleeding, pain or anything else out of the ordinary, after a fall, call your obstetrician/gynecologist.

MEMORY LOSS OR *DESPISTE*

There are two types of memory we use in our daily lives. Long-term memory helps us recall events from a while ago. Short-term memory helps us to store information on an immediate basis, such as "The milk's run out; I have to buy more."

Several studies have demonstrated that pregnant women have difficulties with their short-term memory during the third trimester and after delivery. Scientists still haven't figured out why this happens, but as usual, the prime suspect is the pregnancy hormones. That being the case, the problem usually resolves itself a few weeks after delivery.

> "My memory and concentration failed a lot. I had a mental fog that affected me a lot because I thought it was going to be permanent. *Imagínate la impresión*, imagine the impression you make on people that don't know you."
>
> —*Lorena Asbell*

You can follow various strategies to deal with this problem, but step one is recognizing it exists. Your loss of memory is real and will likely get worse the closer you get to your delivery date. So try some of these:

- Convert a notebook into your "short-term memory." Write down the things you need to do as soon as you remember them, and then review your lists throughout the day.

- Avoid projects and errands that require you to use your short-term memory.

- Delegate household chores. Asking your husband to pay the bills means you don't have to remember to do it.

- Rest. One study showed a lack of sleep also worsens short-term memory.

DREAMS

If you're not accustomed to dreaming a lot, you might feel during your third trimester as though you're going to the movies every night. Pregnancy dreams, especially at the end, are almost like Technicolor films. Some could even win an Oscar. The subject doesn't change much in these movies: you, your baby and likely your husband as supporting actor.

One of the causes of all this mental activity that occurs as soon as you put your head on the pillow is the deep, profound fatigue your body feels. You sleep more hours and dream more. But in addition to the greater opportunity to dream there are also more things to dream about.

> "I had a lot of dreams where I left the baby somewhere. I would leave him underneath the bed and then I was alone in the street. People would ask me, where's the baby? These dreams made me worry because I didn't understand what were they saying about me. With my second baby I didn't have those type of dreams."
>
> —Gloria Villalobos

Pregnancy means great changes for a woman's body and her life. There are doubts and worries about motherhood. All this shows up in the dreams.

First Trimester

This is when the mother-to-be really begins to wrap her brain around the idea she's going to have a baby. On one hand, she's happy because she conceived, and on the other hand, she worries about what's to come. Some of the images that may appear in first trimester dreams are related to fertility, such as seeds, harvest fields, flowers, gardens or even babies that are walking and talking. Your fears are represented by intruders who come into your home or the place where you are. Dreams where you find yourself naked might symbolize your feelings of vulnerability. Dreaming about your mother or about other female relatives is a way to process the fact that now it's your turn to become a mother. And as you take your turn at maternity, you have to deal with figuring out which family values you want to keep and which you don't agree with.

Second Trimester

The idea of your having a baby is even more real in these months, and with that reality come more concerns. One of the most common worries among pregnant women in their second trimester is whether they'll be good mothers. It's normal to dream about having left the baby in the car or at the store, or that the baby is too big or too small or that you don't know how to take care of it. Dreams that involve animals are common. You may dream about water, babies in water or swimming. Some people think the liquid theme refers to the amniotic fluid that will be building up in your belly. Others think it has to do with emotions. More than the mere fact of water, what shows how you are feeling is the type of water that appears in your dreams: dirty, clear, deep, wavy, etc.

Another theme that recurs is the unfaithful husband with a known or unknown woman. The change in your figure and in your sexual desire combined with your sense of vulnerability can easily make a pregnant woman wonder whether her partner will remain at her side.

Third Trimester

During this time, it's normal to have intense sexual dreams about passion with your husband as well as with former lovers or even unknown people. This reflects the change in the sexual relationship you have with your husband and also your doubts about whether you are still attractive. As the delivery date gets nearer, you may begin to dream about babies with a strange, even demonic look. The uncertainty over whether your baby will be born healthy is reflected in these images. Worries about birth and delivery are also symbolized in dreams by erupting volcanoes or collapsing dams.

You may have recognized some of the images described here, or it's possible you're dreaming about other topics entirely. Dreams represent your emotions. If a particular dream makes you feel uncomfortable, first try to figure out exactly what you were feeling during the dream: sadness? fear? happiness? Try to remember the emotion that came with the images. Also think about who else was in the dream and what the objects were. This will better help you identify feelings about your pregnancy that you might not be paying a lot of attention to. For example, if you frequently dream your partner isn't being faithful, perhaps you need to talk to him about your feeling vulnerable and fearful about whether he still finds you attractive. When these feelings are discussed during waking hours, you'll find the fears will disappear from your dreams. But no matter what you dream, remember that this is a normal process that helps you prepare for the next big stage in your life.

PRENATAL CLASSES

If you haven't already done so, this is a good month to take birth preparation classes. The instructor will talk about pregnancy, nutrition, development of the baby and what will happen during delivery, using photographs and videos. You will also learn breathing and relaxation techniques to deal with the pain. Some classes include lessons on how to care for a newborn and breastfeeding.

Although attending one of these classes doesn't guarantee you a pain-free delivery (see page 276), knowing what to expect during the birth of your child will help you a lot. Make sure your husband goes with you to the classes because this is an excellent way to get him to participate in the pregnancy, especially if he's seemed a little distant up to this point. But keep in mind that the recommendations some instructors have for husbands might not really be part of Latino culture. Among Latino couples, the husband may often sit at the side of the bed, hold his partner's hand and offer *palabras cariñosas*, soothing and encouraging words. But some hospital staff may urge the husband to play a more active role, such as giving massages and helping with breathing. Choose the technique and strategy that fits your personality and beliefs. Only do what makes you and your husband comfortable.

Statistics show most babies are born in the United States in July, August and September. If you're expecting your baby during these three months, make sure there will be space in these classes for you, because they fill up quickly. If you can, choose a class with as few couples as possible. The more couples there are, the less time there will be for questions.

The cost varies. Hospital classes are sometimes included in the cost of delivery, or you may have to pay a small fee. Private instructors are more expensive. The Contact List has information on how to find instructors of the different methods.

Lamaze Method

This is the most popular today. It consists of a series of breathing exercises that allow you to focus not so much on your pain but instead on your breathing. The idea is that the mind can only concentrate on one thing at a time, and if your attention is on the air going in and out of your lungs or an imaginary point on the wall, you will feel less pain.

Lamaze preparation classes run about two hours a week for six weeks. This method is taught in most hospitals that offer prenatal classes, and there may be private Lamaze instructors near your home.

Bradley Method

This system teaches you how to accept the pain. The Bradley method is based on the mother relaxing in a comfortable place and position, without much noise or light. The father helps the mother to relax. Dr. Bradley created this method by observing how animals on his farm gave birth: relaxing in a dark, quiet place.

This strategy tries to achieve a delivery without medication, anesthesia or other medical intervention. That doesn't make it very popular in many hospitals. The instructors are often other couples who have given birth under this system. They teach the method in their own homes over a twelve-week period.

Leboyer Method

Here the idea is to make the birthing process as agreeable and pleasant as possible for the baby. Leboyer was a French doctor who believed babies suffered from the sudden environmental change from the warmth and darkness of mother's womb to the coldness and bright lights of the delivery room. Under this system, the birth takes place in a tub of warm water inside rooms with low light and soothing sounds.

International Childbirth Education Association (ICEA)

This group doesn't promote a specific system, but instead prefers a combination of strategies. The association has certified instructors to teach alternative birthing methods that require as little medical intervention as possible.

Hospital Classes

There will likely be a class offered by the hospital or birthing center you've chosen for your delivery. The method generally used to deal with the pain is Lamaze, but you may also be advised about an epidural and the other medical procedures. Your obstetrician/gynecologist can also recommend a class for you.

Doula

This isn't a birthing method but instead a person who will support you emotionally and physically during the birth of your baby. The idea has become popular over the last few years in the United States but has been common among our ancestors for centuries. Traditionally in Latin America, other women joined the midwife to help the mother. The emotional support was considered as important as the physical care. Studies have shown that pregnant women who have the support of a doula or another woman have shorter deliveries and fewer cesareans and use fewer drugs.

The day you give birth, it may help you to have near you your mother, mother-in-law, other women in your family or friends who have delivered a baby and understand what are you going through. Keep in mind that these are emotional times when you'll lose your composure. You'll want to make sure you really feel at ease and trust the person or people you're depending on for help. However, maybe having your mother or another female relative with you will make you more tense and you would rather be alone with your husband. Another option is to find a professional doula (see Contact List). Some advantages of having a doula are:

- They are trained to offer support to the pregnant woman during delivery.
- They will also support your husband, so he can help you.
- They will work with hospital personnel.
- They will help you after delivery with breastfeeding and newborn care.

You may find doulas in training who offer their services for free.

❦

UMBILICAL CORD BLOOD STORAGE

Advances in genetic science have created a new industry: umbilical cord blood banks. This blood contains what are called "stem cells," cells that have yet to decide what they're going to be. These cells are like virgin videotape: Nothing's been recorded on them, so they can pretty much become any type of cell. Recent experiments have shown that stem cells can be turned into red blood cells, white blood cells or even certain muscle cells, which can help to cure a variety of diseases.

Umbilical cord stem cells have been used for years to fight certain types of cancers. You can store these cells so that if your baby develops an illness, such as leukemia, it can be treated with stem cells. But if your family doesn't have a history of these diseases, the chances that it will suddenly appear in your baby are unlikely. And even if it were to show up, the stem cell treatment is no guarantee of a cure. Nevertheless, there is no doubt stem cells hold great promise for the future.

Removing the umbilical cord blood isn't painful for you or the baby. The blood is extracted with a needle after the cord has been cut. The procedure usually isn't covered by insurance companies and can be quite expensive. You'll have to pay an initial fee to recover the blood and then an annual fee to keep the blood stored.

BRAXTON-HICKS CONTRACTIONS

The first time I felt a Braxton-Hicks contraction, I thought my baby was stretching after taking a *siesta*. If you've never felt a contraction before, it's a strange sensation. The muscles of the uterus get hard, and it feels as though your stomach rises. These contractions, called Braxton-Hicks contractions in honor of the doctor who discovered them, help your uterus prepare for delivery. They aren't painful because they don't really affect the cervix and they come at irregular intervals. Generally, they begin during week 20 of pregnancy. The ninth month is when they become common and even bothersome. But changing your posture or walking around and drinking water will probably make them go away. However, if they come very often, you should tell your doctor.

The contractions of delivery are different from the Braxton-Hicks ones. They feel like a pain on both sides of your belly and come at regular intervals (see page 269).

PREMATURE BIRTH

Sometimes, the delivery comes sooner than expected. That can be a traumatic and disconcerting event for the mother. A birth is considered premature if it happens after twenty weeks of gestation and before the thirty-seventh week. Premature births are difficult to predict and prevent. Despite the medical advances of the past few decades, the number of premature deliveries hasn't gone down. The difference is that with modern technology, more babies survive a premature birth. The risks of a premature birth are greater with:

- Premature birth in the past
- A multiple pregnancy
- Vaginal infection
- Use of drugs, alcohol or tobacco
- Being younger than eighteen or older than forty

But many premature births have unknown causes. The signs a premature birth is imminent include:

- Discomfort or pain similar to menstruation
- Discharge of a watery, bloody or gelatinous substance (the mucus that plugs the cervix during pregnancy)
- Regular contractions or hardening of the uterus, with or without pain
- Constant discomfort or pain in the lower back, which is different from what you usually feel
- Pressure in the lower belly, as if your baby were pushing

If you have any of these symptoms, you should call your doctor immediately to figure out as soon as possible if a premature birth is on the way. Your obstetrician/gynecologist will check if your cervix is dilating.

There's also a test that measures what's called fetal fibronectine. This substance is similar to glue and connects the amniotic sac to the uterus. When this glue is detected in vaginal secretions, there's a higher possibility of a premature birth.

To keep your baby from arriving sooner than expected, doctors will prescribe medicines such as magnesium sulfate that completely relax the muscles of the body in order to avoid contractions. It may work, but it is not pleasant. Talk to your doctor to find out what the side effects are of the medicines that may be prescribed.

In addition, to treat your contractions your doctor might prescribe steroids for your baby. Steroids help the baby's lungs mature more quickly in case the delivery indeed does come too soon.

If you're required to lie down for the remainder of your pregnancy, or if the baby comes sooner than expected, try to round up as many of your relatives and friends as you can. You're going to need as much physical and emotional support as you can get.

For people who have never been through a premature delivery, it can be difficult to understand just what the parents are feeling. Ask the hospital if they can put you in touch with couples who have already delivered a premature baby (see Contact List). Talking to them and learning from their experiences can help.

PRENATAL VISIT

After week 28, your obstetrician/gynecologist or midwife may want to begin seeing you every two weeks, instead of once a month. On this visit, you'll go through the usual routine: blood pressure, weight, urinate into the cup, listen to the baby's heartbeat, look for fluid retention in the legs, face and hands. The doctor may also want a blood sample (from a vein or through a finger prick) to see if you're developing anemia. During the last months of pregnancy, the demand for iron in your blood increases, and it's normal to be a little lacking.

FEELINGS

You're totally pregnant. You may not be feeling heavy, but you have a bulging belly. And all that may make you feel great. Also, in this stage of pregnancy, when it is pretty clear that you are pregnant, you'll be the object of *sonrisas y comentarios*, smiles and comments from complete strangers. If the attention doesn't bother you, it can make you feel really special.

You may begin to daydream about what your baby will look like, the places you'll take it, how you'll bathe it and how you'll feed it. These images will be reflected in your dreams.

You're also likely taking prenatal classes during this time. The information you get about delivery will make you feel a little nervous about what's to happen. This is the time to ask all the questions you have. The more information you have, the more comfortable you'll feel when the delivery day finally arrives.

THE *BEBÉ*

Week 26
When the baby is sleeping, its eyes move quickly. Experts think the baby is dreaming at that moment. Brain activity detected during this week shows that the vision and hearing areas are processing stimuli.

Week 27
The lungs are developing a substance called surfactant, which allows the tissues of the lungs to expand so they can take in air and not get stuck together. The eyelids are separating, and soon it will be able to open its eyes.

Week 28
The baby's eyes are formed now (they even have eyelashes) and are able to distinguish the light that passes through your belly to the womb. The baby is gaining weight and accumulating fat. It weighs nearly 2½ pounds (more than 1,100 grams) and measures around 10 inches (25 centimeters). The lungs are now developed enough to allow the baby to breathe on its own if he/she is born prematurely.

Week 29
The baby's skin is less wrinkled than in previous weeks because it is storing more fat. The toenails are formed and the body is beginning to look like a newborn's—the head is no longer so big compared with the rest of the body. The baby can now distinguish noises from the outside and may even react to certain types of music by stopping what it's doing to listen. The baby weighs almost 3 pounds (1,300 grams) and measures 10½ inches (26 centimeters).

Week 30
The baby opens and closes its eyes constantly and has established a regular sleeping schedule. The hair on the head is growing, and if he/she has a lot it can be seen on a sonogram. The fine hairs that up to now have covered the rest of the body begin to disappear.

FOR DAD

Memory

During this month, *el despiste de su esposa*, your wife's memory loss, might be alarming you. She could leave the television remote control in the refrigerator, mail letters without stamps, or not pay the bills on time. All this forgetfulness might become even more severe as the third trimester goes on. The hormones of pregnancy are affecting her short-term memory. So no matter how much you plead with her to pay attention to what she's doing, there's little she can do to resolve the problem. In other words, she's not becoming an airhead—she's really having trouble keeping information in her memory. The best way to remind her to do something is to write it down; leave notes all over the house she can easily find. Or talk to her on the telephone to remind her.

Birthing Classes

One of the best things you can do for your wife and for yourself is to attend a prenatal class together. There are different methods of preparing for a birth, which require different levels of participation from the father. Before signing up for a class, think about what you would like to do during the delivery and if what is taught in the class is something you feel comfortable with. Many Latino men have specific ideas about what their roles should be during pregnancy, and many classes don't follow that game plan. The most common methods taught in prenatal classes are:

- *Lamaze*. Tries to control the pain of delivery by breathing techniques. You will help your wife with the breathing techniques and will give her massages and help her with the different positions for delivery.
- *Bradley*. Promotes natural birth and requires a lot of paternal participation. You should be with your wife at all times, caressing her, talking to her softly and helping her to relax.
- *Leboyer*. Requires a relaxed environment with soft lights and a tub of warm water. The father helps the mother situate herself in different positions and sometimes is in the tub with her.

- *Combination method.* There are classes at hospitals and instructors that mix different techniques and philosophies.

Here's what you'll find at a birthing class:

- Other fathers who are going through the same thing you are.
- Information about how your baby is growing and what's happening to your partner's body.
- How can you help your wife the day of delivery and what to do afterward.
- Instructions on how to change a diaper and burp your baby (very useful for when your wife leaves you alone with the baby).

You might not like the idea of actually watching the delivery. Maybe, following our traditions, your father wasn't present at your birth or those of your brothers and sisters. Or you may not like the sight of blood. But if you're thinking about staying outside the delivery room, I recommend you first attend a birthing class before making your final decision. It's possible what you think is going to happen is very different from what really goes on during delivery.

The classes run from five to nine weeks, for about two hours every week. The classes have flexible schedules for parents who work.

THE EIGHTH MONTH
Weeks 31 to 35

SHORTNESS OF BREATH

During these last three months, you may feel as though you never get quite enough air in your lungs. Sometimes merely going up the stairs or walking a little faster than normal makes you feel exhausted. Your uterus is now pushing up against the bottom of your lungs. Women who are carrying the pregnancy higher or who are pregnant with twins might feel this sensation even more. During the ninth month, when your baby moves further down in your pelvis, you'll be able to breathe better.

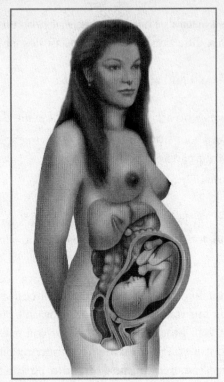

Eighth month

Even though it feels as though you're not getting enough air, your baby isn't suffering from a lack of oxygen. Pregnant women process oxygen more efficiently because they breathe for two. However, watch out to see if you begin to feel more than just out of breath. If your heart begins to race, your chest begins to hurt or you begin to sweat, call your obstetrician/gynecologist or midwife as soon as possible.

A couple of things you might try to ease this feeling include:

- Take your time climbing stairs or avoid activities that make you feel winded.
- Do the relaxation and breathing exercise on page 60.
- Sleep with your torso propped up with pillows if lying down makes the situation worse.

I don't recommend vacations to high-altitude places during these months, unless you're used to it. The feeling of lack of air is only made worse where the air is thinner. I went to the Grand Canyon at seven months and spent the entire time gasping for air *como trucha fuera del agua*, like a trout outside the water.

HEAT INTOLERANCE

If you live in a hot climate, your family and the people who visit your home may find you've converted your home into an igloo. If you live in a colder climate, you may find your husband never takes off his scarf and gloves when he comes in from outside. It's not that the sun is actually hotter during the last months of pregnancy, it's that your body is not tolerating heat as well as it used to. During pregnancy, your body is expending a lot more energy that it usually does, and hormones such as progesterone actually elevate body temperature.

This is the ideal time to pull out that *abanico*, the fan from your great-grandmother that you never knew what to do with. If you want something a little more modern to help you with the heat, some stores sell little portable electric fans that will fit into your purse. Also, try putting cold-water compresses on your neck and wrists. Another option is to get your husband to buy himself an Eskimo suit to wear while he's in the house.

LEAKY BREASTS

During these weeks, you may have noticed a stain on your blouse from your breasts. They're practicing for the breastfeeding that will take place after birth. If you gently press on your nipple with your thumb and index finger, you might be able to squeeze out a little of a yellowish and sticky liquid. This is colostrum, a substance that is produced prior to milk and which has tons of nutrients for your newborn.

Not all women produce colostrum before the baby's born. But that doesn't mean you won't produce it later. Colostrum and milk will eventually show up anyway. If the sudden stains are bothersome or embarrassing, you can insert some absorbent pads into your bra to keep the leaks from seeping through.

INDIGESTION

At the beginning of your pregnancy, indigestion was caused by hormones. The valve that separates the stomach from the esophagus became relaxed, which allowed the digestive acids to leak upward and gave you heartburn. Now your baby is physically pushing your stomach upward, resulting in the same burning feeling. Look at the stomach in the drawings related to this month and the next one. Light and frequent meals can help you avoid these symptoms (see page 171).

HEMORRHOIDS

For those women who have never experienced hemorrhoids, this might be your first opportunity. For those who have, it's likely they'll return or get worse.

Hemorrhoids are swollen veins inside the rectum. Pressure and/or pushing makes them dilate. It's the same as squeezing one end of an inflated balloon. Pregnancy produces exactly the conditions hemorrhoids need to thrive: Constipation and pressure on the rectum. These dilated veins can be found inside or outside the rectum. Some of the most common symptom include:

- Burning or itching in the rectum
- Pain
- Bleeding, especially after a bowel movement
- Swollen veins that stick out from the rectum

Avoiding constipation is one of the best ways to avoid hemorrhoids. Drink a lot of water, eat high-fiber foods such as vegetables, fruits and whole-wheat products and avoid spicy foods, especially ones that contain chiles. To limit the amount of pressure the baby is putting on the rectum, try not to remain seated for long periods of time, and sleep on your left side.

Some people calm the burning and itching of hemorrhoids by taking warm baths. Others do it by applying ice. You can also find hemorrhoid creams in stores. Talk to your doctor before you choose any remedy, because some creams contain steroids that can be absorbed by the rectum, end up in your bloodstream and affect your baby. Be wary of home remedies for the same reason.

In some cases the hemorrhoids just don't get any better, no matter how much fiber you eat and how much water you drink. If you're really getting uncomfortable, go to a proctologist, a doctor who specializes in hemorrhoid treatment. The effort of delivering a baby only makes hemorrhoids worse, and they can become really bothersome after delivery.

One of the ways a doctor will remove a hemorrhoid is to wrap a rubber band tightly around the base of it. That keeps the blood from flowing to it, and the hemorrhoid dries up. This is a nonsurgical procedure and usually works.

FETAL GROWTH

One of the reasons your doctor continues to measure your abdomen in your prenatal visits is to make sure the baby is growing according to plan. When the size of your abdomen doesn't correspond to the growth chart, your obstetrician/gynecologist may order a sonogram to detect any of the following:

- *Delayed intrauterine growth.* This means the baby is smaller than it's supposed to be. The delay can be caused by many things, but the most common is that the placenta isn't providing the baby with the proper amount of nutrients it needs to grow. Your doctor can treat the problem and will check up on the baby's growth over the next months. Sometimes babies with this problem are born via cesarean to limit the stress of birth.

- *Macrosomia.* When a baby weighs more than nine pounds, it's considered to have macrosomia. This isn't a disease, only a medical term used to describe the baby's size. Your obstetrician/gynecologist can give you an idea of how much your baby weighs through a sonogram. But this weight isn't exact. The baby could be as much as a pound lighter or heavier than the doctor's prediction. The problem with the baby's size is that he/she might not be able to go through the mother's pelvis or he/she might get stuck during delivery. Along with the sonogram, your obstetrician/gynecologist will give you an internal exam to determine whether there's a cephalopelvic disproportion. In other words, the doctor wants to know if the baby's head will be able to fit through the mother's pelvic opening.

TWINS OR MORE

"I saw the doctor stop and smile. She said, 'It seems we have not just one, but two!' *La verdad*, truth is that first I was scared, but then I felt very happy. My husband was so proud and happy thinking, look, not only am I capable of making one, but two! But the pregnancy was difficult. I vomited from the day I got pregnant to the day they were born."

—*Elena Nelson*

"My belly was huge. Wherever I went my belly arrived first and then me. It grew a lot after the sixth month and I had to use girdles to support it."

—*Julie Ferrer*

Pregnancies with more than one baby are more difficult than single ones for several reasons:

- The body produces more hormones, and this can mean more morning sickness during the first months.
- The mother needs to gain more weight and the nutritional and iron demands are bigger.
- More weight means more back, muscle and joint discomforts.

Prenatal care is always important, but especially when you are going to have more than one baby. You will need medical attention to make sure that your babies are growing properly and that you are in good health.

WHAT TO TAKE TO THE HOSPITAL

When the moment of delivery arrives, your mind is going to be focused on other things such as contractions, and your husband is going to be focused on you. Having a bag already packed with what you'll need can help you avoid scrambling at the last minute.

Your stay at a hospital for a delivery is usually twenty-four hours, seventy-two if the delivery is cesarean. This is a general list of what you might need that you can modify and personalize.

- Two large nightgowns or shirts that open in front so you can breast-feed your baby. During delivery, you'll probably wear a hospital gown, but after that you can wear your own clothes.

- Big, roomy underwear and sanitary napkins. After having a baby, the size of your belly doesn't immediately return to normal. At first it will be about as big as when you were four or five months pregnant. After delivery, you'll bleed for several days. The hospital will provide you with some sanitary napkins, but take your own to feel more comfortable.

- Socks and a sweatshirt. Even though many women feel warm or hot during pregnancy, the air-conditioning in a hospital can be powerful. Warm socks and a thick sweatshirt will keep you comfortable.

- Pillows, music, candles, etc. Take whatever you use at home to relax. Portable tape and CD players can help you separate yourself from all the hustle and bustle going on around you.

- This book. The chapters on delivery will give your husband a better idea of what's going on and what to expect.

- Toiletries. Everything you take on a trip you should take to the hospital: hairbrush, toothbrush, toothpaste, etc.

- One dress. When you leave the hospital you'll want to have a dress to wear. It's more comfortable than pants, especially if you've got stitches. Choose a size you wore when you were four or five months pregnant.

- The baby's first clothes. During the first twenty-four hours, the baby will wear a little hat to keep him or her warm. The baby still doesn't have a way to regulate its own temperature. The hospital will surely give you one, but you may want to buy something special. Also bring a pajama or overall that opens at the lower end, so it's easier to change diapers (see page 249). You may also bring a small blanket to wrap your baby in as you carry it to the car for the ride home.

- Child seat. This is very important, because the hospital won't let you leave unless you've got the proper safety seat installed in your car. This is the safest way to travel in a car with your baby.

❦

Birth Plan

Establishing a birth plan will help improve communication between you and the people who will give you medical attention during delivery. A birth plan is a list of your personal preferences—for example, a list of the people you want to be with you, how you want to deal with pain, the positions you want to be in to deliver, or what medical interventions you want to avoid during delivery. This list doesn't mean you'll get all your wishes granted. Still, in the middle of the delivery, when you and your husband aren't in the best state of mind to clearly communicate what you want, it's easier to say: "Please take a look at my birth plan."

The birth plan doesn't have any legal implications and is not telling the medical professionals how to do their job. It's only a way to let everyone know what your desires and preferences are. The first person you need to reach out to before writing anything down is your husband, your mother or the person who's going to be with you during the delivery. Prenatal classes along with a visit to the hospital will help you know what your options are. Next, talk to your doctor to make sure your wishes will be respected as long as the delivery goes according to plan. Some of the things to include on your list are:

- *Which people you want to be with you at every moment of the birth.* That could be your husband, your mother and your sister, for example. Or you may want your other children to be present.

- *Ways to alleviate pain.* Perhaps you want to use an epidural or avoid an epidural altogether and rely on other medicines instead. Maybe you want to give it a go without any pain medication at all.

- *Position at birth.* You may want to walk around or be in other positions besides on your back on a bed.

- *Breastfeeding.* Explain if you want your baby handed to you right at birth so you can begin breastfeeding right away or if you don't want the nurses to give him/her formula or other supplements.

These are only a few examples. You can find lists on the Internet all ready to print. All you have to do is fill in a few blanks to personalize the list. Once you've got a plan on paper and you've discussed it with your doctor or midwife, make a copy for them and for you to take to the hospital or birthing center.

The best way to know which procedures you'll be subjected to at the hospital is to ask for an interview with the head nurse on the maternity floor. They're usually pretty busy but will most likely talk to you and your husband for a few minutes about your birth plan. Head nurses are the best source of information on what to expect during your hospital delivery. Also, if you've already established a relationship with the head nurse, you can later tell a *poco simpática*, disagreeable nurse in the delivery room, "The head nurse has already approved my plan, so you can talk to her about it," whatever the problem might be. Nurses in the delivery room follow the doctor's orders, but they work for the head nurse.

BABY LAYETTE

There are all kinds of colors, shapes and materials to choose from when you start to pick out baby clothes and accessories. Because there's so much to choose from, it can be confusing. This list will help you with the baby basics.

- *Diapers.* There are two options: washable cloth ones or disposable. The washable ones haven't changed over the years, but now there are services you can purchase that will take away the dirty ones and replace them with fresh ones on your front doorstep. Among the disposable styles, you can choose ones covered in plastic or covered in an impermeable paper. There are male and female fits, with special absorbent pads in the appropriate places. Don't buy too many diapers in the newborn size, because babies grow quickly in the first weeks after birth.

- *Baby wipes.* These are really useful when it's time to change a diaper, especially if you're away from home. Make sure the wipes aren't perfumed or contain additives, because a newborn's skin can easily get irritated.

- *Pajamas.* The full-body styles that cover both feet will help your baby sleep comfortably, especially in the winter when it's cold. Socks fall off easily. The pajamas that open at the bottom with snaps are easy to get on and off when you're changing diapers. The first size is from zero to three months. Even though these are usually a little big at the beginning, it only takes a couple of weeks before your baby fills them out. Three or four pairs of pajamas will be enough to keep your baby clothed while you're washing the dirty ones.

- *T-shirts.* The most comfortable T-shirts have openings on the sides. That lets the baby's head slide through without hurting its ears. The cotton styles keep the baby cool in the summer and warm in the winter. Three or four will be enough for now.

- *Pants, skirts and dresses.* Pants or a skirt combined with a T-shirt is an easy and comfortable way to dress your baby. Skirts for girls are cute, but make sure the baby's diaper is on tight, because sometimes "accidents" can happen when the baby moves. Underwear helps to keep the diaper in place. Same goes for dresses.

- *Bibs and towels.* You will need bibs because babies frequently spit up a little milk when they burp. Digested milk smells sour and it's easier to change a bib instead of an entire outfit. The towels are for you. Put one over your shoulder when you're burping your baby. Buy just three or four at the beginning. Later, when you figure out how much milk your baby burps up, you may want to buy more. Cloth diapers will work well too.

- *Creams and talcum power.* Babies often get diaper rash and other skin irritations because the skin next to the diaper remains moist. A little baby cream creates a protective barrier between the skin and the wet diaper. Talcum powder dries up the area, but be careful about the powders that contain zinc. It's not good for babies to breathe that metal.

- *Car seat.* This accessory is essential if you want to take your baby anywhere in the car. These seats are generally like portable cribs that face the rear and are strapped in with the seat belt. Newborns aren't old enough to ride facing forward yet, as their necks are too weak to support the stress of a sudden stop. You're going to need one of these to leave the hospital.

- *Baby carriage.* There are all kinds of models to choose from. The first question you should ask yourself is: "How am I going to use this carriage?" If you live in an apartment complex, will you have to go up and down the stairs with the carriage every time you take your baby out? If so, perhaps you should consider a lightweight model that folds up easily. If you live in a house with an elevator or without stairs, or you plan to take long strolls, maybe a larger carriage with sturdy wheels is the one for you. Some carriages come with a baby seat included.

- *Crib*. During the first three months, the baby won't move much and can sleep in a small crib. The good thing about these small cribs is that many of them have wheels and you can push your baby around the house in it to have him/her close to you. But if you don't want to spend much money, you can buy a traditional crib with bars lining the sides. Be wary of older cribs and secondhand ones; not all of them will comply with newer safety regulations. The bars shouldn't be more than 2⅜ inches apart. That's about the width of three adult fingers. Otherwise, the baby's head could get stuck between the bars. An accident like this could be fatal.

All these accessories are only used for a couple of years at most, so you can find many of them in good shape and at reasonable prices at secondhand stores.

CHOOSING A DOCTOR FOR YOUR *BEBÉ*

You're going to visit your baby's pediatrician or family physician a lot during the next years. Between the vaccinations and common colds, you are going to come to know his or her waiting room pretty well. This doctor will be in charge of your baby's health from the moment it's born, so it's a good idea to choose one before you give birth. You can choose a pediatrician, a family physician or even a pediatric nurse.

- *Pediatrician*. This is a doctor who specializes in the treatment of babies, children and adolescents. There are pediatricians with individual practices and others who work in group practices.

- *Family physician*. It's the modern version of the primary care physician. He doesn't have the same specialized education as a pediatrician but is qualified to treat the entire family.

- *Pediatric nurse*. These nurses work with pediatricians and are in charge of general checkups and treating common illness. They've got more time available to see your baby and answer your questions. When there's a more complicated problem, the pediatrician takes over.

You should consider a variety of factors when choosing who will take care of your baby's health. One of the most important is communication. If this is your first pregnancy, taking care of your baby will be a totally new experience and you'll have a lot of questions. You'll feel more comfortable with a doctor you trust and have confidence in; one who answers your questions in a friendly way. You should also think about:

- *Where the office is.* The closer to your home the better. Besides having to go often, if you've got an emergency, you don't want to have to drive across town.

- *What the office hours are.* If you work, you'll need a doctor who has flexible hours and works Saturday mornings.

- *Phone calls.* Ask if the doctor will take calls after hours. If so, how long does it take to respond? When a baby suddenly comes down with a high fever at three in the morning, you want an answer right away.

- *Whether the office has separate waiting rooms.* Some pediatricians have separate waiting rooms for sick children and others for children who are only there for a checkup so they won't get sick. Look closely to see how clean the waiting rooms are.

- *How long the visits and waits are.* Less than fifteen minutes per visit won't give you much time to ask questions and have them answered.

- *Group practice.* If there's more than one pediatrician in the office, ask how often you'll have to see another one because of vacations and on-call shifts.

- *The nurse or receptionist.* How friendly is this person? He or she will be passing your calls on to the doctor. You don't want to deal with attitude when you're worried about your baby's health.

- *Philosophy.* Find someone who shares your ideas on how to treat children. Maybe you're not a big fan of giving children a lot of medicine. Or perhaps you want a doctor who can speak Spanish (see Contact List).

Before you give birth, talk to at least two doctors about their becoming your pediatrician. All you have to say is that you're pregnant and you're looking for a doctor for your baby; you probably won't be charged for this visit. Ask your family members or friends about the pediatricians they used. Your medical insurance company can give you a list of pediatricians who work near where you live.

PRENATAL VISIT

The prenatal visit or visits during this month follow the same routine as the previous ones: blood pressure, weight, urinate into the cup, measure belly, listen to the baby's heartbeat and check to see if there's fluid retention in the legs, face or hands. The last test is important because excessive water retention can indicate preeclampsia. One of the tests done on your urine will also make sure you're not developing this illness.

During one of the visits to the doctor this month, talk about your birth plan (if you've got one) and exactly what will happen during delivery. For example, if you are going to go into labor naturally, ask:

- How long does he/she wait to give medication to speed up labor?
- How many hours of labor will he/she wait before recommending a cesarean?
- How many centimeters must the cervix be dilated before giving an epidural?

Before going to your prenatal doctor visit, make a list of all your worries.

FEELINGS

During this month, many women are convinced they couldn't be any more pregnant. The eighth month makes you feel as though your belly just can't get any bigger. However, it will. Your body will continue to adapt to and accommodate the baby growing inside it. The baby's movements are now stronger, and sometimes you can see a baby's foot or elbow pushing from the inside. This may fill you with joy and at the same time may make you feel concerned about how your life is going to be now that you will be responsible for a little baby, or if you will be a good mother. In case you have to or want to go back to work, you may worry about who will take care of your baby, or maybe you're having second thoughts about returning to work. All these feelings are normal. As with many of the emotions brought on by pregnancy, they're only a way to help you prepare to deal with a new situation.

Try to talk to friends or relatives about how they felt when they gave birth to their children. Ask them what scared them. Ask them how it turned out. You'll be surprised at the stories they tell.

THE *BEBÉ*

Week 31
The movements of the hands are now obvious and intentional; he/she can grab the umbilical cord. The brain is developing rapidly and the digestive system is already functioning. The only thing that remains to develop is the lungs. The baby weighs 3½ pounds (1,600 grams) and measures 11 inches (27.5 centimeters).

Week 32
Your baby doesn't have as much room to move around anymore, so its movements will feel a little different to you. The baby will recognize voices, perhaps the father's, definitely yours. If your baby is a boy, its testicles are making their way out of the abdomen to their final position. The baby weighs nearly 4 pounds (1,800 grams) and measures 12 inches (30 centimeters).

Week 33
During this week or the next one, the baby will turn itself around to put its head toward your pelvis. You'll notice if he/she has moved depending on where you feel the kicks (in the ribs or the pelvis). Its skin is now taking on a rose-colored tone, as the fat deposited underneath the skin's surface has taken away some of the reddish color. The pupils dilate and reduce with the amount of light entering the eyes.

Week 34
Your baby is constantly swallowing amniotic fluid and urinating it. It's practicing the movements of breathing with its lungs. The fingernails have reached the fingertips and they keep growing, but they're still delicate. The baby weighs nearly 5 pounds (more than 2 kilograms) and measures 13 inches (32.5 centimeters).

Week 35
The baby is gaining weight quickly. The arms and legs now have the little rolls of fat that newborns have. Since there is not much space left in your uterus, the baby's arms and legs are crossed.

❦

FOR DAD

Un Mes "Pesado," a "Heavy" Month

The stage where your wife felt radiant and happy about her pregnancy may be long over. The baby continues to grow, and the discomforts of having a 5-pound person inside her might be showing up in her mood. During these weeks your wife needs all the physical help you can offer for household chores.

Energy

At the same time, this is the month when many pregnant women feel a newfound sense of energy as they work to prepare the baby's room, a crib, clothes, put closets in order, clean and many other tasks. She'll wear herself out doing all this if you don't help her. Don't let her climb ladders to paint the baby's room or do other heavy chores. Her balance isn't what it used to be.

Attention from Strangers

During this month your wife is obviously very pregnant. She's likely to get a lot of attention from family members, friends and even strangers. That attention might be more than you can stand. It might make you uncomfortable to watch people reach out and touch your wife's belly without even asking. Don't interpret it as a *falta de respeto*, a sign of disrespect, especially if your wife doesn't mind. People are fond of pregnant women, and they like to share stories and talk about their experiences.

Your Hospital Bag

Sometime during this month, you should prepare a bag with the things *you* will need at the hospital or birthing center. You might include:

- Coins for drink machines and pay phones
- A list of telephone numbers to call
- A camera or video camera
- This book

- Magazines, books, a deck of cards or games (if your wife gets an epidural, she might feel like playing)
- Crackers and snacks (you might need them if the labor goes on for hours and there's no place to buy food—the vending machines usually aren't all that good)
- Your toiletries and a change of clothes

Add anything else that will make you feel more comfortable (music, radio, your favorite pillow) because if the labor drags on for hours or the pregnancy gets complicated, you may find yourself in the hospital for a while.

If you and your wife have established a birthing plan, put a copy in your bag. You'll be in charge of making sure everyone follows it.

THE NINTH MONTH
Weeks 36 to 40

VARICOSE VEINS

Varicose veins have lost their elasticity and have become distended. Blood accumulates inside them because they are not strong enough to force the blood out. During pregnancy, varicose veins may appear in your legs and sometimes even on the vagina.

Varicose veins form mostly during the third trimester because of the pressure the uterus puts on the vena cava, a vein that runs back to the heart from the lower body. Varicose veins in the legs look bluish, and some are quite painful. Also, the pressure of the baby's head on the veins that allow blood to flow to the pelvis may cause varicose veins on the vagina. In addition to the pressure on the veins, pregnancy hormones force the veins to relax, which makes it difficult for the blood to be forced through them. If your mother or father has or had varicose veins, you're more likely to get them. After birth, most of them disappear, but sometimes not all.

The best thing to do to avoid varicose veins is to improve your circulation by:

- Walking frequently. This combats not only varicose veins but also leg swelling, which is so common during the final months of pregnancy.

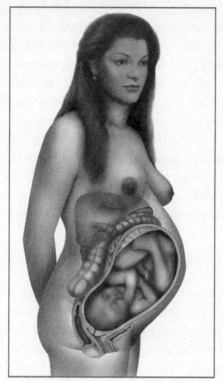

Ninth month

- Elevating your legs whenever you can to keep blood from pooling in your legs.

- Avoiding having heat blow on your feet while you're in the car. Also avoid hot baths, because they will only make the veins relax even more.

- Asking your doctor about using special socks that squeeze the lower legs and improve circulation.

BLADDER CONTROL

Trying to delay going to the bathroom during the last months of pregnancy is a real feat, especially in places where a bathroom might not be available immediately. On top of that, many times you'll feel like going again just a few minutes after you've left the bathroom. Take a look at the illustration above, and compare the shape of your bladder now with its shape during the first months of pregnancy. As you can see, your bladder is sandwiched between your pelvic bones and the weight of your uterus. That's why it seems like it's time to empty it no matter how little liquid is inside.

If you laugh really hard or have to sneeze, there may not be any way to keep a few drops of urine from leaking out. Laughing, sneezing, coughing or doing something strenuous puts pressure on the bladder. A panty liner will help absorb the moisture, but make sure you change them often to keep that area clean and to avoid infections. You can also do Kegel exercises to strengthen the muscles of the lower pelvis (see page 59).

When your baby drops toward your pelvis during the final weeks, this pressure on your bladder can increase. The good news is when that happens, you'll have more space around your stomach and lungs.

Yeast Infections

Vaginal yeast infections find pregnant women easy targets. The hormonal changes that have taken place make the vagina an ideal place for growth. This means burning, itching, irritation and other discomforts in the vaginal area. Typically vaginal yeast infections produce a white discharge similar to cottage cheese. These infections are caused by a yeast called *Candida albicans* that actually lives in the vagina under normal conditions. It's also in the rectum, stomach and mouth. But because of the hormonal changes during pregnancy, this yeast may grow uncontrollably. There are many medicines you can take to battle this problem, often without a prescription. Ask your doctor before taking anything, because some of them aren't advisable for pregnant women.

Yeast infections can appear several times during pregnancy. Some of the things you can do to prevent them and to improve the symptoms are:

- Dry your vaginal area well after taking a shower or bath.
- Don't use feminine sprays or panty liners that have perfumes or deodorants.
- Wear cotton underwear.
- Don't wear tight pants. Change out of damp bathing suits as soon as you can.
- When you go to the bathroom, wipe from front to back to avoid contaminating the vagina with organisms that live in the rectum.
- Avoid eating sweets—yeasts love sugar.

Yeast infections won't affect your baby, but on occasion they can give the baby a mouth infection during delivery (*algodoncillo* or thrush). This infection can then be transferred to your breasts when you breastfeed.

MOVEMENTS

During the final weeks of pregnancy, the baby doesn't have much space to move around inside your uterus. Its movements change and you can feel them more intensely and less frequently. But this change in movement is gradual, not from one day to the next. If you think your baby is too quiet, do a movement count (see page 132) and call your doctor if you fear something's not right.

LIGHTENING

Although not all women go through it, when it does happen, it's usually with four to six weeks to go before delivery. Lightening is when the baby drops into the pelvic cavity in preparation for delivery. This has its advantages and its disadvantages. On one hand, you're likely to breathe and digest better, as the baby has moved out of the way and there's more space for your lungs and stomach. On the other hand, your bladder is going to be more squished than ever. The baby in the illustration on page 257 has dropped, and as you can see, there's not much space for the bladder. You may feel some pressure in the area of the vagina or a sense the baby *como que se va a salir,* could come out at any moment. Rest as much as you can and try to stay off your feet.

If you are one of the women who experiences lightening, you will be able to tell the difference in your abdomen by looking in the mirror. Your clothes will feel different, as will your balance.

Lightening most often happens during the first pregnancy. It can also happen without the mother noticing at all because she carried the pregnancy low to begin with. If this isn't your first baby, lightening will likely happen during the first stages of labor.

INSOMNIA

Even though you're exhausted, falling asleep may be difficult. Or you may find yourself waking up several times a night. Your insomnia might be due to the baby's movements, since he or she might have a different sleeping pattern from yours (and will probably continue with this nocturnal lifestyle after it's born). You may also be having intense dreams that wake you up from time to time. Or you may not be able to sleep just because you can't ever find a comfortable position to lie in.

> "My baby moved a lot at night. I had to find the right position for my belly so she was comfortable, because otherwise she moved a lot."
>
> —*Dana Morales*

Staying awake for much of the night won't put you in a good mood, especially if you have to get up early to go to work or take care of the rest of your family. A relaxing bath before going to bed, listening to soft music or reading might help you get a little shut-eye (see page 159).

But maybe, no matter what you do, you won't be able to get to sleep. Don't get upset. Even though you're not actually sleeping, stay in bed and try breathing exercises. Your body will appreciate the chance to wind down. Try to take brief *siestas* during the day.

SEX

With a belly as big as ever, nights of passion with your partner may not be at the top of your list of fun things to do. The last weeks of pregnancy are difficult for almost every couple. The size of your belly makes most sexual positions complicated or uncomfortable. Also, the pressure of the baby's head on your pelvis might make penetration uncomfortable, too. With all that, you may have more difficulty achieving orgasm. In addition, having sex can cause a yellowish liquid called colostrum to leak from your breasts.

Despite all that, some couples enjoy having sex during this month. Many men find their wives to be most attractive at the end of their pregnancies. As long as your obstetrician/gynecologist says it's fine, sex in the ninth month won't affect your baby at all, though you may bleed a little after sex or even feel contractions after an orgasm.

YOU'RE OVERDUE

Those last days or weeks after your due date can be an exasperating time. It's like the clocks don't keep time. Days drag on and on, and so do the discomforts of pregnancy. And as if that weren't enough, you'll get the usual comments like "*¿Todavía no?*" "Not yet?" and "So when are you due?" It's as if you were keeping the baby inside you on purpose.

Many things can cause a delay in delivery. It may console you to know that only 4 percent of women actually give birth on their due dates. Most babies are born between weeks 38 and 42 of pregnancy.

A doctor in the nineteenth century made up the way the due date is determined. This man figured a normal pregnancy lasted 244 days from the moment of conception or 280 from the first day of the last period. But this formula was only for women with a 28-day menstrual cycle who ovulated on day 14. We still use the same formula today, even though many women have longer or shorter menstrual cycles. Also, studies show that food, the number of prior pregnancies and your ethnic background influence due dates. Sometimes the delay is just because of a mistake in the calculations. In other words, it's very common to be overdue.

Generally, if there are no complications, obstetricians/gynecologists wait until week 42 before inducing labor because babies born after that time tend to have more problems, such as gaining too much weight or swallowing meconium.

During these last weeks maybe your obstetrician/gynecologist will want to do some tests to make sure the baby is doing fine (see page 132).

I don't recommend you try home remedies to induce labor. In a normal pregnancy, the time of delivery is decided by the baby, not you. Herbs and other home remedies may cause strong, unexpected contractions or diarrhea and may be toxic for the baby. Relax as much as you can and try to enjoy these last few days. Believe me, soon after the delivery, you'll miss those quiet moments by yourself.

WORK

If you've got some project hanging over your head at work, this is the time to put other people in charge of it, or at least give a co-worker some of the details of how to get it completed. Depending on what type of work you do, you may have left your job with two or three weeks to go. For example, if you work on your feet, the last weeks can be trying. Your doctor may write a note to give you temporary disability if your workplace doesn't offer maternity leave (see page 27). But if you prefer to work until the end so you can take off more time after the baby's born, try some of the things on page 218 to avoid having your legs swell too much.

Energy and Preparations

Even though you feel tired, you may also feel a renewed energy to clean the house, wash clothes, reorganize the closets—all in preparation for the arrival of the newest member of the family. There are some who believe this need to prepare the house is equivalent to the instinct some animals have to prepare a nest for their newborns. They even label this spurt of energy the "pregnancy nesting instinct." You may want to save part of this energy to make some other preparations that will help you in the long run.

- Figure out now with whom you're going to leave your other children when you rush to the hospital, and what you will do with your pets. If it's a relative who will take charge while you're at the hospital and he or she is not familiar with the area, make sure to give that person a list of telephone numbers to call in an emergency. If he or she doesn't speak English, provide the telephone number of a friend or neighbor who can help. Also, ask at the hospital if there's a nurse who speaks Spanish whom your family members can call in case you don't have a phone in your room.

- This is a great time to begin cooking meals you can eat when you get home with your baby. When you're all together at home, you won't have much spare time to cook. Having a whole week's worth or more of meals already made can be a big help.

- If you want to get a passport for your baby, ask the county offices where you live where can you get the required forms before the baby is born. It's easier to pick them up while you're pregnant than when you've got a newborn in your arms. The hospital where you deliver or the birthing center will give you forms to get your baby's birth certificate and Social Security number.

- If you want to baptize your baby during the first weeks after you get home, talk to your church or religious center about it now. Sometimes they require you to fulfill certain requirements ahead of time or you have to reserve a space and date.

- If you're going to send out announcement cards, have the envelopes stamped and ready to go.

More than anything, *no se agote*, make sure you don't wear yourself out. Your husband or any other family member can help you with all these projects. When the due date gets close, you're going to need all the energy you can muster.

PRENATAL VISIT

During the last month of pregnancy, your doctor will want to see you once a week to make sure everything is okay. As always, the doctor will check your weight, urine, blood pressure, measure your belly and listen to the baby's heartbeat.

Between weeks 35 and 37, the doctor might also take a vaginal swab to make sure you don't have any Group B Streptococcus bacteria (see page 103). This infection can be passed on to the baby during delivery. It can be treated with antibiotics.

If you are overdue or you've got gestational diabetes, high blood pressure or any other complication, your doctor might also want to take a close look to see how the baby is doing. That's done with a fetal stress test (see page 133), which makes sure:

- The baby is getting enough nutrients and oxygen
- The baby's heart is beating properly
- There's enough amniotic fluid

Talk to your doctor about when it may be necessary to induce labor and what methods would be used to do it (see page 299). Also, ask what is the number to call if your labor starts after office hours, and when you should go to the hospital.

FEELINGS

One of the things that got me most nervous during the last weeks of my pregnancies was looking at my belly and wondering how something that big was going to fit through something so small and how much was it going to hurt.

Worries about how the birth will progress and how much it will hurt are inevitable. I'm sure you've heard some horror stories from your relatives and friends that don't do much to calm you down. But getting as much information as you can about pain during delivery and the ways to control it can help to assuage your fears, especially if this is your first baby. A big part of the worries of first-time mothers is based on fear of the unknown. "What will it feel like? How will I react? What will happen to the baby?" Chapter 10 has a section about pain, with the experiences of other Latina mothers during their deliveries.

Besides these worries, you may also feel irritable during the last weeks of pregnancy. You might feel tired of being pregnant, your legs are swollen, time goes by slowly, you've had it with everyone asking you when the baby is due and you can't sleep at night. And if your due date has already passed, you're probably not going to want to deal with anyone. *Creáme que la comprendo,* I understand what you are going through.

One way to make it through these last weeks is to focus on completing a project. Perhaps you want to sew something for your baby to wear, finish up a photo album or do anything else that won't make you too tired but will distract you from some of your worries. Enjoy these last few days to go out to the movies or to dinner with your husband. In just a few days, you're going to be too busy for things like that.

THE *BEBÉ*

Week 36
This is when the baby usually descends into the pelvis in preparation for birth. The baby is now completely formed and only needs to gain a little weight. It now weighs nearly 6 pounds (almost 3 kilograms) and measures a little more than 13 inches (32.5 centimeters) from crown to rump (from the top of the head to the buttocks).

Week 37
During this time, the baby will gain between half a pound and a pound a week. Its lungs continue to produce surfactant, a substance that will help them open up during the first breaths of air.

Week 38
Your baby now weighs almost 7 pounds (a little over 3 kilograms). It's not growing longer, as it did during past weeks. The lanugo, the thin hairs that covered the body, has nearly disappeared, although some may remain on the shoulders and back.

Week 39

The white covering that protected the baby from the amniotic fluid, called the vernix, is also disappearing. A good amount of meconium is inside the intestines. This is the green-colored feces the newborn will discharge soon after birth.

Week 40

The amount of amniotic fluid is slowly diminishing, as are the supportive functions of the placenta. The baby is ready to be born at any minute.

FOR DAD

Sex

Some couples have better sex than ever during this last month, but that is more the exception than the rule. Sexual relations with your partner may now become complicated. The belly is very big and she might feel very uncomfortable. Talk to her about what positions are better. The baby is putting pressure on her vagina, and what was pleasant before might not be now.

Communication

Communicating is very important this month. Some fathers feel left out and alone during these last months because they are not having as much sex as they would like or because their partners are somehow distant and absorbed in preparing for the baby arrival. The majority of affairs occur around this time in the pregnancy. The consequences of an action like that are devastating. Not only will you betray her trust, but it comes at a time when she feels most vulnerable. Keeping close contact with your wife will dissipate those ideas, if they were ever present.

Hospital Preparations

There's not much time left now before the big day, and you might be feeling a little nervous. Here are some things you can do to get ready:

- Practice your trip to the hospital. Figure out the best place to park.

- Now that you are at the hospital, get registered. You will be able to calmly fill out the forms that require your insurance information, name, address, etc., instead of rushing while your partner is in labor.

- Prepare the car to place the infant seat, and make sure it will be properly secured with the seat belt.

- Put a roll of quarters in the car in case you have to use a parking meter.

- Make sure the gas tank is full all month long; fill it up as soon as you reach half a tank.

- Explain what's going on to your boss and look for someone who can take your place if you have to leave on the run.

You may want to read Chapters 10 and 11. They will help you get a better idea of what the labor symptoms are and what your wife might be feeling.

Feelings

Some fathers-to-be don't face the reality of fatherhood until this final month or until after the baby has actually been born. Realizing all of a sudden that there's going to be another member of the family for whom you're responsible—forever, no less—can provoke some contradictory emotions: You may be immensely happy, or you may want run and hide, or both. Don't feel ashamed or alarmed if you begin to have doubts about whether you really want to be a father at this late date. It happens to many men. Ask other fathers whom you trust what they felt just before the births of their babies.

10

Labor and Delivery

After waiting for nine months, the long-awaited and yet feared event has arrived. On one hand, forty weeks of pregnancy (or more) have left you wanting only one thing: To deliver the baby! Now! On the other hand, facing the birth of your baby can make you pretty nervous. If this is your first child, you will not know what to expect, and some stories that you've heard by now will probably concern you. Even if you have had other children, if your previous labor was difficult or if it ended in an emergency cesarean, you could be wary of what's going to happen this time.

The physical part of a normal delivery process is the same for all women: The cervix dilates through (usually painful) contractions and the baby comes out as you push. But the way each woman deals with and experiences delivery is different. It depends on a lot of things, such as your tolerance for pain, the environment in which you give birth, who is with you and the medications you decide to use. What may be ideal for one woman (delivering in a hospital with the aid of an epidural) may not be appealing to the next woman. This chapter will explain exactly what happens to your body during delivery and how to prepare yourself mentally and physically for delivery.

SIGNS THAT LABOR IS GETTING CLOSER

At the end of pregnancy, or even sooner if we're talking about a premature birth, there are certain signs that will tell you your body is preparing to deliver the baby. Except for the contractions, not every mother-to-be feels all of these signals. Just because you begin to notice some of the tell-tale signs doesn't mean the delivery will be right away. It could take hours, days or even weeks. Still, if you're beyond your due date, any one of these signals will give you hope.

- *Lightening.* Some women, but not all, experience a "dropping" of their bellies. That means the baby is positioning itself to get ready for birth by moving lower into the pelvic cavity. This can happen weeks or days before delivery (see page 259) or even during the delivery.

- *Nesting instinct.* Days or even hours before delivery, some mothers feel a burst of energy, which they spend on cleaning the house, organizing closets and even finishing up photo albums. More about this on page 262.

- *Irritability.* This is a different irritability from the regular one. The sensitivity that affects women just before birth is caused by the hormonal changes the body is going through to prepare for delivery.

- *Diarrhea and nausea.* The new hormones that are running through your veins are getting your body ready for the task of delivery. Just as at the beginning of pregnancy these changes can affect your stomach and intestines, they can make you feel nauseous or give you diarrhea now too.

- *Back pain.* We're not talking about the typical back pain of the last few weeks of pregnancy. This is a pain that runs across the lower back like a band and extends down to both sides of your belly. It can be a slight sensation or a significant pain.

- *Abdominal pain.* These pains are similar to menstrual cramps. They may feel like slight contractions or a nearly constant pain.

- *Braxton-Hicks contractions.* They get more intense as birth approaches (see page 236). But if they go on for more than an hour, you should go to the hospital, especially if this is your first baby. They might be labor contractions.

- *Mucous discharge.* During pregnancy, a thick plug of mucus plugs the cervix and protects the baby from the outside. In some women, this plug is released before delivery, as the cervix begins to dilate. It can be watery or dense, and sometimes it's accompanied by a little blood. This is normal. However, if the color is a bright red and there's more than a teaspoon, you should talk to your doctor right away.

• *When the water breaks*. During the last weeks of pregnancy some women fear their water will break right as they're walking down the street or in the supermarket or at work. Even though the sac containing the amniotic fluid may indeed rupture while you're in public, probably it won't look like a puddle below you. When you're standing, the head of your baby is pressing on the cervix, and that will keep the fluid from pouring out. However, it is possible that you will feel a constant dripping. If your water breaks while you are lying down, maybe you will feel it more, as it happened to Leticia Gutierrez:

> "I was lying down and I felt a menstrual cramp. I was going to turn around when I felt something wet. I made it to the bathroom just in time. Lots of water came out. Shortly after, my contractions started."

Usually the water breaks during delivery. But if happens before, it's important you pay close attention to the look and smell of the liquid. If it's green or brown and smells bad, it likely contains meconium. Meconium is the first feces the baby produces. Normally there is no meconium in the amniotic fluid, but if there is, the baby could breathe it in or swallow it, which could cause an infection. The liquid should look clear and without blood.

Once the sac that is protecting the baby is broken, bacteria now can get to the baby's environment. That's why it's a good idea not to take a bath or have sex after the water breaks. Generally, contractions begin just a few hours after the sac is broken. But if more than a day goes by before the contractions start, the risk of infection is higher and your obstetrician/gynecologist may have to induce labor.

• *Contractions*. Contractions are the most common sign birth is near, but there are exceptions. A phenomenon called "false labor" is where the contractions come at regular intervals and are painful but don't make the cervix dilate. But you don't go through these contractions for nothing. They may actually help the uterus to soften up and may efface or thin out your cervix (see page 278). Sometimes it's difficult to tell false labor from the real thing; however, false labor contractions have certain characteristics:

- They are irregular and don't follow any specific pattern.
- They do not get more intense.
- They are felt more in the abdomen than in the uterus.
- They decrease in intensity with walking or a change in posture.
- They go away after a few hours.

Real labor contractions are regular, don't lessen no matter how much you walk around or change position and get more intense as time goes by.

If your contractions are more or less every five to ten minutes and last about a minute, it's most likely your baby is on the way. The frequency of the contractions and their duration aren't the same for all women. What's key is figuring out whether there's a pattern. To track your contractions, get out a pencil and paper and mark when each contraction begins and how long each one lasts, or ask your partner to write it down. Digital watches that include a stopwatch option are also helpful to track what's going on.

The chart below gives you an idea of how my contractions went during my last pregnancy. At first I thought I was going through another series of Braxton-Hicks contractions, but after writing down their frequency and duration, I saw the pattern. And when the pain started to get worse, there was no more doubt that my second child *estaba en camino*, was on the way.

Hour	Duration	Interval between contractions
10:43 A.M.	50 seconds	
10:52 A.M.	53 seconds	9 minutes
11:00 A.M.	30 seconds	8 minutes
11:07 A.M.	48 seconds	7 minutes
11:14 A.M.	30 seconds	7 minutes
11:23 A.M.	60 seconds	9 minutes
11:30 A.M.	70 seconds	7 minutes

By the time the next contraction came, I was on the phone with my husband telling him to hurry home. At ten that night, my daughter Patricia was born.

When you are in the middle of active labor, contractions will be every two to three minutes and will last for sixty seconds or more.

Even though you may not write down your contractions, it's possible your intuition, your sixth sense, is telling you something is going on. Still, if you're not sure and you want to be reassured, call your doctor or go to the hospital, especially if your due date is weeks away, if you're bleeding and if your water has been broken for hours. The worst that will happen is the hospital will tell you to go back home again. No one's going to think you're exaggerating your symptoms or that you're silly for not knowing when you're about to deliver.

WHEN TO GO TO THE HOSPITAL

You should go to the hospital when you think your labor has begun or when you notice the signs of labor. Your doctor or midwife may be able to tell you over the telephone how are you doing, but the only real way to know if you've begun to dilate and the baby is handling the contractions well is by doing an internal exam and listening to the baby's heartbeat. If you are not admitted, you can go back home or go for a walk.

Arriving at the Hospital

Generally, if you talk to your doctor ahead of time, pack your bag and pre-register, your arrival at the hospital could even be calm. Each hospital has a different routine, but this is more or less what you can expect:

- If you've got serious pain or you don't feel well, you'll be put in a wheelchair before you're taken to the maternity ward. If you've already registered, your husband can be with you the entire time. Otherwise, he'll have to stay behind to fill out the paperwork.

- At the maternity ward, you'll go to a room or an examination room. One of the nurses or doctors on duty will ask you how you feel, if your water has broken and the frequency and duration of your contractions, and he/she will check your blood pressure and make sure you are not retaining excess water. Then they'll likely fit you with a monitor to measure the strength and regularity of your contractions and determine how well the baby is tolerating them (see page 133). Most hospitals now have sonogram machines in the examining room. A sonogram can tell the doctor if there's enough amniotic fluid, the condition of the placenta, if the baby is coming feet first and its approximate weight. This information is vital for the doctor if you've had any complications during pregnancy. In addition to the sonogram, the doctor will also check to see how many centimeters your cervix has dilated. The norms are different from hospital to hospital, but you probably won't be admitted until your cervix has already dilated to three centimeters. If your cervix still isn't dilated enough and you don't want to go back home, you can walk around the hospital to see if dilation progresses, and the nurses can check you again after a while.

• If you have dilated three or more centimeters, you will be officially admitted to the hospital. You'll be given a gown to put on, and it's likely you will be hooked to a monitor to keep track of the contractions and the heartbeat of the baby. You'll also be given a plastic bracelet with your name on it; your husband or companion will get one too.

• Some hospitals routinely insert an intravenous catheter in each mother-to-be's hand to give her liquids so she doesn't get dehydrated during delivery and also to give her medicine quickly in case of an emergency.

• Unless you're about to deliver right away, it's possible your doctor won't be at the hospital yet. If the hospital you go to has an obstetrician/gynecologist and anesthesiologist on hand all the time, those doctors will see you until yours arrives. The on-duty anesthesiologist can give you an epidural as soon as it's been authorized. At hospitals that don't have an obstetrician/gynecologist or an anesthesiologist on duty all the time, the nurses will take care of you and you'll have to wait until the on-call anesthesiologist arrives for an epidural if you want one.

These and other procedures are common in many hospitals. But you can ask if they'll change some of them. It's easier for them to accommodate your wishes if you have already spoken with your obstetrician/gynecologist or the head nurse or if you've prepared a birth plan.

• If you want to move around and you're not relegated to bed rest, it may be possible to have your contractions monitored at intervals. When you are connected to the monitor you will not be able to walk. But some hospitals are using cordless monitors that allow you to move around freely (see page 297) while your contractions and your baby's heart rate are being monitored.

- You can walk around with the intravenous catheter because the fluid bag is hung from a metal post on wheels. Another option is to choose a heparin lock. That means you'll have the catheter stuck in the back of your hand but you won't be constantly attached to the drip bag.

Depending on the nurse you get, your delivery may be more or less *agradable*, enjoyable. Even though this will be one of the most memorable and important days of your life, for the nurses who work on the maternity ward, this is just another delivery, one of hundreds they'll do every year, and as you know, we all have bad days at work. Try to establish a nice and friendly rapport with the nurses who are attending to you. But if you've gotten stuck with a disagreeable nurse who isn't in step with your wishes, tell your husband to talk to the head nurse or doctor about what's going on.

Be courteous but insist on having your wishes respected. However, *no se enoje*, don't get upset. You and your husband need all your energies to deliver your baby. The best way to avoid arguments and tension during delivery is to make sure ahead of time that the nurses are on the same page as you about your birthing plan. Visits and interviews ahead of time will help you get an idea of what can you expect on your delivery day.

Arriving at the Birthing Center

A midwife will take care of you at a birthing center. When you arrive, you'll be given an internal exam and the baby's heartbeat will be checked. Unless the birthing center is inside a hospital, it's unlikely the center will have a sonogram machine to see how the baby is positioned, the condition of the placenta, or the amount of amniotic fluid in your belly. Many centers have warm bathtubs you can get into as soon as you arrive if you like. The midwife will monitor the baby's heartbeat on a regular basis. Your family members can stay with you or they can wait in a room nearby.

LABOR PAIN

For the great majority of women, delivering a baby hurts—it hurts a lot. What to do about the pain is another matter, but the pain is for real. Many prenatal classes, videos, pamphlets and books will talk about "a lot of pressure," "strong contractions," or "intense sensations." And for many years, many prenatal classes were given under the heading "painless labor." The only problem with these descriptions is that when a woman feels pain during labor, she may think that she did something wrong, that she failed or that she's been tricked into thinking it was supposed to be easy.

The fact that labor hurts doesn't mean you have to suffer the unbearable pain some of your friends may have told you about. Fortunately, there are many ways for you to deal with the pain. Also, different women feel different amounts of pain depending on their physical condition, their mental state and their cultural background.

You're going to find yourself unpleasantly surprised if you haven't thought about what you want to do if the pain becomes really intense during delivery. Even if you've decided to use an epidural, that doesn't mean you're not going to feel anything. Here's why:

- Often you won't be given an epidural until you've dilated a few centimeters, and it may take hours for this to happen.

- Even though the doctor has authorized you to receive an epidural, the anesthesiologist may not be available immediately.

- If you ask for the epidural soon after you've completely dilated, you may not get one because the time for pushing is just around the corner.

- When the time to push arrives, the anesthesiologist will lower the amount of painkilling medicine you're receiving so you can better feel your pushing and the contractions.

- The epidural might not have any painkilling effect on you, or it may take on the left or right side of your body only.

You might consider the following points regarding pain. (Try writing your answers down on a piece of paper. It helps.)

- When something hurts, do you take some medicine right away to get rid of the pain, or do you wait for the pain to go away on its own? What is your tolerance for pain and how have you reacted when something really hurts you?

- How do your surroundings affect you when you're in pain? Do you prefer to be alone or to be with others? Would you rather sit in silence no matter who's around? During delivery, you're going to have several people nearby. How will you feel with people coming and going from the delivery room? For some women privacy during delivery is important.

- What do you think of women who scream during delivery? Will you care what others think if you shout in pain? This has a lot to do with how your family deals with pain. In general, we Latinos are more expressive than other cultures. Still, in your family, *los gritos,* a lot of screaming may be interpreted as hysterics or an exaggerated reaction. If your idea of delivery is a woman in control but you can't help screaming, you might feel tense or embarrassed.

- Will you think you're less of a woman if you use an epidural? Our grandmothers and some of our mothers didn't have many options when they gave birth. In some families, the woman who delivers a baby without anesthesia is seen as more valiant. Perhaps you want an epidural as soon as possible, but does that match up with what your family thinks?

- How do you imagine your delivery will go? How will you manage the pain of contractions (even if you're choosing to have an epidural)? Do you see yourself doing your breathing exercises? Do you see yourself just putting up with the pain by yourself? Are you even thinking about pain at all?

After answering the previous questions, you may have discovered your idea of delivery and your true reaction to pain are different. If you haven't thought about it at all, try to imagine at least how you'll respond to the pain. Maybe you don't want to think about it because it scares you.

- Have you chosen the people who will help you during your delivery? Your mother? Sister? Relatives? A doula? What kind of relationship do you have with them? How do they react when you suffer? Some studies show that women who have another woman to rely upon during delivery have an easier time. Birth is a moment when many women feel very vulnerable. The person who is supporting you can help you feel better, especially if you both agree what type of support you need. For example, if you want to try a delivery without an epidural but your mother can't bear to see you suffer, she's not going to give you much support when the contractions begin. And if the reverse is true—you want an epidural and your mother doesn't think it's a good idea—the delivery can be even more tense. Some women choose a doula (see page 235) because she's a professional.

• How will your partner help you during delivery? Some studies show that a husband, even if he is *un amor*, a really sweet one, doesn't provide the same quality of support as a woman who has had children herself. Talk to your partner about what you expect of him during delivery. He may have a completely different picture in his head. Many men are great at providing emotional support, but it's difficult for them to understand exactly what's happening and what you're feeling because they have never delivered a baby.

• Will you appreciate or be annoyed by people shouting encouragement at you during the final pushes before birth? In many hospitals, it's customary for a cheerleader team of nurses and family members to encourage the mother to push. Even though this may be done with all the best intentions, some women can't stand the idea of a group of people standing over her and shouting, "Push!" "Push!" "Push!" How would you feel in that situation? Tell your doctor, your husband and your family members what they should do.

How Much and Why Does Labor Hurt?

Answering the previous questions will have given you some ideas of how you'll react to labor pain. Still, if you haven't had children, it's difficult to imagine. Below some Latina mothers describe their labors.

"It's like a menstrual cramp but many times stronger. It starts in your back and it moves forward and down. It's a kind of pain that it doesn't go away no matter what."

"As if someone were cracking my bones. *Es un dolor del diablo*, a very strong pain, a pulsating pain that gets in this place and you can't seem to get rid of, no matter how much you squirm or move around."

"I cannot describe it. It's like an extreme menstrual pain, very, very, strong. *Te duele la espalda que no lo soportas*, you can't stand how your back hurts."

"Very strong and intense. I was able to *aguantar*, to take it, because the contractions didn't last for hours."

"The pain was strong and intense. I had like thirty minutes of that but *se hace eterno*, it lasted an eternity."

Why Does Labor Hurt?

To understand why labor hurts, think of a blown-up balloon stuck all the way into the end of a sock. The long part of the sock that goes up your leg above the ankle is the cervix when it's closed. But for the balloon to come out, the sock has to stretch and open up. That's what your cervix does during labor. You can also think of a lightbulb and an empty glass. Your uterus is shaped like a lightbulb, and during labor it has to take on the shape of a glass. At the beginning of labor, the narrowest part of the lightbulb is the cervix. For the baby to pass out completely, the cervix has to open like a glass.

The uterus is a muscle made up of long fibers that run from the cervix upward. During contractions, these fibers pull the cervix and stretch it until it is opened. The muscle fibers of the uterus are connected to nerves that feel those contractions—like when you feel a leg cramp, only in your uterus. The contractions continue for hours and usually get more intense as time goes by.

Stages of Labor

Labor is divided into various stages, depending on what your uterus is doing at each moment. The stages of labor are like a map professionals use to monitor where you are and how much further you have to go.

- *First stage.* The cervix goes from being long and closed to thinning out and opening completely so the baby can come out. The cervix is slowly opening thanks to the contractions, which continue to get more and more intense as the hours go by. There are several periods in this stage:

  * The cervix effaces or thins out and then opens two to four centimeters. This is called the latent phase. If you look at the illustration on page 278 you'll see that the thickness of the cervix has to "flatten" in order for the opening to start separating. This period can begin days before delivery and may not be painful. Or it can happen right before birth with sensations that range from bothersome to painful.

* The contractions become more intense and more frequent. This is called the active phase. It's the most rapid period of dilation; the cervix could open up to seven centimeters in a matter of hours. Halfway through this period is when women usually ask for an epidural or other pain reliever.

* The last period of dilation is called the transition. This is the most difficult one because the contractions are powerful and they come almost on top of each other. This period doesn't last very long—about an hour. The epidural isn't usually given at this stage because it's about time to begin pushing.

When this stage goes on for too long, it might mean the baby is too big. This condition is called dystocia or "failure to progress." It's one of the more common reasons for having a cesarean.

Cervix dilation

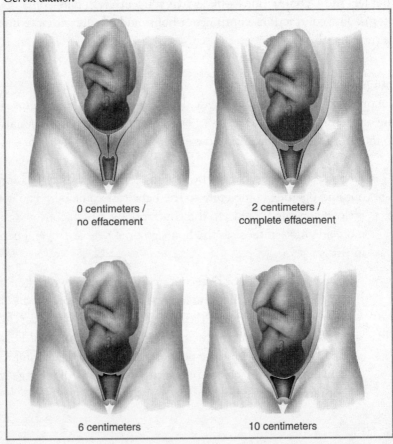

0 centimeters /
no effacement

2 centimeters /
complete effacement

6 centimeters

10 centimeters

- *Second stage*. This is when the baby is born. It goes from ten centimeters to the delivery of the baby. The contractions are long and powerful but they might be less painful. Now you can begin pushing on each contraction. This stage can last a few minutes or a few hours. Sometimes, even though the doctor can see the baby's head (it's crowning), the rest of the baby just won't come out. Doctors can choose to use forceps or a vacuum to help things along. In some births, the baby's head comes out first but a shoulder will get stuck on the pubic bone. That requires a special maneuver to get the baby out.

- *Third stage*. This is the period it takes for the placenta to come out once the baby is delivered. You will still feel contractions, but they're much softer. They help the placenta detach from the wall of the uterus and come out. It's very important that the entire placenta be expelled from the uterus. Any pieces left inside may cause an infection. Sometimes the obstetrician/gynecologist will pull it out by gently tugging on the umbilical cord. In this stage doctors make sure that you are not bleeding too much because there is an open wound on the inside of the uterus, where the placenta was. There are some rare situations where the mother can bleed a lot, such as when the placenta will not come out (placenta accreta) or when the whole uterus turns inside out (inverted uterus). Neither of these conditions is common, but they need immediate medical attention.

If this is your first baby, your labor may run from eighteen to twenty-four hours. On average, first-time mothers dilate 1.2 centimeters each hour. Women who have previously had children dilate 1.5 centimeters an hour.

YOUR STAGES OF LABOR

Has It Really Started or Is It Something I Ate?
If this is your first pregnancy, you're not going to have anything to compare what you're feeling to. You could feel some of the symptoms described on page 268, but you might not know if your labor has started.

"Around one or two in the morning, I thought my stomach was upset from one of the desserts I'd eaten at a party earlier that evening. *Me sentía inquieta*, I was unsettled. The doctor assured me: 'You'll know when it starts.' That was not true; I had no idea. My mother woke up and asked me: 'What's the matter? You're going to the bathroom a lot. Lie down with me and let's count.' And sure enough, that was it."

—*Laura García*

"At night I started to feel this back pain. It was so uncomfortable. I turned to one side, then to the other. I couldn't sleep. I made myself a tea, but it was not happening. I couldn't sleep."

—*Sandra Hernández*

Mi Amor, It's Time to Go to the Hospital

At this point you have no doubt something is happening. The contractions could still be light, and you might be wondering whether it's time to go to the hospital.

"I'd always heard it was better to stay at home for as long as possible because there's a greater chance of cesarean if you haven't dilated much right when you arrive at the hospital. *Así que, aguanté toda la noche*, I held out all night long, and we didn't go the hospital until the next morning. When I arrived, they asked me: 'Why didn't you come sooner?' "

—*Elena Nelson*

"I drove four times to the hospital and three of them I was sent back home. We drove there, they put me in a wheelchair, gave me an internal exam and sent me home. I was having pains but as soon as I saw the Emergency sign, *se me quitaba todo*, everything disappeared. I was scared I would not make it on time."

—*María Teresa Díaz-Blanco*

"I didn't want to go to the hospital too soon, but it got to a point where all I was doing was walking around and I was not feeling better. My husband told me: *estás muy mal*, you are not doing well, so we went to the hospital and my baby was born a couple of hours later."

—*Gloria Villalobos*

AT THE HOSPITAL

Many women are disappointed when they arrive at the hospital only to find out they haven't even dilated three centimeters.

"I was crossing my legs in the car because *yo juraba que se me salía el niño*, I could swear the baby was coming out. I was screaming like crazy. They checked me and they told me I was not dilated at all."

—*Ana María Caldas*

"I arrived at the hospital in the morning after spending all night turning around, taking baths and reading newspapers. They gave me an internal and said, 'You are not there yet, go back home.' I said, 'I can't go back home!' So they sent me to walk."

—*Nhora Estella Gómez-Saxon*

The Pain

Once labor has started, the pain and intensity of contractions grow. If you want an epidural, it is given generally after three centimeters of dilation. Any sooner and it could slow down the contractions. This is when the support of another woman or your partner comes in very handy.

"I had my husband's support and a doula. We had both taken prenatal classes. It was a very strong pain but I was thinking that it was normal; it was not the pain of being sick and it was not constant, *iba y venía*, it came and went. With each contraction they applied pressure to my back and my husband helped me remember it was only a temporary pain and that I was able to control it."

—*Gloria Villalobos*

"I was told about the many supposed disadvantages of an epidural, and how wonderful it was to give birth naturally. I thought, *listo, lo tengo natural*, I will have a natural delivery. I handled it up until I reached four centimeters and then the pain was unbearable. *Grité hasta que me cansé.* I screamed until I couldn't anymore. And when I finally gave in and asked for an epidural, it was too late."

—*Laura García*

"I was amazed at how well I handled the pain. Sure, it hit me hard, but it wasn't all that bad. You just deal with it. At the moment of truth, I guess God gives you the strength to make it through the pain."

—*Leticia Gómez*

"After all the stories I'd heard, I imagined that I was going to feel some pain, but when those contractions started to get stronger, the only thing in my mind was, how far does this pain have to go before they give me *la bendita epidural*, the blessed epidural? I just couldn't believe that I had to go through that because I wanted an epidural from the very beginning."

—Julie Ferrer

Before Pushing

If you've been given an epidural, they will reduce the dosage so you can feel your muscles and begin pushing. If you are having a natural labor, you may go through a difficult stage now. The final centimeters of dilation happen when you're most tired. In this stage you may feel like quitting and going home, or you may say some pretty irrational things.

> "I was always told I'd know when it was time to start pushing. What a lie. I had no idea, and what I really wanted to do was *levantarme y salir corriendo*, get up and run away. No one ever said that was the sign to begin pushing."
>
> —Margarita Gaviria

Pushing

Some women worry that when they start pushing out the baby, feces will come out too. Sometimes that happens, but if that's the case you probably won't notice and a nurse is there to clean it up right away.

> "From one moment to the next I had this urge to push. I thought that I wanted to go to the bathroom and I thought, 'Oh my God, the last thing I need now is poop *con todas estas viejas encima mío*, with all these women on top of me!' But then I though this must be the *pujadera*, the pushing urge."
>
> —Nhora Estella Gómez-Saxon

> "I dilated from six to ten centimeters in no time. I was already feeling the urge to push, but the nurse told me not to until the doctor arrived. *Tenía que pujar como fuera*, I needed to push so badly, I just needed to push. When I saw her coming and putting the mask on I just pushed like there was no tomorrow. I let it all out. He came out like a football."
>
> —Leticia Gómez

> "The nurse told me, 'I can see his hair,' and I forgot all my pain. I pushed three times. I was feeling the pain but it didn't hurt because the moment of meeting my baby had arrived."
>
> —Teresa Díaz-Blanco

The Baby Comes Out

When the baby comes out, it can burn a little for a few moments. Make sure your doctor knows if you want him/her to give you a cut in the tissue surrounding the vagina (episiotomy) or not (see page 319).

Baby delivery

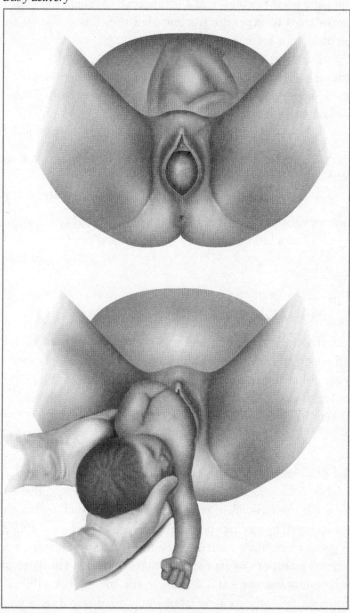

"When my baby came out I didn't feel any pain. The feeling was like a wet fish slipping out of your hands. The doctor cut me, but I didn't think it would have been necessary."

—*Lorena Asbell*

My Bebé

Once the baby is born, you'll feel a great sense of relief. You'll still have some contractions to expel the placenta, but they'll be a distant thought once you have your baby in your arms.

"It was such a relief. I didn't have to do it anymore, there was not going to be more pain, and on top of that, my baby was born. They put him on my belly. It was such a joy."

—*Gloria Villalobos*

"It was such a relief when the baby came out. I had him in my arms while they stitched me up."

—*Leticia Gómez*

"When my baby was born, I didn't hurt anymore. I didn't feel a thing, only that I had a lot of energy and was full of joy."

—*Laura García*

MANAGING LABOR PAIN NATURALLY

The ideas that follow are physical and mental techniques to help you make it through labor without medication. Even if you've planned on using an epidural at the first sign of pain, these techniques will help you in case the anesthesiologist doesn't arrive right away, the epidural takes a while to kick in, or the dose is reduced so you can push.

Practice

The basic principle of all these exercises is relaxation and practice. The pain of labor is caused by the contractions of the muscle fibers of the uterus. If the other muscles in your body are tense, you'll feel even more pain because you'll be forcing your uterus to work against a resistance. Your uterus is going to contract no matter what, because unless you have a cesarean, there's no other way for the baby to come out. So the more you can work with your uterus instead of against it, the easier labor will be.

Of course, that's all easy to say, but the normal response to pain is to tense up. That's why the secret to the success of these relaxation techniques is practice. The exercises that you'll read about seem very simple and even a little boring because there's no real way to replicate what a labor contraction is like. That's what happened to me during my first pregnancy. After going to prenatal classes and practicing the breathing exercises three or four times, I was convinced I knew what I was doing. But, *me esperaba una sorpresa,* boy, was I in for a surprise. When the stronger contractions started, one after another, the breathing techniques didn't help me a bit. Neither did the instructions my midwife or my husband gave me. My body was totally tense, and my mind fixated on the pain and when each contraction was going to end. By the time one contraction ended, I was already tense thinking of the next one.

If you want to avoid this situation, you should practice your relaxation techniques as often as possible. That's the only way they'll be of any use when you need them. But not all women relax in the same way. You should search for a method or a combination of methods that works for you. Try to recall what you did in the past to relax yourself and to ease pain. For example, the next time you get a headache or your back hurts or you feel tense or any other discomfort of pregnancy, try a different technique and see what works. Yoga classes can teach you to relax in very uncomfortable positions.

In the end, make sure you've got a relaxing environment to go to when you begin labor. Soft lights, silence and a comfortable room temperature will help you create a relaxing environment.

Breathing

One of the body's first responses to pain and fear is shortness of breath. When we breathe quickly, in short breaths, it's a message to our bodies that something isn't right, that it's time to go into fight-or-flight mode. Your heartbeat accelerates, your blood pressure goes up, and your blood goes to your arms and legs, which have also tensed up in case you have to run away. This reaction is one we've developed over millions and millions of years of evolution, to escape predators. Good then, not so good during labor. That combination of reactions will not help you because, on one hand, a tense muscle hurts more than a relaxed one, and on the other, the baby needs oxygen and must get it from blood in your uterus, not in your arms and legs.

But there's a way to trick your body so it doesn't resort to its instinctive reactions. If we breathe deeply and calmly, the body thinks everything's okay and the tension disappears. That's why all those prenatal classes put so much emphasis on breathing.

Take air in through your nose slowly, concentrating on how it's filling up your lungs and expanding your abdomen. Then let the air out slowly through your mouth, focusing on that alone. Push aside all other thoughts from your mind and put all your attention on how the air enters and leaves your lungs. Your body will relax and the pain, although still there, moves to the background. While you breathe out, you may choose to use sounds or other mental techniques explained below.

Sounds

The Latino culture is much more vocal than others. You only have to go into a Latino restaurant at lunchtime to figure that out: We talk joyfully, passionately discuss last night's soccer game, wave our hands around wildly. All that with a healthy dose of Latin music blaring in the background. The expression of pain is also more vocal in Latino cultures. *Llorar a gritos*, crying or screaming over the loss of a loved one, is common at burials.

So logically, during labor, we also express ourselves vocally. Modulating your voice along with the severity of each contraction is another technique that can help you to relax. In fact, this practice has its beginnings among our ancestors centuries ago. Practicing this technique can even be fun. First try to make long sounds by pronouncing vowels. The "a" is a good one because you have to open your mouth and throat wide in order for it to sound right. That will help you to relax. The "e" and the "i" also work because you don't have to close your lips as much as you would pronouncing "o" or "u." You can also try combining letters, using syllables or phrases or even howling like a wolf (I'm serious—this works for some women). The secret is not to shriek with your throat but to let the sound come from your abdomen as you exhale. These types of sounds are very common in martial arts to help release energy.

If you're giving birth in a hospital with non-Latino staff, some people may feel uncomfortable with this form of expression. In some cultures, pain is kept inside. Or the staff might worry that you'll upset other women delivering in rooms nearby. If you find yourself in those circumstances, you can do two things: Use a paper bag or other object that will help to minimize the volume of your sounds, taking it off when you need to breathe in; and/or hand out earplugs to all the assistants who are in the room with you. If you find this method helps you to relax and there aren't any other mothers nearby who might be getting upset, *haga oídos sordos*, just don't pay attention, and shout all you want. And if someone shouts with you, as a show of support, so much the better.

Visualization

These techniques work well when they're practiced along with slow and relaxed breathing. You can concentrate on a mental image during your contractions. Here are some images you may think of:

- How your cervix is opening up a little more with each contraction, or any other image of something opening slowly, such as a flower in bloom.
- How your baby is pushing little by little with its head, trying to get out.
- A place you'd like to go and all the details of that beautiful scenery.

You can also use a picture or drawing or photograph that you like to focus your thoughts upon. Just as with the breathing techniques, the key is being able to eliminate from your mind any other thoughts except the mental image.

Concentrating on the Pain

This is a difficult method, but for some people it works. The idea is to explore your own pain and concentrate on how the sensations change. You assign a color or image or sound to each feeling of pain. The pain of a contraction doesn't feel the same all the time. It changes in intensity and location. According to this theory, instead of avoiding the thought of pain altogether, you should focus on the details of the pain. That way you don't feel as much. Once again, the key is to put all your thoughts on the sensations you're feeling and not allow any other things to enter your mind. For example, you may think, "My uterus is contracting more on the right side than the left," or "Now I feel a sharp pain, kind of cold like the color blue," or "This feeling is warm and heavy like the color red." You should avoid thoughts such as *"No aguanto este dolor,* I can't stand the pain much more, because it keeps getting more intense," or "This is hurting more than before," or "I don't want to feel this anymore." Maybe this technique will work for a while, but then you may need to switch to another one.

Music

This is similar to the mental imaging technique, but instead of focusing on visual details, your mind concentrates on each sound in the melody. Soft music usually works. You can listen with headphones to isolate yourself even further from your environment. Listen to different types of music to see which ones help you to relax the most, or create your own labor tapes. This method can be combined with others.

Massage

For women who feel back pain during labor, putting pressure on that point or massaging it can help a lot. It's hard to know before labor begins which type of massage will work best or even if you want anyone to touch you at all. Still, it's a good idea to practice ahead of time with your husband or the person you've chosen to be with you during delivery. Massages during pregnancy feel wonderful. Intense pressure during labor helps better than soft massage. You can also give the massage using warm compresses or bags of ice. It all depends on what works best for you. Take a cream or oil with you to the hospital so the massager's hands slide more smoothly over your skin.

Muscle Relaxation

In this exercise, your mind concentrates on each individual muscle in the body. You should find a posture in which no muscle feels tense. Begin with a toe. Feel how that toe is so relaxed, it's as though it's floating. Imagine all the tension evaporating from that area of your body. From there, continue with the entire foot, your calf muscle and your thigh. Then go to the next toe and do the same thing. Some stores sell muscle relaxation tapes where a voice will tell you which body part comes next and how to relax. You can also make your own tape to listen to during labor.

Water

Water is a wonderful thing during delivery because it helps muscles to relax in a natural way. Floating in a tub or taking a warm bath can help a lot if you get really tense during labor. If you're going to deliver in a birthing center, they're sure to have a tub you can get into. Some hospitals that don't have tubs will allow you to rent one. Once you're in the water, you may find it's easier to practice the other relaxation techniques. Some headphones are waterproof, so you can listen to music while you're soaking.

Labor Positions

Pain during delivery helps us figure out which position is best. Move around and try different positions during delivery. Not only it will help you relax, it will help labor progress. The force of gravity is one of the best aids when you're trying to get the cervix to dilate and get the baby to descend.

If you're giving birth in a hospital, you'll be able to move as long as they haven't given you an epidural or connected you to a monitor. Lying down on your back in a bed is

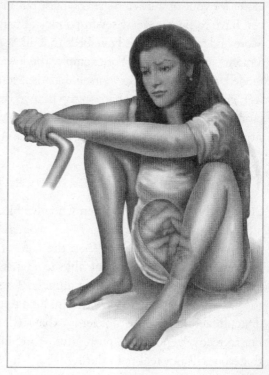

Delivery position: squatting

Delivery position: sitting

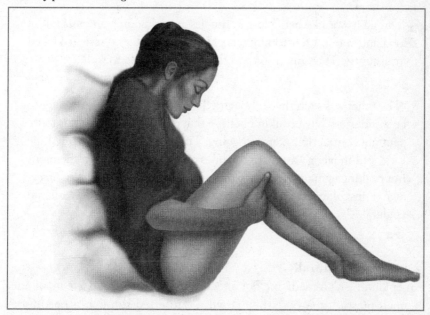

easier for your obstetrician/gynecologist but more difficult for you because you have to push at least seven pounds of baby uphill for it to come out. More and more hospitals have beds that allow a mother-to-be to deliver in a more natural position. For example, the lower part of the bed can be extended, and you can prop yourself up. Also, you have platforms to rest your feet, and some beds have bars on top that you can hold on to if you wish to push while you squat. Ask around and talk to your doctor about which positions are possible when you go into labor.

THE EPIDURAL

Six to eight of every ten women who give birth in a hospital use epidural anesthesia to ease labor pain. Many women don't even imagine giving birth without an epidural. When the pain of the contractions starts increasing and a woman is not able to manage it by other methods, an epidural is the closest thing to a miracle. A few babies have the name of the anesthesiologist who gave the epidural to their mothers. In a long and difficult labor, when the mother is exhausted, this can be the only way for her to recover enough to push later. An epidural is not a total warranty that you will not feel pain during labor, and sometimes it can have side effects. However, an epidural can turn a nightmare of a labor into a wonderful experience in a matter of minutes.

"For me it was like being lost in the desert and finding an oasis full of food and water. I felt totally relaxed and I was able to rest. It kicked in instantly. The only thing was that I was not able to walk."
—*Laura Loustau*

"The relief was such that I thought, 'From now on this is just going to be wonderful!' I just couldn't believe that after feeling such an intense pain my contractions kept on going. The only thing that assured me I was still in labor was to see the lines on the paper sheet in the monitor peaking up like crazy. I saw them and thought, '*No me quiero imaginar*, I just don't want to imagine how would this be without an epidural.'"
—*Julie Ferrer*

What Is an Epidural?
An epidural isn't a medicine but a technique for giving you the medicine. A small plastic tube (a catheter) will be inserted through a needle be-

tween the vertebrae in your spine. The catheter goes into the space surrounding one of the layers of your spinal column.

Through that catheter, the doctor can administer anesthetics, analgesics or both. Anesthetics eliminate all feeling in the area, just as when
the dentist gives you a shot in your mouth. You don't feel a thing for a
while. Analgesics only eliminate pain; you remain able to move your
body parts, and you will still have feeling in that area. It's like when you
take an aspirin to get rid of a headache.

Anesthetics are the drugs that keep you from feeling your legs and the
rest of your lower body. That's why the dosage of anesthetics has to be reduced when you begin to push the baby out. Today, many hospitals use a
combination of anesthetics and analgesics, which allow you to still feel
the muscles in your lower body without pain. These combinations are
called "walking epidurals," even though you don't really walk around
much because you're connected to a bunch of machines.

The medicine is pushed through the tube by a pump that gives you a
constant dosage during labor; they give you a new dose every time you
need it, or you can regulate how much you get depending on how much
you hurt.

Epidural

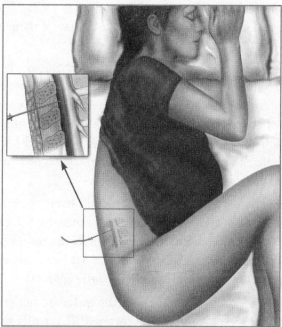

What Does an Epidural Feel Like?

The anesthesiologist is the doctor who will give you the epidural at the hospital. To open the space in your spine to insert the needle, you may have to lean forward. Generally, the needle is inserted while you're sitting down on the bed, bending forward while someone supports you. Your back will first be disinfected, and they might apply a local anesthetic, too. When the needle goes in, you'll feel a prick, like when blood is taken from your arm. When the catheter is pushed through the needle you will feel not pain but pressure. The epidural can be bothersome, but it's a lot less inconvenient than a strong contraction. You'll begin to feel gradually less pain in ten to twenty minutes, accompanied by a heavy feeling in your legs. At this point, the contractions will feel more like pressure than pain.

Nine of ten women feel a great relief, although in some cases the epidural doesn't have any painkilling effect or it may work on only one side. In these situations the other pain control methods will help you.

The doctor will usually wait until you've dilated three or four centimeters before administering the epidural because the drugs slow down the progression of labor. When a cesarean is done, the anesthesia is pumped through the same catheter as the epidural.

Possible Complications

In some cases, the epidural causes side effects. Some of them are:

- *Headaches.* These happen frequently and are caused when the needle makes a small hole in the layer that covers the spinal column. The liquid that's inside escapes and may cause a strong headache that can last for several days. When this happens, sometimes the doctor will inject some of the mother's own blood back into the space where the spinal fluid is leaking, to try to create a plug when the blood coagulates.

- *Back pain.* Some women say the epidural hurts their backs, right where the needle went in—sometimes for months. Still, the women who don't use an epidural also say their backs hurt after delivery. Several studies done on the subject have not been able to prove any significant increase in back pain due to the epidural.

- *Fever.* No one knows why, but sometimes the mother's temperature will rise after the epidural is administered. This really isn't good for the baby and can require tests and monitoring and even other types of procedures to make sure the baby doesn't have an infection.

- *Low blood pressure.* Because the veins are relaxed with the epidural, blood pressure drops. This is dangerous for the baby because it means less blood and therefore less oxygen is reaching the placenta. It's easy to treat by increasing the fluids given to the mother.

- *Length of labor.* Many studies have been done to investigate the relationship between cesarean deliveries and epidurals, but there is no agreement. Some studies say that women who get an epidural have a greater chance of the delivery ending in a cesarean, and others say that's not the case.

- *Effects on the baby.* Some of the medicine that is given in the epidural reaches the baby. Although it doesn't have as strong an effect on the baby as it does you, it's possible the baby will be less alert when it's born. In some cases, the baby can have trouble breastfeeding right after birth.

Other drugs are also used to deal with the pain of labor, though they're not as effective. But they can make the pain less intense and help the mother to relax.

THE LATINO FAMILY DURING BIRTH

We Latino families like to attend the births of our relatives and be near our loved ones as the family grows. Your hospital may have a limit on the number of people who are allowed in the delivery room with you. Some of your relatives may have to wait outside. Maybe even the number of people who can be at the hospital is limited. Make sure you know how many people are allowed and where before you show up at the hospital with the entire clan. Plan the role each person is going to have. If your mother or husband will be helping you during labor, make sure another family member is in charge of going outside the delivery room to tell the people waiting there. Also, you may set up a visit rotation, where people come and go in turns, but make sure they know you might not be in the mood for *plática* or chatting.

Your Support Person
Among Latina women, it is common for our mothers, mothers-in-law or other women in the family to be the ones helping us breathe and relax

during labor. Other times this person will be your husband or partner. Before labor begins, talk to the people who will support you about how you want to try to manage the pain and what your preferences are.

If for some reason you can't find a member of your family to be your support person, consider hiring a doula (see page 235). Even though your husband is going to be with you, the assistance of a professional doula will be a great help. Many doulas still in training don't charge for their services.

FOR DAD

It may seem unbelievable after all these months, but you're about to get to know your baby!

You may not know how to react when you see your wife in pain, or you may feel responsible for all she's going through. But you're not alone. Many fathers feel the same things. Maybe you will be confused because one moment your wife may not want you to leave her side and the next she won't want you to touch her. Just this once, do what she says and don't take it personally. She knows what she needs at each turn.

You should also do what makes you feel comfortable. Some Latino men offer comfort to their wives during labor in ways that aren't expected by the hospital employees. According to a study, Latino fathers-to-be speak in sweet terms to their wives during labor, and they take their hands and offer support. Perhaps the nurse in the delivery room expects you to give your wife a massage or help her with her breathing exercises or something else you may not feel comfortable with. Tell the nurse that in our culture, things are done differently. The woman who's helping your partner can be responsible for the breathing exercises and the massages during contractions.

If you want to play a more active role in the labor, don't look at your mother-in-law or a doula as someone who's getting in the way of you and your wife's special moment. The support you can offer to your partner is something no one else can provide. Just fulfill her needs and be a guardian. Make sure there aren't too many people in the delivery room and that the birth plan both of you have written up is followed.

Emergency Labor

Babies born in cars and elevators aren't all that common, but sometimes it happens. If you find yourself in this situation, remember to do these things:

1. Put the mother in a position she finds comfortable. Lay some clean towels or at least some clothes underneath her. Don't put her on the edge of a bed or a place where the baby might fall once it's been delivered; newborn babies are really slippery and can be difficult to hold on to.

2. Call 911 or the emergency services unit in your area. If you can, put your telephone on speaker mode so the person who's on the other end of the line can give you instructions clearly and you can follow them with both hands free.

3. Let the mother push when she wants; don't pressure her. When the head of the baby appears, *do not* pull on it. Instead, support the head and let it come out on its own. If the water hasn't broken, puncture the amniotic sac yourself with your fingers or something pointy. Be careful not to hurt the baby. If the umbilical cord is wrapped around the baby's neck, stick a finger underneath it and lift it over the baby's head.

4. Support the head while the shoulders and arms come out and then the rest of the body. The baby should begin to breathe on its own. However, if the baby is blue, massage his/her back. If there is still no breathing, give mouth-to-mouth resuscitation.

5. Tie off the umbilical cord with a strip of clean cloth; if you've got nothing else, a shoelace will do. The knot should be about 3 inches (7 or 8 centimeters) from the baby's belly button. *Don't* pull on the umbilical cord to get the placenta to come out of the mother. The placenta will be expelled on its own five to twenty minutes after delivery. Save it if you can so the doctor can inspect it. Don't cut the umbilical cord.

6. Once the baby's out give it to the mother and cover them both with a blanket or clothes. Don't pull on the cord. Wait until help arrives.

Medical Interventions

The debate has been going on for years between those who say birth is a natural process that doesn't require medical intervention and those who say modern delivery technology saves babies and should be used whenever possible, including cesarean deliveries. I think both sides have their points. On the one hand, pregnancy isn't an illness and the human race has progressed through thousands of years without internal fetal monitors and cesarean deliveries. On the other, just a few decades ago babies and mothers could die during delivery because our modern technology was not available yet.

However, there is a medical intervention that has grown out of proportion. The United States has more cesarean deliveries than any other country in the world. Nearly one in every four women who has a baby in this country delivers via cesarean. The United States is also the country where more people sue their doctors for malpractice than anywhere else.

Lawsuits are a serious problem for doctors in the United States. It's changing the way they practice medicine. When an obstetrician/gynecologist ends up facing a judge or a jury, he/she will have to prove that the best care possible was given. And today, that means the doctor used whatever technology was available at the time.

One example of this mind-set is the practice of performing a cesarean delivery the moment an irregular heartbeat is detected in the baby. Even though this has caused the number of cesarean deliveries to skyrocket, the number of babies born with symptoms of cerebral palsy (caused by a lack of oxygen to the brain during delivery) hasn't gone down. Still, an obstetrician/gynecologist can say that everything possible was done to protect the baby's health if he/she used all the technology available and performed a cesarean.

With problem pregnancies, there's no doubt medical interventions save lives. But with pregnancies that are going according to plan, the intervention of a doctor may only complicate the natural birthing process. For example, if your doctor thinks labor is going too slowly, you may be given Pitocin. That means you'll also have to be fitted with a monitor to see how the baby is reacting, and you'll be confined to a bed. Perhaps the pain is a little too much for you to handle, and then you'll have to be given an epidural. When you get an epidural, it may be difficult for you to urinate, and a catheter will be inserted in your bladder for that. Or with the epidural, you may not be able to push as well and the baby will have to be pulled out with forceps or suction. Or the delivery may be slowed down even further with the epidural and after several hours your doctor may decide a cesarean is necessary. After delivery, the baby might not be as alert due to the epidural and it will be difficult to start breastfeeding. It's important to note that this chain of events doesn't happen in all cases, and there are millions of women who have had happy deliveries and healthy babies thanks to Pitocin, epidurals, monitors and all the rest.

The important thing is to have a clear idea of what you want during your labor and what you can expect of your doctor and your hospital. The more information you have about how your doctor delivers babies and what the policies are of the hospital where you're going to give birth, the less likely it is you'll be surprised about what happens on delivery day. Ask as many questions as possible ahead of time, and keep in mind that if there's something you don't like, you may be able to change hospitals or doctors, even at the last minute.

MONITORING CONTRACTIONS AND THE BABY'S HEARTBEAT

During labor, doctors and midwives keep an eye on how the baby and mother are doing by monitoring the baby's heartbeat and the duration and intensity of the mother's contractions. Doctors can use a variety of machines to listen to the baby's heartbeat. One of them you're familiar with, the Doppler; it's the same machine the doctor used during your prenatal visits. Internal and external monitors register the baby's heartbeat on a piece of paper. Doctors review the results to see if the baby's heart rhythm is going up (acceleration) or going down (deceleration). An acceleration is a good sign. That means the baby's heart is reacting to movement, just as your heart rate goes up when you exercise or do any other activity. During labor, the baby's heartbeat will go up and down. This is normal. But if the baby's heart rate goes below 90 beats a minute, doctors will begin to worry something's not right.

Fetal monitors are great for detecting a healthy baby's heartbeat. They're not so precise when it comes to figuring out whether anything really is the matter with the baby. Sometimes the baby's heart rate goes down, or decelerates, and the doctor will decide to do an emergency cesarean. But after all that, the baby ends up being just fine; nothing was ever wrong. However, other babies have been saved by an emergency cesarean after an abnormal reading. Talk to your doctor about what will be done if your baby's readings aren't normal.

Other monitors keep track of the duration and intensity of your contractions to make sure they're effective and are dilating the cervix.

External Fetal Monitor

This device measures the intensity of the contractions and the baby's heart rate. The goal is to see just how the baby responds to the contractions. The monitor uses two straps or belts placed around your belly (see figure on page 133). One of them keeps track of the contractions, the other the beats of the baby's heart. It's very important that it be placed right. The external monitor isn't as precise as an internal monitor (described below), because the heartbeats are measured through an ultrasound. Sometimes the ultrasound can mistake the mother's heartbeat for the baby's or will only pick up portions of the baby's beat.

If you want to move around or walk during contractions, you can ask to be monitored only for twenty to thirty minutes every two hours to make sure everything is fine. Some hospitals are using newer equipment that measures the contractions and heartbeats with mobile monitors (telemetry). Those will let you move around while the monitoring goes on.

Internal Fetal Monitor

An internal monitor keeps track of the baby's heart rate. It consists of a very fine filament in the shape of a spiral that is inserted in the baby's scalp. It is connected to a cable that sends the cardiac rhythm to a machine. The internal monitor can be used only once the water has broken and there is enough dilation to be able to reach the baby's head. This device gives data on how the baby is responding to the contractions because it registers the cardiac rhythm directly. There is a small risk that the baby will develop an infection where the filament was inserted.

Some obstetricians/gynecologists use the internal monitors routinely, and others use them only in cases where there are problems that have to be looked at more closely. Ask your doctor when and how he/she uses them.

Intrauterine Catheter

This catheter is placed inside the uterus, between the baby's back and the uterine wall. It measures the force of the contractions on the baby. Sometimes even regular contractions aren't enough to dilate the cervix, and an external monitor using a strap around the mother's belly isn't precise enough to measure the force of the contractions.

When the contractions press on the umbilical cord, it could cut off the supply of oxygen to the baby. In those cases, an obstetrician/gynecologist can inject a saline solution into the uterus through this catheter. The saline acts like a pillow that reduces the pressure and allows labor to continue.

INDUCED LABOR

A hormone called oxytocin produces the uterine contractions. The artificial equivalent of this hormone is called Pitocin. This substance can be given to the mother intravenously to speed up delivery. There are various reasons to induce labor. The most common are:

- Preeclampsia, diabetes, an irregular fetal heartbeat or other complications that could put your life or the baby's life in danger.

- A due date that's past. After week 42, the risk of complications for the baby rises, but it is common for the obstetrician/gynecologist to want to induce at 41 weeks, since the risks go up as the days go by.

- The mother wants to have the delivery coincide with the availability of a certain obstetrician/gynecologist, with the presence of family members or for other reasons. This type of induction is not encouraged by obstetricians/gynecologists but does occur.

The number of induced labors, especially those requested by mothers, has doubled in recent years. Some studies show that induced labors, especially in a first pregnancy, often result in a cesarean. Other studies show there is no increase in the likelihood of a cesarean. In either case, it's important you talk to your obstetrician/gynecologist about inducing labor so you know the risks it might have for you and for the baby.

How Labor Is Induced

The best way to induce labor is to make sure the cervix has thinned out sufficiently. Before it can begin to dilate, the cervix must get thinner (see page 278). The most common ways to make this happen are:

- *Stripping the membranes.* The obstetrician/gynecologist uses a finger to manually separate the amniotic sac from the uterus, reaching in through the cervix. That stimulates the thinning of the uterus and birth.

- *Vaginal gels or suppositories*. They contain prostaglandins, substances that help the uterus to soften up.

The degree of effacing or thinning of the cervix is measured in percentages. You'll be given a percentage of, say, 50 percent or 75 percent. One hundred percent is the maximum. The cervix can keep dilating as it thins. For example, the doctor may say you have dilated 1 centimeter and that your cervix has effaced by 50 percent.

Once the thinning of the cervix has begun, you'll be given an intravenous catheter to start you with the Pitocin. Along with the drip bag, the nurses will set up the fetal monitor (see page 133) to follow just how you are responding to the Pitocin and how the baby is responding to the contractions. The monitor measures the frequency of the contractions and the baby's heart rate.

What You Feel During Induced Labor

Induced contractions could be more difficult to tolerate than natural ones. When they're caused by artificial means, the rhythm and intensity can be stronger than normal. You will be connected to several monitoring devices, so you will not be able to walk around or change positions with as much freedom. Generally, in an induced labor an epidural is used only after the cervix has dilated to 4 centimeters. If it is given before that, the contractions won't be as strong and efficient.

Amniotomy or Artificial Amniotic Sac Break

Puncturing the amniotic sac the baby is floating in is a way to induce labor or hurry up one that seems to be taking too long. The procedure is called amniotomy. It's not painful for you or the baby. The obstetrician/gynecologist inserts a little hook through the cervix to break the sac. This is usually a successful way to speed things up because the baby's head can now push against the cervix. An amniotomy can also let the doctor see if there is any meconium in the amniotic fluid or insert an internal fetal monitor to determine if there are signs of fetal stress.

Amniotomy has some small risks. On occasion the umbilical cord can come out through the cervix and be compressed (prolapsed cord). This will cut off oxygen to the baby. There is also a risk of infection if the labor continues for many more hours, as once the sac is punctured, the baby is no longer protected from outside germs.

CESAREAN

A cesarean is a surgical operation where the doctor extracts the baby through a cut in the uterus. Just a few decades ago, the cesarean was an operation to be used only in emergencies, but today it's the most common surgery in the United States. There are many reasons why a cesarean is recommended:

- Insufficient or slow dilation of the cervix
- Irregular baby heart rate or other problems
- Previous cesarean sections
- The baby is too big or is positioned feet down or any other abnormal way
- Other reasons (placenta previa, twins or more, etc.)

We Latinas, especially the ones who develop gestational diabetes, have a greater chance of delivering a big baby, and such a baby might get stuck on its way out. Doctors will often recommend a cesarean to avoid this problem. Each obstetrician/gynecologist follows different standards when deciding whether to deliver a big baby by cesarean, but the following will give you an idea of when a C-section is recommended:

- 9 pounds (a little more than 4 kilograms): You'll likely be given a chance to deliver naturally
- 10 pounds (4.5 kilograms): You'll be offered the choice of having a cesarean
- 11 pounds (nearly 5 kilograms): The doctor will probably encourage you to have a cesarean

The baby's weight is determined before delivery through an ultrasound, but the reading isn't exact and could be a pound above or below what you're told. So unless the baby's weight is way off the charts, you'll likely be given the chance to try a vaginal delivery first.

How a Cesarean Is Done

The procedure is the same for planned and emergency cesareans with the exception that if it's an emergency cesarean, you may be given general anesthesia instead of an epidural to allow the doctors to intervene more quickly. If you're having a planned cesarean, you must not eat eight hours before surgery.

- *Preparation*. When you arrive at the hospital, you'll be given an intravenous catheter and have a blood test done. The nurses will outfit you with several devices that measure your blood pressure, pulse, the amount of oxygen in your blood and how the baby is doing. Once that's ready, you'll be given an epidural for the surgery. The doctor will also insert a catheter to empty your bladder. This catheter will be left in for twenty-four hours or more after the surgery. You will probably be shaven in the area where the cut is to be made.

- *Partner*. Most hospitals allow your husband or another person to be with you during the operation. This person will have to leave you for a few moments to put on a surgical gown. Then he/she will sit next to you as you lie on the operating table. There will be a curtain that separates you two from the doctor who's operating.

- *Surgery*. Before making any incisions, the doctor will pinch you to make sure you don't feel anything. If you do, you'll be given more anesthesia. Once the anesthesia takes effect, you should feel pressure as the baby comes out, nothing more. The cut is usually done horizontally and is made where the pubic hairline begins. After extracting the baby, the doctor will manually pull out the placenta, then sew up the uterus with stitches and the outside skin with staples. The stitches used to close the uterus are absorbed by the body and don't have to be removed.

- *Your bebé*. You'll probably hear your baby before seeing it. If all goes well, the nurse will let you see him or her for a moment, and then the baby will be taken to be evaluated and bathed. On your way back to your hospital room, you'll be given your baby back and you can begin breastfeeding if you want to.

- *After surgery*. You'll still have to have the catheter in the back of your hand until you can eat on your own. The pain medication will also be given through the catheter at first; later you can take pills for it. Don't forget to ask for medication if you hurt, because sometimes it is given only on demand. Your stay at the hospital will last three to four days if there aren't any complications. The staples will be removed before you go home.

Recovery

Recuperating from a cesarean birth takes longer compared with a vaginal delivery. That's because there's a deep injury to the abdomen that needs to heal. However, recovery is different for every woman. The first days you may feel pretty bad, especially when you try to stand up. If you plan to breastfeed your baby you will need all the help that you can get in those first weeks. The baby will probably want to eat every two to three hours. This won't give you much time to rest at the time when your body needs to recuperate. Try to rest as much as you can because the better you feel, the better care you'll take of your baby. It takes about six weeks before you begin to feel more or less as you did before the surgery. It may take several months more before you can regain a sense of feeling around the scar.

You should call the doctor if you suffer any of the symptoms explained on page 325 (When to Call the Doctor).

Emotions After a Cesarean

If you'd planned on a vaginal delivery and wanted to do everything in the most natural way possible, you may be sad after a cesarean. Some women feel as though they've failed by not delivering vaginally. Others feel as though the cesarean could have been avoided if only they'd done this or that during pregnancy. Still others *le agarran antipatía*, get angry with the obstetrician/gynecologist for ordering an unnecessary surgery when they could have given birth naturally. Others have the same feelings because the doctor made them go through the whole labor process only to give them a cesarean at the end anyway.

Those who are near to us can often ignore these feelings. After all, we've got a healthy baby, don't we? In particular, some men have a hard time understanding what there is to complain about when mother and child are healthy.

Of course we mothers are concerned about the health of our babies, and we are grateful everyone is doing well. Still, that doesn't mean we won't have feelings about what happened. Don't blame yourself. The cesarean wasn't your fault and there really wasn't much you could have done to avoid it. Cesareans are usually ordered based on circumstances you have no control over. Also, express your frustrations; try writing a letter to your husband or your doctor explaining just how you feel. You may never mail this letter, but writing down your feelings will help.

Vaginal Birth After a Cesarean (VBAC)

At one time, doctors thought that once a mother had delivered by cesarean, all future pregnancies had to be delivered the same way because
the scar on the uterus would rupture with the contractions of a vaginal
birth. Even though the controversy still rages, many doctors will allow a
mother to try a vaginal delivery if she's had a cesarean before. One thing
is for sure: Vaginal births are less risky, take less time to recover from and
are less painful. My first delivery was cesarean and my second one vaginal. The difference in recovery was *como del día a la noche*, like night and
day. It took me six weeks after the cesarean before I began to feel better.
After the vaginal delivery, I felt great after four days.

Vaginal birth after a cesarean isn't for all women or for all obstetri-
cians/gynecologists. Generally, if you fulfill the following characteristics,
you're a candidate:

- You're not suffering from the same physical condition that caused
  the cesarean the first time (your pelvis is too small, the baby's
  breeched, placenta previa, etc.).
- The incision made during your prior cesarean was not vertical but
  horizontal.
- You're delivering at a hospital capable of doing an emergency cesarean if the uterus does indeed rupture.

The risk of rupturing the uterus during a vaginal delivery after a cesarean birth is small (between 0.5 and 1 percent). And even if the uterus
does rupture, everything can still turn out fine if you are in a hospital.

Episiotomy

An episiotomy is a cut in the tissue around the vagina (called the perineum).

A few years ago the episiotomy was done routinely. But lately doctors
are performing the procedure much less. In general, episiotomy is used:

- When forceps or a vacuum is required
- When the head or the part that appears first is too big and the tissue will tear anyway

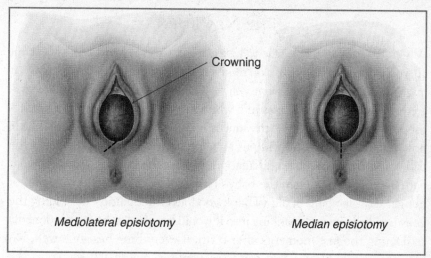

Mediolateral episiotomy · Crowning · Median episiotomy

Episiotomy

Some doctors feel that it's much easier to repair a clean cut compared to a ragged tear when the perineum rips by itself during delivery. Certain studies show the majority of episiotomies complicate things more than they help. Some of the disadvantages include:

- Creates more bleeding than a normal tear
- Bigger risk of infection
- Pain after delivery
- May produce pain during sex even after it has healed
- Could cause fecal incontinence because the perineum tissue has been weakened
- Can cause more tearing at the point of incision as the baby begins to come out

There are things you can do to make your perineum stronger before delivery to avoid tearing. Massage is the best way to get this tissue used to the pressure it will feel during delivery. First, wash your hands well. Using a little mineral oil, introduce your fingers into the vagina and apply pressure, stretching the tissues as far as they will go, as if the baby's head were coming out right now. Then massage the tissue, taking it between your thumb and forefinger. Don't press too hard. This area is delicate and you don't want to hurt yourself.

THE NEWBORN

When you see your baby, *se le va a olvidar todo*, you're going to forget about all you've been through. If you're given your baby as soon as it's born, it might not look quite like what you've imagined. Newborn babies are covered in mucus and sometimes in a white substance called vernix. The doctor or midwife will suck out the mucus from the baby's nostrils with a little nose pump. Then he/she will put a clamp on the umbilical cord near the belly button to stop blood circulation and cut the cord. If you wish, your partner can do this. Then the baby's back will be massaged to help him or her get that first gulp of air. (Thank goodness the tradition of holding the baby upside down and spanking it so it would breathe has been abandoned!)

During the first moments after birth, if everything has gone well, babies are usually alert. They can't see very far, but they'll see your face clearly when you hold them in your arms. Ask the nurse to let you hold your baby for a few moments before it is bathed. This first meeting is unforgettable for many parents.

Apgar Score

Soon after delivery, the nurse or midwife will give your baby an Apgar test. This determines just how alert the baby is, what color it is, its pulse and if it's breathing well. This test is repeated five minutes later. Zero, 1 or 2 points are given depending on how well the baby is responding in each one of these categories: Breathing, heart rhythm, color, muscular tone and movement. If the score is 7 or higher, everything's fine. When it is less than 7, doctors will take a sample from the umbilical cord blood to see how well the baby is processing oxygen. They may also want to have the baby under observation in case there's a problem.

NEWBORN SCREENING TESTS

Shortly after birth a nurse will take a blood sample from the umbilical cord to see what the blood type and Rh factor are. They will also take a little blood with a lancet from your baby's foot to check if there is a hereditary or metabolic illness. These tests vary from state to state, but the most common are:

- *PKU.* Detects a disease called phenylketonuria, where the lack of an enzyme could cause mental retardation. It is treated through diet.

- *Congenital hypothyroidism.* Babies who don't have enough thyroid hormone have delays in their development. Thanks to this test they can get a treatment to prevent it.

- *Galactosemia.* Babies with this condition can't tolerate dairy products or some other foods. If it's not treated, the baby can have mental retardation and other problems.

- *Sickle cell disease.* This is an inherited disease that affects red blood cells. It's common among Caribbean Latinos.

- *Cystic fibrosis.* In some states this test is given routinely. Cystic fibrosis is a hereditary disease that causes dense clots of phlegm to form in the lungs.

Antibiotic Eye Drops and Vitamin K Shot

A routine procedure in hospitals is to put some antibiotic eyedrops or cream in the baby's eyes. This is done to prevent the baby from developing an eye infection in case the mother had chlamydia or gonorrhea (see page 104). Often these venereal diseases don't produce symptoms in the mother, but the baby can get infected through the vaginal canal. These types of eye infections are serious and cause blindness in the baby.

Vitamin K is necessary for blood clotting, and newborns have very low levels of this vitamin. In case the baby had any kind of hemorrhage after birth, his/her blood might not be able to coagulate. That is why it is routine in many hospitals (it's the law in some states) to give the newborn a vitamin K shot.

Hepatitis B Vaccine

Hepatitis B is one of the diseases that can pass most easily from mother to baby during birth. It's pretty common to vaccinate babies right after birth, unless it was checked through a recent blood test that the mother didn't have this disease.

The First Breastfeeding

After you meet your baby for the first time, a nurse or midwife will give him/her a bath and will weigh him or her. Because the baby still can't regulate its temperature very well, it'll wear a hat for the first twenty-four hours. They have clothes in the hospital for the babies, as well as diapers. When you leave the hospital, you will be able to dress him or her up with the clothes you brought.

This is a good time to breastfeed your baby for the first time. Even if you're not producing milk, the baby will be taking colostrum, a yellowish substance that is just the best thing right after birth. Colostrum contains minerals and amino acids customized for your baby and antibodies that will help him/her develop the immune system.

It might not feel as though anything is coming out of your breasts, but your baby really is suckling small amounts of colostrum. At the moment, that's all he/she needs because the baby's organs still have to learn how to digest. During the next two to three days, colostrum will become even more abundant, and later the milk will begin to be mixed in, too.

In addition to being good for your baby, breastfeeding is also very good for you during the first days after birth, because it will cause contractions that help your uterus return to its normal size and shape. You will find more advice on breastfeeding in the next chapter.

11

After Birth

I remember after my daughter Adriana was born, I spent hours looking at her little fingers, the shape of her lips, the curve of her eyelashes, the size of her ears. It was incredible to me that from nothing, a human being had developed inside me. But what really amazed me was knowing that she was *mi bebé*, my baby, my very own baby.

No matter what you've read or heard, there's no real way to describe what you feel knowing the baby in your arms is yours and that it will depend entirely upon you for survival. There's a big difference between being pregnant and holding your own baby. You might need a little time to realize you're actually a mother now.

Our grandmothers and mothers knew about this big shift, and for generations our ancestors went through the *cuarentena*, or quarantine, after giving birth. While other family members took care of the household chores and other children, the mother spent nearly six weeks focusing entirely on the newest member of the family and on her recovery. During this time she would recover from labor, learn to breastfeed if she hadn't done it before, and establish a close, loving relationship with the new baby. After the six weeks, the mother was feeling almost like before giving birth and the new baby was part of the family routines.

Today in the United States, few Latinas can enjoy a *cuarentena como Dios manda*, a traditional period of recovery. We usually live far away from our families, we don't have much time off from work and the rest of our family needs us to take care of things. Still, despite all the demands on the modern Latina mother, there is a way to recuperate properly and to give to your baby the best possible care.

STAYING IN THE HOSPITAL OR BIRTHING CENTER

The time you spend in the hospital will be one or two days if there weren't any complications during labor and delivery and three or more days in the case of a cesarean, depending on the state. Some insurance policies only cover a twenty-four-hour stay for normal deliveries and forty-eight hours for cesareans. Make sure you find out ahead of time how much your policy covers. The rules at birthing centers are different. Some only allow you to stay a few hours after delivery. At others you can stay the night.

Despite the strong physical and emotional demands on your body during delivery, you may not necessarily feel worn out afterward. Many women enjoy a burst of energy after giving birth, even if it's just at the thought that *ya pasó todo*, now it's all over. Depending on whether you've had a vaginal delivery or a cesarean, you'll be given different types of care after birth.

- *Vaginal delivery (with or without epidural)*. When the excitement of birth has ended, you'll likely hurt. This is because of the huge effort your body has made—with nearly all the muscles you've got—to push the baby out. If you've had to have your vagina stitched up, that will hurt, too. The nurses will give you bags of ice you can apply to reduce swelling, a container or sitz bath with warm water to sit in or a painkiller if the pain is really getting to you. You may also find it difficult to urinate because the muscles in your pelvic area might have been strained during birth. In addition, the bladder has suddenly found there isn't a baby squishing it anymore and it can hold a lot more liquid.

- *Cesarean*. You'll still have to keep the intravenous catheter in your hand for another twenty-four hours. Same goes for the urinary catheter. When the effects of the epidural begin to wear off, you'll probably feel discomfort or pain in your abdomen. But, through the IV, the doctors can give you a painkiller. Also, your intestines won't be working properly yet, and gas might bother you. One of the things nurses will recommend is that you get on your feet and begin walking as soon as possible. Even though it might be tough to do, make the effort because that will speed up your recovery. Just before you leave the hospital, the nurses will take out the metal staples holding your incision. This doesn't hurt.

Rest

In the old days, newborns went to a special room in the hospital with the rest of the babies. They stayed in there except when their mothers needed to feed them at certain times of the day. Fathers and other family members would arrive and look at the newborn through the window. Today, most hospitals have abandoned this system and allow the babies to be in the same room with their mother. It's called rooming-in. During the visit you made halfway through your pregnancy, the hospital will have explained what its policy is. Depending on the hospital, it's possible your husband, your mother or some other relative can spend the night (in a chair or on the couch in the worst of cases); some hospitals don't allow overnight visitors. Whatever the case may be, I recommend you take advantage of your time in the hospital after delivery and try to rest as much as you can, because when you get back home, you won't have all this help.

If your hospital offers a breastfeeding consultant, make an appointment. You'll have a much better start to your breastfeeding experience and you'll get better at it more quickly.

As far as visits go, it really depends on how you feel. But in my experience, it's easier to receive well-wishers at the hospital than at home. Once you're home, you'll feel obligated to *atenderles*, entertain them. Still, if you don't feel up to having people come visit you at the hospital or even to talk by telephone, tell your husband or your mother to excuse you.

Leaving the Hospital

You won't be allowed to leave the hospital with your baby unless you have an infant car seat. Usually you'll be put into a wheelchair and wheeled out of the hospital, even if you feel capable of walking. A nurse will accompany you to the car to make sure you've got a car seat for the baby.

This might seem a little extreme, but infant car seats have saved many lives. The only place your baby can travel safely in the car is strapped into a special seat. If you want to be closer to your baby in case it cries during the ride home, sit in the backseat. No matter what you do, don't take the baby out of the seat and hold it. Comfort your baby while it remains strapped in. In a crash, no matter how small the impact may seem, the baby will be flung from your arms if you're holding it. And a bang to a newborn can be fatal. So even if you're only going around the corner, make sure your baby is always in the proper seat and buckled in.

RETURNING HOME

If everything went well, you've only been away from home for twenty-four to forty-eight hours, less if you delivered at a birthing center. The days when a woman stayed routinely in the hospital for a week or more after a normal delivery are long gone. What hasn't changed is the Latino tradition of having your mother or mother-in-law come live with you for a while. Either one will help you take care of the baby and give you a chance to recover.

Don't even think about doing this alone. If you have a good relationship with your family, buy your mother-in-law, sister, aunt or any other relative a plane ticket for the longest stay you can! Your husband can help you with chores and the like, but if you need to get up every two to three hours day and night to feed your baby, you're going to need as much help and rest as you can get.

❧

Having someone around to help you during the first weeks after delivering a baby can make the difference between a happy adjustment to the new member of the family experience and a battle against fatigue and depression.

If your mother-in-law or other family members also want to pitch in, set up a system whereby one person relieves another. That way, instead of having all your help for only two weeks, you can stretch it out for a couple of months. If you don't have any relatives who are close enough to help, or you would rather not have them around, try the following:

- *Friends*. Ask your friends if they can come over to help you out at least a couple of days a week. This will give you a few hours of rest. Your friends who are mothers will know exactly what you're asking for.

- *Doulas*. If you hired a doula during your delivery (see page 235), she will visit you at home to ensure everything's going fine. She may even be able to help you for a few hours at your home during the first few weeks after birth. That way you'll be able to nap for a couple of hours while an experienced person watches the baby.

- *Housekeeping*. Hiring a housekeeper may seem like a luxury you can't really afford right now, but if you're alone, you might consider it for a couple of weeks. In these circumstances, help isn't a luxury but a necessity. Even though you may not actually leave the baby with the person you hire, the key is letting you get off your feet while someone does the chores.

Lack of Sleep

For many new parents, the most difficult part of caring for a newborn is dealing with the accumulation of fatigue from not sleeping enough. During the first few days or even weeks, it's possible to survive on only a few hours of sleep a night. But after sleeping only four to six hours a night for several months, the body just can't take it. You begin to malfunction. A lack of sleep causes the following problems in humans:

- Fatigue
- Less brain activity
- Lower production at work
- Irritability
- Impatience
- Anxiety
- Depression

These symptoms get in the way of your recuperation and of your relationships with other family members, including your baby. That's why having enough help so you can rest is so important.

❦

"You are so tired after going through all that. You don't sleep at night, you worry about the unknown, having a new baby, checking to see if he is breathing at night . . ."

—Ana María Caldas

"Lack of sleep was not good for me. I think I didn't have enough milk because at night one breastfeeding session was right after the other. My family and friends told me *duerme cuando ella*, sleep when she does, but I just couldn't."

—Ana María La Salle

After three months, the baby usually begins to sleep more hours at night. After six months, it may even begin to sleep the whole night through. But until that happens, here are some ideas to help you get the proper amount of sleep for yourself:

- If you're breastfeeding, buy a breast pump so that someone else can feed the baby with a bottle at least once during the day or night. That way you can get several consecutive hours of sleep.

- Take turns with your husband or with another family member to care for the baby so you can sleep all the way through the night at least once every two or three days.

- Try to take *siestas* when your baby does. If you've got other children, make them take naps at the same time or sleep while they are at school.

- Unplug the telephone and lower the volume on the answering machine.

- Establish a routine. Feed your baby before going to sleep so it doesn't wake up hungry half an hour later.

Make your sleep time a priority. Remember, the more you sleep the more rested you'll feel and the better the mood you'll be in. That will allow you to finish other chores more easily and to get along better with your family.

Feeling Overwhelmed

Taking care of a demanding baby plus the fatigue of giving birth combined with several nights in a row without much sleep and all the household chores can make any woman feel overwhelmed. How can anybody do laundry and make dinner when it's already two in the afternoon and you still haven't had time to take a shower and get dressed? Feeling overwhelmed by the house chores and the baby care is common among women who have just given birth.

> "Once all the help was gone I felt pretty overwhelmed. *Tenía que dar para todo*, I had to do everything and I just couldn't do it like before. I had to balance my priorities: Either I clean the house and make lunch or I take care of this baby."
>
> —*Gloria Villalobos*

> "When my mom left I thought, now what? My husband is wonderful, he takes turns with me taking care of the baby. However I felt this emptiness. . . . My mother was the one who took care of him, fed him . . ."
>
> —*María Teresa Díaz Blanco*

It's not just a lack of time that can be overwhelming. It's knowing that you are one hundred percent responsible for the feeding, health and wellness of the new baby. If you're far away from your family or if your baby has some health problems, this feeling of being overwhelmed can be even greater.

The first thing to remember is that you're not alone. It's normal to feel this way. This isn't about your being an incompetent mother. This is just one of the many changes your life will go through now that you're a parent. It's natural for you to take a while to adapt to your new circumstances. You'll see how in a couple of months everything will change. In the meantime, take some steps to make the transition as easy as possible.

Priority List

The secret to surviving these first few weeks is accepting the idea that, at least for a while, you're not going to be able to keep the house as clean as you like, you're not going to be able to attend to your husband as you used to and you're not going to have time to cook up those wonderful family dinners everyone enjoys. The priorities for you during this time are taking care of your baby, getting yourself some rest and eating right. Everything else can be put on hold.

Write down exactly what your priorities are on a piece of paper and stick the sheet on the refrigerator where you can see it every day. This list might seem a little silly or obvious, but seeing your priorities on paper will make them seem more real. For example, in addition to the first two (taking care of your baby and getting some rest for yourself) the list might include doing laundry, cooking, going to the supermarket, cleaning the bathrooms, etc. Each day, try to do only one thing on your list, in addition to taking care of your baby and getting enough rest. When you do laundry, try using a frozen food for dinner instead of working in the kitchen. When you cook, forget about cleaning the bathroom and going to the store. Little by little, you'll find you have more time and energy to take on more chores. And the more you are able to do, the less overwhelmed you'll feel. If you feel rested and in control of the situation, you'll find it's easier to deal with your changing hormones after delivery.

Visits

Both expected and unexpected visits from friends and family are a true Latino tradition. After the birth of a baby, they're even more frequent. Friends, family and neighbors all come by to take a look at the little one and congratulate the new parents. But it's also a Latino tradition to entertain and attend to guests. No one likes to have *la casa patas arriba,* a messy house, or not to have anything to offer guests to eat and drink when company arrives.

Under normal circumstances, a visit from a friend or relative is a chance to sit down and chat and relax. But on days when you've barely had a chance to take a shower or do the chores, attending to a visitor might not be one of your priorities. Plus, you may not feel comfortable breastfeeding your baby in front of some people, and you might feel it is not polite to leave them alone while you take care of your baby.

One way to keep your doorbell from ringing every half hour is to organize a baptism or get-together soon after the birth. That way many people can get to know your baby at once. When your friends or relatives call you to say they want to come by, you can tell them you've got a party planned within a few days. Your husband and other relatives can help you to get ready for the gathering. Think of it: You get help preparing for the party, many people get to say hello to the baby and congratulate you and it all happens when and where you want. Another way to solve the unexpected-visitor problem is to set aside one day a week for guests. That way you only need to have the house spotless on certain days.

If you don't feel well or you are starting to get really tired, tell your visitor honestly. Anyone who's had a baby will understand that you're not being rude.

PHYSICAL RECOVERY

Whether you had a cesarean or a natural birth, with each day that goes by you are going to be feeling much better. There are some things that will help you get better faster:

- Walk and move around. If you had a cesarean, this might be a bit difficult. However, it is the best thing that you can do to avoid blood clots in your circulatory system.
- Eat well, especially if you are breastfeeding. You should add to your diet 200 calories more a day. Eat vegetables, fruits and grains, and drink a lot of liquids.
- Keep an eye on pain, bleeding and fever.

Bleeding

After delivery, you may bleed for three to six weeks. That is your body's way of eliminating what was accumulated on the walls of your uterus during pregnancy.

During the first few days after delivery, the bleeding may be as intense or more so than during menstruation, and red in color. Afterward, the amount of bleeding lessens every day and the color changes to pink, brown and finally yellow. These secretions are called lochia, and they can last for up to six weeks after giving birth. Sometimes blood clots will appear in the flow.

Often, after you have begun to bleed less, the amount of blood flow then increases again. This is because the body is getting rid of the layer that forms where the placenta was attached to the uterus. Even though this flow can be heavier, you shouldn't go through more than one pad an hour. You should talk to your obstetrician/gynecologist if you start to bleed more. It's not a good idea to use tampons for at least six weeks after delivery, to avoid getting infections.

One way to know if you're getting enough rest is the color of the bleeding during these first few weeks after birth. If the color of the flow begins to get redder again after turning lighter, you may be pushing yourself too hard. Remember, you've still got an injury in your uterus, where the placenta was attached, that has to heal.

Size of the Uterus

Right after birth, the uterus weights about 2 pounds (1 kilogram) and it runs from your vagina up to the belly button. Six weeks after, it will have returned to almost its prepregnancy size.

Breastfeeding your baby is one of the best things you can do to reduce the risk of bleeding too much and to guarantee that your uterus returns to its normal size as soon as possible. When you breastfeed, your body produces a hormone called oxytocin (this is the same hormone that caused contractions during labor) that will make your uterus contract again. But don't worry—even though you may feel these contractions, they don't have anything to do with the ones you felt during labor.

If the incision from the cesarean section bothers you, you can use a girdle to get some support, but it shouldn't be too tight.

Swelling

After delivery your feet and ankles might get very swollen. During the next few days you will be eliminating all the liquid you accumulated during pregnancy. But meanwhile, because of gravity, this liquid goes to your feet. In the days following your delivery you will urinate very often and a lot each time, and sometime later you'll see your feet start going back to the shape they had before pregnancy. If you feel uncomfortable because of the swelling, try putting your legs up, the same thing you did when you were pregnant. However, if the swelling is not going down or you are having trouble urinating, you should talk to your doctor as soon as possible.

Abdominal Cramps or *Entuertos*

Sometimes the uterine contractions that help the organ return to its normal size can be strong. Generally, mothers who have given birth by cesarean and mothers in their second pregnancy feel them more. One of the functions of these cramps or contractions after delivery is to close off certain veins in the uterine wall. Once the placenta becomes detached from the uterus, all the blood vessels that were supplying it with nutrients during pregnancy need to be closed down. As the size of the organ decreases, the tissue contracts and slows down the bleeding.

Going to the bathroom to urinate before you begin breastfeeding will help you to avoid further discomfort from the contractions. A full bladder gets in the way. If these cramps or contractions are getting too bothersome, use the same relaxation and breathing techniques you employed during labor. The contractions usually go away after a couple of weeks.

Also, your intestines and other abdominal organs are reorganizing themselves after being pushed aside for the past nine months. Sometimes this readjustment can cause some abdominal pains. But it's all temporary.

Tears and Episiotomies

You might not recognize your own anatomy the first time you take a shower after delivery, especially if you had an episiotomy. The perineal tissues, which are located between the vagina and the anus, will be swollen because of the pushing and because of the stitches, if you had them.

If the doctors did an episiotomy on you, you may not have many stitches, but if you tore, you may have a lot. There are four types of tears that can happen during delivery. They are classified depending on their length and depth.

A first-grade tear is superficial and usually heals by itself or only requires a couple of stitches. The rest of the tears affect deeper layers of tissue and require more sutures to close the wound. Third- and fourth-degree tears can affect the muscles of the rectum and result in a slower and more painful recovery.

Here are some things you can do to lessen the swelling:

- Apply ice wrapped in a plastic bag or in a rubber glove to the swollen area during the first three or four days after delivery.

- Rinse the swollen area using a special plastic bottle. You'll likely get one while you're in the hospital. To wash the affected area, use water or a mix of water and some type of disinfectant such as Betadine. For example, mix one part Betadine with three parts warm water. This will help the stitches to dry out more quickly.

- After going to the bathroom rinse with warm water before you pat dry. Keep a few paper cups in the bathroom for this purpose.

- Sit in a warm sitz bath. If you're not given a special portable container for this at the hospital, you can buy one in any pharmacy. It's

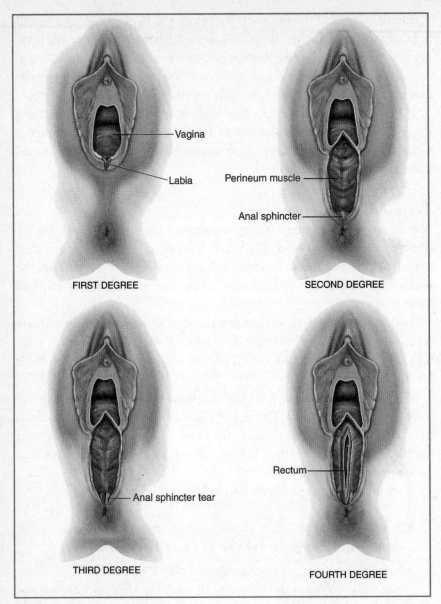

Labels on figure:
- Vagina
- Labia
- Perineum muscle
- Anal sphincter
- Anal sphincter tear
- Rectum

FIRST DEGREE

SECOND DEGREE

THIRD DEGREE

FOURTH DEGREE

Degrees of perineum tearing

placed on top of the toilet. You can add rosemary leaves to the water. That will help you heal more quickly. Pour boiling water over
two or three teaspoons of dried rosemary leaves in the container and
give yourself a bath when the tea is steeped.

- Use an inflatable ring while sitting. These are inflatable cushions in the shape of a doughnut that keep you from putting too much pressure on the stitches while you're seated.

- Use anesthetic creams or sprays. If you feel a lot of pain in this area, your doctor may prescribe you a painkilling cream or spray.

The discomfort usually begins to subside after five or six days. After ten days, you may feel much, much better. During the healing process, it's normal to feel itching in the torn area.

Hemorrhoids

Because of the force you used to push the baby out during delivery, you may have gotten hemorrhoids or you may have worsened the ones you already had. There are some over-the-counter creams that can help. You can also use a mild laxative such as milk of magnesia or glycerin suppositories. Be careful with laxatives, because if you are breastfeeding, your baby can get diarrhea.

Hemorrhoids are veins that are distended because of all the pressure put on them (see page 244). Generally they get back to their normal size after a few days. But if you've tried the creams and other over-the-counter remedies and they don't work after several weeks, talk to your doctor. Some surgical procedures are quite simple and effective.

Constipation and Gas

You might find yourself terribly constipated after delivery, especially if you've had a cesarean. The intestines don't recuperate for a few days after the operation. Sometimes gas gets trapped inside, which can cause pain. If you've also got hemorrhoids to deal with, you'll not be looking forward to going to the bathroom. Drinking a lot of water, eating high-fiber foods, making small, easily digestible meals and walking will help you to overcome the constipation and put you back on a regular schedule. A mild laxative can also help, but be careful if you are breastfeeding.

Urinary Incontinence

One of the things you may have noticed after delivery is that you're no longer capable of controlling your urine as before. This is because the muscles in the pelvis are stretched out after pregnancy and birth. Kegel exercises (see page 59) are an excellent way to recuperate pelvic muscle tone, especially if you've had an episiotomy.

Most women get back their muscle tone and control over urination after a while. But mothers who have had several children may find they don't get all their control back. If the bladder is full, it is not uncommon to have a few drops leak out after straining, sneezing, coughing or laughing.

Baths

Traditional Latino culture says you shouldn't bathe yourself in a tub during the first few weeks after birth. The fear was that dirty water would get back inside the woman and cause an infection. More recently, scientists have learned that's not true and there's no reason not to take a bath almost as soon as you arrive home from the hospital. Nevertheless, check with your doctor. If he/she approves, go ahead and *disfrútelo*, enjoy a bath, because the warm water is ideal to help sore muscles feel better.

However, if you have had a cesarean or have stitches in your vagina, it is better to use the shower instead for the first few days. Bacteria could get in the wounds and infect them. Make sure when you are washing your hair that the dirty water does not go on top of your cesarean section scar. Rinse the scar with lots of warm water before getting out.

Weight and Nutrition

As soon as you give birth, you'll lose the weight of the baby, the placenta and the amniotic fluid. That could be as much as 10 pounds, but still, you won't have gotten rid of all the other fluids that have accumulated in your body over the past nine months. During the next few days, you'll see how the numbers on the scale keep going down each time you step on. However, some of the weight won't come off yet. In fact, if you're going to breastfeed your baby, you'll have to add an extra 200 calories to your diet. You need to eat as healthily as possible and drink a lot of fluids to make sure the milk you're giving your baby is of the highest quality (see Chapter 3).

Sex

Your doctor will likely recommend you abstain from penetration for four to six weeks after delivery. Everything else is fine.

If you had an episiotomy or you tore a great deal during the birth, you might worry how sex will feel. The tissues of the perineum heal quickly, and after four to six weeks you'll feel almost totally recovered. Nonetheless, you're the one who should decide when you're ready.

Experimenting with different positions may allow you to find a way to avoid putting pressure on the areas where the stitches were. If you're breastfeeding, you may also need to find new positions because pressure on your breasts could be uncomfortable. And the hormonal changes your body continues to go through may mean you don't get as lubricated as before. Lubricating creams, sold in most pharmacies, can help.

In addition to the physical recuperation, it's important to keep the romance alive with your spouse. That's one of the toughest things for new parents to do. A baby demands a lot of time and attention, day and night. But connecting with your partner will help you in this time of family adjustment. Between taking care of the baby and returning to work and your husband's work, weeks could go by without you two having any time to yourselves. Try to make a *cita romántica*, a romantic date with your spouse at least once a week. You don't necessarily have to go out anywhere, but create a romantic mood by lighting candles or playing music. Talk, enjoy each other, and reconnect, even if it's only for a couple of hours.

Birth Control

A popular belief is that a woman can't get pregnant while she is breastfeeding. And it is true that many women who breastfeed don't have their periods. But that doesn't mean breastfeeding is a reliable birth control method. A woman who is breastfeeding can ovulate at any time, without having her period beforehand.

Getting pregnant again right after you've already delivered one baby isn't a good idea. Your body needs time to recuperate from the huge effort it's just made. The ideal time between children is two to five years.

Talk to your doctor about what method of birth control you can use. With the pill, small amounts of hormones can pass through the mother's milk to the baby, especially if you take pills with high levels of estrogen. All this depends on what type of pill you take and how often you breastfeed the baby.

EMOTIONAL STATE

Two or three days after giving birth you may begin to feel a little sad and even cry at the drop of a hat. You may also have sudden mood swings—after feeling happy and energetic, you will start to cry for no reason. The huge hormonal changes combined with fatigue are doing a number on your body. Many mothers go through what's called the baby blues. These are natural changes in a woman's body, and the best thing for you to do is accept them and open up to them. Cry when you feel like it. In a few weeks, at the most, you'll feel a lot better.

Even though this is only a temporary stage, you should still try to rest as much as you can and eat as healthily as possible. The lack of sleep and a poor diet will only make the emotional problems worse.

"With the second one I was depressed. It was difficult with the two kids, *lloraba a la nada*, I cried about everything and the lack of sleep made it worse. I didn't have any family here or anybody I could leave the children with so I had to carry the load myself. The good thing is that I recognized what it was and I asked for help. If you don't recognize it, that's when it gets bad."

—*Leticia Gómez*

If you think your sadness isn't going away after a couple of weeks and you begin to have thoughts of harming the baby or yourself, talk to your doctor immediately. This could be the start of postpartum depression (see page 341).

ADVICE AND TRADITIONS

One of the best Latino traditions during the time right after birth is *la cuarentena,* or the quarantine. The mother will spend forty days resting with the newborn after delivery and only worry about taking care of the baby. Other members of the family will keep house and watch over the other children. If you've got relatives who live nearby, I'd suggest you try to follow some version of this tradition. You'll feel like a new woman after those forty days of recuperation (or even twenty).

In the olden days during this time some other practices were performed. Depending on how traditional your family is, there might be relatives who insist that you take *purgantes* or laxatives and try not to eat cold foods or fruits. Here are some of the traditions you might have to watch out for:

- Purgantes *or laxatives.* Traditionally these were taken to clean out the uterus after delivery. But the truth is, strong laxatives don't work on the uterus, they work on the intestines. At the least, they'll give you terrible diarrhea, which can be dangerous if you're breastfeeding your baby.

- *Avoiding cold food and drink.* This tradition goes back to the sixteenth century, when illnesses and the symptoms they caused were divided into two categories: *Caliente o frío*, cold or hot. The time after birth is a "hot" period, according to tradition, so you needed to avoid cold foods and drinks so as not to upset the balance. The only problem with this tradition is that you'd have to give up eating fruits, vegetables and other foods that are considered "cold." Those are some of the healthiest foods you can eat after delivery.

- *Frío en la matriz or cold womb.* The belief was that the womb would get cold if the mother didn't rest. Damiana teas were used to treat a woman with a cold womb. But be careful with them because they can make you bleed.

If you've lived for a while in the United States and you've got family members who still believe in these traditions, you may have a difficult time reconciling the two ways of thinking. In fact, this doesn't have to be a choice between the traditional and the modern. You can pick up the best of both worlds. Don't dismiss out of hand the advice your family members give you. Listen and thank them for the knowledge and concern they're showing you. Sometimes grandmothers, aunts, mothers and neighbors who aren't yet integrated into U.S. society may feel you're rejecting them personally because you are rejecting what they have to offer. After all, as far as they're concerned, these traditions have worked for generations. Ask them questions about how things were done in the olden days—the family stories can be fascinating. And also share with them what you've learned. Set limits *con cariño*, with love.

WHEN TO CALL THE DOCTOR

As recently as the 1800s, bleeding or an infection after delivery caused grave danger to the mother, often ending in death. Thanks to the advances in medicine, tragedies like this are rare as long as you get immediate medical attention. In the case of severe bleeding, the mother can become gravely ill in a matter of minutes. Even if you don't have medical insurance, it's very important to get to a clinic or emergency center right away if you have any of these symptoms:

- *Severe bleeding.* In the first few days after delivery, the blood flow will be heavy. But talk to your doctor right away or go to the emergency room if you are soaking one sanitary napkin an hour for several hours in a row. Also, call your doctor if the blood is bright red.

- *Blood clots.* It's normal to discharge blood clots in the first few weeks after birth. But they're cause for concern when they're larger than a nutshell.

- *Bad smell.* If your discharge has a bad smell, this could be a sign of an infection. Perhaps a piece of the placenta wasn't discharged.

- *Fever.* Fever and chills are indicators that something isn't right. It's normal for your temperature to be a little high after giving birth, but if it's higher than 100.4 degrees Fahrenheit (38 degrees centigrade), you should talk to your doctor.

- *Infected stitches.* If the area where you were given stitches for a cesarean, tearing, or an episiotomy looks red, has a liquid discharge, has a bad smell or hurts, you can have an infected stitch. Check if the incisions are healing properly.

- *Difficulty urinating.* It's common for a new mother to have a little trouble going to the bathroom right after birth, but if this condition goes on for several days and you feel pain when you urinate, talk to your doctor, because you may have a bladder or kidney infection.

- *Abdominal pain or swelling.* The cramps or contractions after birth should last from two to five days, and you'll feel them more when you're breastfeeding. But a pain that doesn't get better or that gets worse when you push on your abdomen could be cause for concern.

- *Breast pain.* Sometimes the ducts that carry milk out of the breast get clogged. If the milk doesn't come out, it can result in an infection. You may feel it like a little bump that's warm, pink and painful to touch. Breast infections of this type are called mastitis and can cause a fever.

- *Sharp chest pain.* This type of pain can be caused by a clot in the lungs. This is a dire emergency—call your doctor right away or go to the emergency room. Even if it turns out to be nothing, you shouldn't wait and see if this symptom passes.

- *Thigh or calf pain.* This can also be caused by a clot. If you feel there's a certain sensitive spot that hurts to touch and it's red or hot, put your legs up and call your doctor or emergency services.

- *Deep depression, fear of harming the baby.* Sadness is typical after birth. Many mothers feel like crying for weeks afterward. But if you feel extremely depressed and strange thoughts get into your head, you should talk to your doctor right away. Read the section about postpartum depression (see page 341).

Even though it may seem to you the symptoms you feel *no son nada,* aren't really much, some of these conditions can get worse in a matter of hours. Don't wait until the last minute. It's better to call or go to the hospital than to have an emergency that's not treated. Now you've got another person who's counting on you to be around for a while.

Six weeks after delivery, your obstetrician/gynecologist will want to see you again. During this visit, you'll be given an internal exam to make sure the uterus is returning to its normal size. The doctor will also take a look at the cesarean incision or the vaginal stitches. And as usual, you'll have your blood pressure taken and you'll step onto the scale. If you had gestational diabetes, this is also a good time to see how your blood sugar levels are doing.

THE *BEBÉ*

Appearance

Most mothers don't think their newborn babies are anything less than beautiful. However, when you first hold yours in your arms, it won't look like the ones you see in the diaper commercials on television. Don't worry; the baby's appearance will change a lot during the next weeks and months.

- *Head.* The shape may be a little pointed. That's because it was "molded" to fit through the birth canal. Mother Nature is smart and has allowed the baby's skull bones to bend and fold slightly on top of one another so the head will fit through the vagina. In other babies, there's a little swelling on the back part of the head or on either side. The baby has two soft points on its head called fontanels where the bones still haven't closed.

- *Face.* The eyelids may be swollen. Sometimes there is a flap of skin below the eyes, like bags under the eyes, because the nose still hasn't fully formed yet and the extra skin collects there. Some babies have pink marks on the facial skin that gradually disappear or small white pimples that are later absorbed. The newborn's eyes are a gray-blue color that will change over the coming months.

- *Skin*. Some babies are born with a light layer of hair on their shoulders, back and arms. These are the remains of the lanugo that protected them during their time in the uterus; it will disappear in a few days. The baby may also have areas where the skin looks as though it's peeling. This is the skin that was in contact with the amniotic fluid and is now adapting to being in contact with air. The nails are thin and fine, almost like paper, and they may be long.

- *Genitals*. The genital organs tend to be swollen at the beginning because of the mother's hormones running through the baby before birth. For the same reason, baby girls may have a whitish vaginal flow that may include a little bit of blood for a few days. The breasts of baby boys and girls may be inflamed.

Your pediatrician or the pediatrician at the hospital will take a look at your baby soon after it's born or will come for a visit within the first twenty-four hours. Talk to your doctor about anything that worries you.

Weight

The average weight of a newborn baby at the end of a normal pregnancy is around 7 pounds. We Latinas have big babies that usually weigh about 8 pounds or more. Still, during the first few days after birth, most babies lose weight. This is normal and you shouldn't stress out thinking you're not providing enough milk for your baby. Your pediatrician will confirm whether your baby is progressing normally.

What Does a Newborn Do?

Generally a newborn will dedicate itself to these activities, in order: *dormir, comer y llorar*, sleep, eat and cry. During the first hours after birth, babies are alert and look attentively at their parents. Later newborns can sleep up to sixteen hours a day. However, those sixteen hours aren't in a row. After breastfeeding, the baby may sleep for three or four hours until it's time to eat again. Newborns don't have a regular sleep pattern and sleep in shorter periods. At the beginning it may not be able to distinguish between day and night. Sometimes it will take long *siestas* during the afternoon and then stay up all night. To help your baby get adjusted to a more normal sleep schedule, do your night feedings with only a little light and hardly any noise. *Cántele suavecito*, sing softly to your baby, but don't look into its eyes or do anything that will excite or arouse him/her.

Maybe your baby is not sleeping much or is fidgety even if he/she is fed and changed. A baby's cry is a sound designed to get a reaction from adults. There aren't many people who can just ignore it. And that makes sense, because that's the only way the baby can communicate at the moment. A baby will cry for all kinds of reasons, but the most common are: it's hungry, it's got a dirty diaper, it's uncomfortable. Think about how much the baby's environment has changed. He/she was in a safe, secure, warm, dark place where it never had to ask for food or worry about wet diapers, loud noises or temperature changes. Your baby is adjusting to all kinds of new stimuli during the first few days.

Have you ever noticed how most mothers carry their babies with their heads resting on the mother's left arm? That's because the mother's heartbeat is easier to hear on the left side. That beating has been a comforting and familiar sound for the baby during the past months. If your baby is fidgety, try to hold it as much as possible. You're not spoiling your baby; you're taking care of him/her. There will be plenty of time in the future to set limits.

Sleeping Positions and SIDS

SIDS, or sudden infant death syndrome, is the sudden death, without explanation, of an apparently healthy baby. The baby dies in his/her sleep without the parents or the caregiver noticing anything. SIDS is still a medical mystery, but in the last ten years, since doctors have begun recommending that babies sleep on their backs, the number of deaths from SIDS has gone down more than 40 percent. Along with placing your baby on his/her back to sleep, you can also take other measures to reduce the risk of SIDS:

- Don't use any stuffed animals, fluffy bedding, pillows or any other object in the crib that can cover the baby's face, and use a firm mattress.
- Make sure that the baby is not overheated.
- Don't allow anybody to smoke when your baby is around.

Meconium

Meconium is the first feces the baby passes. The color will be a dark green, almost black, with a pasty texture, like tar. Meconium usually appears in the first twelve to forty-eight hours. When your baby was still inside you, it swallowed amniotic fluid to practice. Floating inside that fluid were dead skin cells, hair and other secretions that have been stored inside the baby's intestines. This is what creates meconium.

The consistency and color of the baby's feces will change in the next few days to a more yellowish green color that looks like mustard seeds, if the baby is breastfeeding. If the baby is eating formula, the color will be more greenish.

Belly Button

What's left of the umbilical cord will start to dry out and will eventually fall off about a week or two after birth. The best way to help this process along is to keep the area clean and dry. Clean it a couple of times a day with a cotton swab dipped in alcohol. Fold the waist part of the diaper down for a few days, so it will not be covering the baby's belly button. The *fajeros* or girdles *para meter el ombligo,* to push the belly button in, could cause infections (see page 331).

If you see the area around the belly button becoming red or if it starts to smell bad, call your pediatrician, because it may be infected.

Advice and Traditions

Our mothers and grandmothers raised us with a lot less scientific information than we have available today. Some of the customs followed for generations are based on traditions that may be thousands of years old. Your mother, mother-in-law or other relatives may still follow some of them. But if you think the way things were done then doesn't apply now, there could be some family arguments in your future when it comes to taking care of the new baby.

The best weapon against these conflicts is information. If the tradition is a spiritual one that doesn't threaten the baby's health in any way, and it will please your mother or mother-in-law, why not? Many Latinas in the United States use a combination of modern medicine and traditional spiritual practices. A good *limpia o barrida,* a cleansing around the house before taking the baby home or a quick ceremony to scare away the *ojo* or evil eye can actually be good experiences, if for no other reason than that they keep the peace. Customs that may harm the baby are the ones you have to watch out for.

Caída de Mollera or Sunken Fontanel

Describes the indentation in the fontanels, which are the areas in the skull that still haven't closed up. When there is a sunken fontanel the baby usually is irritable and sluggish, has digestive problems and can cry frequently. According to popular tradition, this can happen when the baby gets scared or falls, or if the mother's nipple is removed from the baby's mouth too quickly (when the baby sucks without a nipple the fontanel sinks). A sunken fontanel can also happen if somebody has *vista fuerte*, a "strong sight" that could give *ojo* or evil eye to the baby. As you can imagine, a sunken fontanel has little to do with this. The traditional cure for the problem is to grab the baby by the feet, hold it upside down and pat the soles of the feet so the fontanel will pop back out. Another common solution is to push on the baby's palate. These remedies can hurt the baby.

A sunken fontanel really means the baby's dehydrated and needs medical attention as soon as possible. As the pressure of the fluids around the brain goes down, the fontanel sinks in. Grabbing the baby by the feet and holding it upside down or pushing on the palate is dangerous and it can cause other problems, but the real danger is not treating the dehydration. The baby needs more than just liquids. You need to talk to your pediatrician immediately if you see a sunken fontanel in your baby or if he or she acts differently.

Umbilical Hernia

A common Latino custom is to put a *fajero* or little girdle on the belly button or tape to prevent an umbilical hernia or a belly button that sticks out. The belly button is the scar that the umbilical cord leaves behind after it's fallen off. This is where all the baby's nutrients entered its body during pregnancy. A little hole in the middle of the baby's abdominal muscles allowed the cord to go through. After birth, the muscles grow and cover the hole up. Sometimes this process takes a while or it doesn't happen at all and part of the abdomen can come back out through the hole, like a little balloon.

The pressure of a girdle or bandage around the belly button won't affect whether the internal hole closes up. In fact, it can cause more problems than it can help. First, the extra pressure around the waist may make it difficult for the baby to digest food; it may even cause vomiting. Second, if you put a coin or marble on top of the belly button with the intent of keeping everything inside, the wound can get infected. The best way to help this wound heal is to treat it like any other wound: Periodically disinfect it and expose it to air. Don't interfere with the normal process of the muscles covering the internal hole back up. Hernias usually heal themselves in a couple of months. If not, a doctor will take care of it with surgery.

Air Currents

There is no scientific study or pediatric manual that will change my mother's mind regarding the dangers of air currents for babies. While it's true babies don't regulate their temperatures very well, that's only during the first twenty-four to forty-eight hours. The fear of air currents is a mix of Aztec traditions and the temperature-balance theories of medicine from the sixteenth century. The baby may get uncomfortable or sweat too much if it has too many clothes on.

Susto or Fright

Babies and adults can be equally affected by *susto* after they've seen something that scares them or after a fall or accident. When a baby has suffered *susto* or fright, it may cry frequently, appear anxious, not want to eat or display any number of other symptoms. A folk healer may try to get the spirits to help calm the baby and may also try giving it a special herbal tea. Anything that has to do with spiritual beliefs is just wonderful, but giving babies teas can be dangerous. A baby can get diarrhea or have other problems. Talk to your pediatrician about the symptoms your baby has; they may be caused by something other than a scare.

Mal de ojo or Evil Eye

Someone with *vista fuerte* or "strong sight" can cause *ojo* or evil eye in other people, especially babies and women. The symptoms of *ojo* include continual crying, fever and/or a scared look. To protect babies from this problem, tradition says, the baby must be outfitted with a red or pink bracelet or *ojo de venado*, a seed that's sold in a lot of Latino markets. The seed is hung around the baby's neck or on the wrist. This treatment is harmless, although you should never hang things around the baby's neck or arms because it can choke him/her or cut off the circulation. You can place it with a safety pin on the baby's clothing. Also, be on the alert because symptoms that are considered to be *ojo* might be caused by another, more serious illness.

SWADDLING

This practice makes a lot of sense and it's customary at many hospitals. The idea is to wrap the baby like a tamale in a little blanket or light cloth. In certain Latino cultures, it's important to keep the hands from flailing in front of the face, especially when the baby cries, because the baby could get scared if it sees them. Although this hasn't been proven, what we do know is that when the baby is wrapped up like a *tamalito*, a little tamale, it feels safe and secure, as though it's back in the uterus; that can calm the baby down, especially during the first few days after birth.

HOME REMEDIES AND HERBS

In Latino culture, home remedies are used to treat babies who have colic or who don't eat or sleep well. The remedies include everything from baths with lettuce leaves to drinking teas made of oregano. Herbs are not innocuous. They can be harmful to adults and much more so to babies, who have undeveloped digestive systems that aren't used to anything other than mother's milk. These teas can cause diarrhea, vomiting and dehydration, even if they get to the baby through the mother's milk. Don't ever let anyone give your baby a home remedy without first talking to your pediatrician.

When to Call the Doctor

Pediatricians are accustomed to receiving numerous calls from mothers who have just brought their babies home from the hospital after birth. This is normal. After all, babies don't come with an instruction manual. They look so fragile at the beginning that anything is a cause for concern. It's always better to ask—no matter how simple the question may seem— than to deal with an emergency. You should call your pediatrician if your baby has any of these symptoms:

- *Fever.* The normal temperature for a baby is between 96 and 98 degrees Fahrenheit (35.5 to 36.6 degrees centigrade), taking the temperature in the armpit.
- *Difficult breathing.* The baby has a difficult time breathing and is flaring the nostrils.

- *Diapers*. Fewer than six wet diapers and three with stools after the first forty-eight hours.
- *Loss of appetite*. The baby doesn't have any interest in eating. Newborns usually nurse eight to twelve times a day.
- *Yellowish color*. This is known as jaundice. The skin or the whites of the eyes take on a yellow color because of an excess of bilirubin.
- *Sleep*. Not enough or too much sleep. More than six hours in a row after eating or periods of six hours without sleeping are cause for concern.

BREASTFEEDING

Study after study over the past decades has confirmed what Mother Nature has known for millions of years: The best food for a newborn is *la leche de mamá*, mother's milk. Breastfeeding is good for you, too. When you breastfeed for at least six months, you reduce the chances of getting breast cancer, ovarian cancer and osteoporosis. For your baby, the benefits are almost too many to count. The positive aspects of breastfeeding have been documented in many studies:

- Breastfed babies have fewer chances of developing cancer, as long as the breastfeeding continued for at least six months.
- Babies who are breastfed are three times less likely to die from sudden infant death syndrome (SIDS).
- Breastfed babies have fewer respiratory infections, blood pressure complications and weight problems.
- Breastfed babies have better sight during the first months of life and higher IQs later in life.

Infant formula is inferior to mother's milk. It's impossible to reproduce in a formula what you are giving your baby through your milk.

The yellowish fluid that comes out of your breasts during the first few days after birth (called colostrum) helps to develop your baby's immune system. You are giving your baby antibodies to fight against illnesses you've already had. The milk also gives your baby the right amount of fats, proteins, amino acids and other elements necessary for the best development possible. Besides, it's just the right temperature. The benefits of breastfeeding are so irrefutable, the American Academy of Pediatrics recommends all mothers breastfeed their babies for at least a year.

This isn't a new idea in Latino culture; breastfeeding is the norm. Still, as more and more Latinas become accustomed to the way of life in the United States, fewer and fewer of us are breastfeeding, or we do it for only a few months. Only three of every ten women continue to breastfeed their babies for longer than six months.

Schedules

There are different theories regarding whether it is better to feed the baby on demand or on a schedule. At least during the first few days doctors recommend you feed the baby every two hours, day and night. Later the baby will start feeding every three to four hours. Even if the baby is sleeping, you should wake him or her up for a feeding.

A baby that sleeps for hours on end without asking for food is not a good baby, it's a sick baby.

One of the advantages of having a feeding schedule is that the baby will probably start sleeping at regular times. You will be able to plan your life and your rest around his/her schedule. However, if your baby is hungry before the next feeding, don't hold him/her off. If your baby wants to eat, it's because he/she needs to.

Newborns can dehydrate easily. If you live in a warm climate, ask your pediatrician if you can give the baby water in addition to the milk. The best way to know if your baby is getting enough liquid is to count the wet diapers.

Every twenty-four hours your baby should have at least six wet diapers and three soiled ones with mustard-colored feces if it is being breastfed and greenish ones if it is having formula.

Disposable diapers today are very efficient, and sometimes it is difficult to know if they are really wet. Check carefully because this is the best way to know if your baby is doing well.

Breastfeeding Difficulties

Even though breastfeeding is the best thing you can do for your baby, saying it and doing it are two completely different things. The idea of breastfeeding your baby may be appealing before you give birth. But when you get home from the hospital or birthing center and your breasts are sore, the baby only wants to be at your nipple, and there is no way to get some rest at night, the idea of heating up a bottle might not look so bad after all.

> "The baby only wanted one breast, not the other. It started hurting because there was no rest for that nipple. It didn't matter if I put her *así o asá*, in this or that position. I had to take the milk out of the other breast with a breast pump because it would get full of milk."
> —*Ana Miriam La Salle*

> "I broke two chairs *de los brincos que yo pegaba*, from jumping every time I put her to the breast. The first month was horrible. Two weeks after birth my nipples cracked and it hurt a lot, so much I thought about stopping the breastfeeding. *Pero poco a poco*, a little at a time it started getting better. She actually healed my breasts."
> —*Victoria Long*

Don't give up if you feel sore or unmotivated. The majority of mothers go through this phase. To begin with, many of us don't have the support network our mothers and grandmothers relied upon.

Breastfeeding isn't automatic. It's a process you and your baby have to learn how to do together.

Just because breastfeeding is a natural process doesn't mean you'll necessarily know how to do it. Some of the common problems new mothers experience include:

- *Milk doesn't appear.* A mother's breasts don't produce milk as soon as the baby has been born. It usually takes two to three days after a natural birth and up to five after a cesarean. The first thing your breasts produce is called colostrum, a yellowish substance that's like gold for your baby's nutrition. This liquid isn't only nourishing, it's also got antibodies that will protect your baby from illnesses. At first, colostrum appears in such small amounts that you'll think your breasts aren't producing anything. Even if you don't see anything, it's there. You may only produce a few spoonfuls during the first days after birth, but that's all your baby's digestive system can handle at the moment. A newborn can cry a lot during the first few days and it may appear as though it's hungry all the time. Your baby is adapting to a brand-new environment. Rest assured that what your breasts are producing during the first days is sufficient. The best thing you can do to keep increasing your production of milk is to breastfeed frequently. In no time you'll begin to actually see the colostrum and then the yellowish color will change to the white of milk. And by the way, the size of your breasts doesn't have anything to do with how much milk you produce.

- *Breast swelling.* When the milk finally appears, it may cause your breasts to swell to an uncomfortable size. The best way to hold down the swelling is to breastfeed as frequently as possible. That still may not be enough to stop the discomfort. A milk pump can help to empty out your breasts more quickly than breastfeeding. This milk can be stored in the refrigerator or even frozen. But if your breasts continue to hurt, try this: Buy some purple cabbage, wash and dry the leaves well, cover your breasts with them and hold the leaves in place with a bra. Leave them there for a few hours and you'll see how the swelling goes down. But only try this if the frequent breastfeeding and the breast pump don't work.

- *The baby doesn't latch on properly.* Breastfeeding is a learning process for your baby too, and it requires patience and practice. The best position to start breastfeeding is to hold your baby in your arms with a pillow underneath so your baby rests at the level of your breast. The most important thing is that the baby opens its mouth enough to take in the entire nipple. To get the baby to open its mouth, touch its lips with your nipple, touch the cheek with your finger or push down on its chin gently. When the baby opens it mouth, quickly pull the baby toward your breast. Don't pull on your breast to get it to the baby. The entire nipple should be inside the baby's mouth. If it nurses only on the tip of the nipple, the nipples will quickly get sore. If your baby doesn't take in enough nipple on the first try, stick a clean finger into its mouth to break the suction seal and try again. You may have to try six to eight times or more before the fit is right. But don't give up. Take your time. Both you and your baby will get better with practice.

- *Sore nipples.* Sometimes, soon after you begin to breastfeed, your nipples might become painful or cracked. Having a baby sucking on them with the force of hunger is hard work for them. Generally, nipples are most sore when babies latch on. Once they start feeding, the discomfort lessens a bit. Sometimes your nipples will become sore or cracked because the baby isn't nursing correctly. To alleviate the pain of irritated nipples, put a few drops of milk over

Right position of nipple during breastfeeding

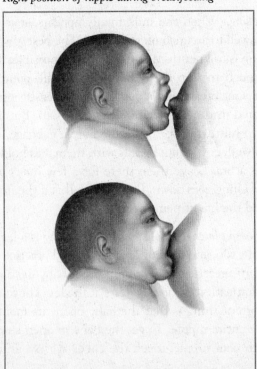

the entire nipple and let it air dry. Don't use creams because they will cover the nipple's pores, and because the baby can swallow them. Remember to be patient. This will get better, too. If it is really too uncomfortable for you to stand, use a breast pump to empty your breasts of milk. You can control the intensity of the suction in a breast pump.

- *Fatigue.* At first, babies eat every hour and a half to three hours. But the clock begins ticking the moment the baby begins to feed, not when it finishes. That means if your baby eats every two hours and it takes a half hour to eat, then it'll only be one hour and a half after you've finished before it's time to start again. This schedule will make anyone tired, not to mention a woman who has just been through labor. Taking care of a newborn can be exhausting, but it is possible to breastfeed your baby and survive. Try using a breast pump. That will allow your husband or other family member to feed the baby while you take a nap. Also, you can try breastfeeding in bed. Believe me, *cada vez le será más fácil,* it will only get easier.

- *Returning to work.* It's more difficult to breastfeed while you are working, but it is feasible. Many mothers do it. To continue your production of milk you'll have to use a breast pump two to three times a day for at least ten minutes during work. Milk should be stored in a cool place. Some breast pumps allow you to empty both breasts at once and store the milk in a cooler. But the most important thing to figure out is if your workplace has the right space to do this in. Some breast pumps will work when plugged into the car's cigarette lighter.

- *Medicines.* Some drugs pass through the mother's milk to the baby. That's why many women stop breastfeeding when they take a medicine. Before deciding whether to quit breastfeeding, talk to your doctor about drug alternatives that won't affect the baby.

Support
One of the keys to successful breastfeeding during the first months after birth is getting support from friends and family. If you can't find people who encourage you and help you out while you're tired and uncomfortable, you might resort to using formula instead of breastfeeding. So it's best to try to set up a support network ahead of time. That will make things a lot easier.

- Talk to your husband and relatives. Try to figure out how important it is to them that you breastfeed and what they think they can do to help you. Breastfeeding requires time and dedication. This means that until all of you get on a set schedule, you won't be able to pay as much attention to your husband and the rest of the family.

- Rent or buy a breast pump. This will allow you to empty your breasts if they fill up with milk and will also let other people participate in feeding the baby.

- Search for a breastfeeding support group. There's nothing like sharing your experiences and difficulties about breastfeeding with other mothers who are doing the same thing. Also, you won't feel so alone as you make your way through the tough times. That will encourage you to keep trying. There's an organization called La Leche League dedicated to promoting breastfeeding. That group will help you find a support group near where you live (see Contact List).

- Make an appointment with the breastfeeding consultant at the hospital. She can tell you how to prepare for breastfeeding, what you need to do if you have inverted nipples, where to rent or buy a breast pump and how to find a support group.

Formula

Despite the best intentions and efforts, sometimes breastfeeding just isn't possible, or it isn't possible for too long or maybe there just isn't the desire there to do it. Fortunately, today there are many formulas on the market that will allow a baby to get its nourishment.

Any supermarket will have formulas for all circumstances and situations: With soy, with iron, without iron, without lactose, for the first months, for later, in travel size or economy size, in powder form or liquid. The powdered milks are cheaper than the ready-made ones, but at the beginning you might find it easier to use the more convenient ones for a few weeks. Be careful heating the milk in a microwave oven because there could be "hot spots" that will burn the baby's mouth.

Baby bottles come in all shapes and sizes. Orthodontic bottle nipples in theory promote proper tooth formation because they mimic the shape of a mother's nipple. They've become really popular in the past few years. If you get confused with so many options, talk to the breastfeeding consultant at the hospital for some advice.

POSTPARTUM DEPRESSION

It's not all that uncommon for new mothers to feel sad or feel like crying from time to time. This stage usually goes away after a couple of weeks. The only thing you need to get through it is *un buen pañuelo de lágrimas*, a good strong hanky and someone to listen to you and support you.

However, sometimes the hormonal changes along with the stress and fatigue of caring for a newborn can cause serious chemical imbalances in the brain that result in postpartum depression.

Postpartum depression is a serious illness that needs treatment; it doesn't go away on its own.

This illness usually shows up about six weeks after birth and can last for months or even years. It will get worse if the mother doesn't get medical help. Below you'll find a psychological test that will help you figure out if you've got postpartum depression. Some of the most common symptoms of this illness include:

- Sadness or a lack of happiness during most of the day, almost every day for two weeks straight
- Difficulty concentrating or making decisions
- Anxiety or apathy
- Fatigue
- Extreme changes in appetite or sleep patterns
- Feeling guilty or that you're a bad mother
- Thoughts of suicide or death
- Thoughts of harming the baby

Latinas who have postpartum depression face a few other difficulties in addition to the illness. Our culture values maternity and usually doesn't understand how a woman who just had a baby could be sad, reject the baby or not want to do anything.

Some of the ideas that run through a mother's head when she has postpartum depression can make her feel guilty. It may make her think

342 %2 WAITING FOR BEBÉ

she's going crazy. Sometimes a depressed new mother might have fantasies about how to harm the baby or herself. They are thoughts *que se meten en la cabeza*, that appear from nowhere. The mother may decide to distance herself from the baby because she's afraid of hurting him or her. Other times a depressed new mother may suffer from anxiety or panic attacks.

In many Latino cultures, mental illness doesn't inspire a lot of sympathy. It is considered something shameful and taboo that shouldn't be talked about. It's more acceptable to have a physical ailment than a mental one. The perception is that depression is a problem of will; the mother just isn't trying hard enough to overcome her sadness.

Therefore, a Latina mother who is suffering obvious symptoms of postpartum depression may choose to ignore them *para ver si pasan*, to see if they go away. Other times depression or anxiety are labeled as *nervios*, or a case of "nerves." *Nervios* are understood as a normal reaction to a situation that causes stress or anxiety. The traditional way to treat a case of the *nervios* is with teas or a visit to the folk healer.

Postpartum depression doesn't respond to those type of treatments. That's because this is an illness, not a reaction to what's going on in the mother's life. It's actually a real chemical imbalance in her brain. A doctor has to rebalance her brain chemistry. Moreover, postpartum depression is common. Four of every ten women in the United States suffer some type of postpartum depression. It's more common than diabetes or high blood pressure.

Some circumstances promote postpartum depression, such as having had some type of depression before, previous postpartum depression, having been depressed during pregnancy, being in an abusive relationship or not having enough family or social support.

Consequences of Postpartum Depression

The effects of postpartum depression can be grave depending on the stage the disease is at. In every case, however, the health of the mother is affected, and in many cases so is that of the baby. The most common consequences are:

- The mother gets physically sick. Because mental illnesses aren't well accepted in Latino culture, it's normal for a depressed new mother to find another way to express the effects of her illness. It's common to have physical problems such as headaches, back pains or whatever other type of discomfort that will help her to justify how she feels emotionally.

- Physical symptoms of depression itself, such as insomnia, lack of appetite, anxiety, fatigue and irritability. The fatigue of taking care of a newborn can make these symptoms worse.
- The mother has a negative attitude toward the baby, which could have negative consequences for the child.
- The mother's relationships with the rest of the family are affected.
- In severe cases, the mother can lose control and contact with reality, resulting in her physically harming the baby or herself.

Postpartum depression is devastating. Many women who suffer through it decide not to have more children in order to avoid the possibility of experiencing it again.

Treatment

Just as with ordinary depression, postpartum depression can be treated successfully. The sooner treatment begins, the better. Postpartum depression is most commonly treated with drugs and therapy, just as ordinary depression is (see page 106). Selective serotonin reuptake inhibitors (SSRIs) are usually effective drugs, although a different medication might be given to breastfeeding mothers. One treatment that's currently being investigated is a mix of antidepressant drugs and estrogen and progesterone.

The first step to getting treatment is reaching out for help. Talk honestly with your doctor about how you feel. The Contact List has other places you can look for help. Despite feeling bad about what you're going through because you're not being the mother you thought you'd be, remember that many other mothers have gone through the same thing. They got the right treatment and their lives went from black and white back to color. They resumed their joyful lives, loving their babies and their families and relishing their roles as new mothers.

Postpartum Depression Test

This psychological test has been used for years to see if a woman has postpartum depression. Take the test by yourself. Circle the answer that corresponds to how you've been feeling over the past seven days and at the end add up the points in parentheses near each answer.

1. I have been able to laugh and see the funny side of things.
- a) As much as I always could (0)
- b) Not quite so much now (1)
- c) Definitively not so much now (2)
- d) Not at all (3)

2. I look forward with enjoyment to things.
- a) As much as I ever did (0)
- b) Rather less that I used to (1)
- c) Definitively less that I used to (2)
- d) Hardly at all (3)

3. I blame myself unnecessarily when things go wrong.
- a) Yes, most of the time (3)
- b) Yes, some of the time (2)
- c) Not very often (1)
- d) No, never (0)

4. I have been anxious or worried for no good reason.
- a) No, not at all (0)
- b) Hardly ever (1)
- c) Yes, sometimes (2)
- d) Yes, very often (3)

5. I have felt scared or panicky for no good reason.
- a) Yes, quite a lot (3)
- b) Yes, sometimes (2)
- c) No, not much (1)
- d) No, not at all (0)

6. Things have been getting to me.
- a) Yes, most of the time I haven't been able to cope at all (3)
- b) Yes, sometimes I haven't been coping as well as usual (2)
- c) No, most of the time I cope quite well (1)
- d) No, I have been coping as well as ever (0)

7. I have been so unhappy that I have had difficulty sleeping.
- a) Yes, most of the time (3)
- b) Yes, sometimes (2)
- c) Not very often (1)
- d) No, not at all (0)

8. I have felt sad or miserable.
> a) Yes, most of the time (3)
> b) Yes, quite often (2)
> c) Not very often (1)
> d) No, not at all (0)

9. I have been so unhappy that I have been crying.
> a) Yes, most of the time (3)
> b) Yes, quite often (2)
> c) Only occasionally (1)
> d) No, never (0)

10. The thought of harming myself has occurred to me.
> a) Yes, quite often (3)
> b) Sometimes (2)
> c) Hardly ever (1)
> d) Never (0)

If your total is more than twelve, you may be suffering from postpartum depression and you should call your doctor right away.

RETURNING TO WORK

You may not have any other option but to return to work just a few weeks after you've delivered your baby. Or you may go back because you don't want to abandon the professional life you led before you got pregnant. In both cases you'll have to leave your baby in the care of someone else. Some Latinas have the good fortune of having a mother, mother-in-law or other relative who can live with them for the first few months. There's nothing like leaving for work knowing your baby is in the hands of a trusted relative. And then there's the added benefit of saving lots of money. One thing to think about is how your husband will deal with and relate to the person who's coming to live with you. He may not be as enthusiastic as you are about having your mother in the house for a year. But even if your baby is cared for by a relative, it is normal to feel worried at first about leaving him or her.

"I feel sad and worried. My sister stays home with her two kids and is going to take care of my baby until my mom comes in a few months. But I worry if he will get enough attention, if he is going to be okay.

She has two kids, she should know how to take care of a baby and she is my sister, *pero me sigo preocupando*, but still I worry."

—*Leticia Gutiérrez*

When there aren't relatives or friends who live nearby to help, some couples decide it's cheaper and easier for one of them to stay at home and stop working until the children are old enough to go to school. Another option is to take the baby to a day care center or leave it in the care of a person who is trained and authorized to take care of children. Or you can hire someone to come to your house to take care of your baby. In these cases, you should investigate thoroughly the security and cleanliness of the day care center as well as the prior record of the person who will take care of the baby.

If someone is coming to your house, whether it's a relative or a stranger you're hiring, you should ask that person to take a Red Cross infant emergency course. These courses are also offered in Spanish. This will make you rest easier, knowing that if there's an emergency your caregiver will know how to react. Call your local Red Cross chapter about these courses—and take one yourself too.

If you've hired someone to come to your home to care for your baby, you will be able to establish the rules from the start about what you expect to be done and not to be done. But if the person who is coming to live with you is your mother or mother-in-law or other relative, you may not agree with their way of doing things. It's easier to explain from the start in a caring way what you want done with your baby rather than to criticize afterward about the care that's being given. For example, you may want to explain that you want the baby to fall asleep in the arms of an adult or in the crib. You may say the baby needs to be fed at a certain hour and what things should not be given to him or her. If your mother or mother-in-law comes to live with you, take her along when you go to the pediatrician so she's included in the baby's care. Ask her how she took care of you or your husband. There will be a lot more harmony in the household if your mother or mother-in-law feels *respetada*, respected.

If you don't have maternity leave, see page 27. Your doctor might be able to request that you receive temporary disability, giving you a few more weeks to spend time with your baby.

FOR DAD

Congratulations! Not only are you a dad, but you've also survived your wife's pregnancy and labor. There are still a few intense but precious months ahead of you, however. Now is when your wife most needs your physical support and caring. This a transition period for both of you and the rest of your family. *Tenga paciencia*, be patient, because as the days go by, all the things that seem so complicated and difficult now will only become easier. Keep in mind the following:

Fatigue

Your partner will feel exhausted during the first months after delivery, especially if labor was long and difficult. She'll feel even worse if she had a cesarean. It's important for you to plan together how she can get the most rest. The baby will need to eat every two to three hours. Believe me when I say the more rest your wife gets, the better it will be for both of you. So for a while, another member of the family will have to take care of some of the chores around the house, such as cooking, doing laundry and cleaning. Take turns feeding the baby so she can rest for a few hours straight, or do the night shift every two to three nights so she can have a whole night's sleep. She can use a breast pump and you can feed the baby with a bottle filled with her milk. You'll help your wife and you'll feel closer to your new child.

Sadness or Tears

Many women cry or feel sad for two to three days after delivering a baby. This usually goes away after a couple of weeks. If after two weeks the symptoms are still there, or if you see your wife has become more irritable, can't sleep, has changed her eating routine or is distancing herself from the baby, you should take it upon yourself to call the doctor. Your wife may have postpartum depression. This is an illness as serious as diabetes or high blood pressure; your partner has no control over it. And it gets worse if it's not treated; the whole family will be affected. Postpartum depression is caused by a chemical imbalance in the brain that can be treated.

This illness makes some women have anxiety attacks or strange thoughts. Your wife may tell you she's having fantasies about harming the baby. Take your partner to the doctor if you see her acting strangely, even though she may insist everything's fine.

Problems Breastfeeding

Even though breastfeeding is a natural process, mothers and babies have to learn how to do it. Sometimes there can be problems such as irritated nipples, or the baby may not learn how to nurse properly. These difficulties can be frustrating for a new mother, and she might decide to use formula to avoid feeding problems altogether. However, mother's milk is the best thing you can give your baby to help it grow up healthy and intelligent (see page 334). The attitude you have toward breastfeeding will influence the effort your wife puts into it. If you support and encourage her to keep trying no matter what the problem is, she'll likely continue. Many studies have shown that the support the father gives toward breastfeeding is the determining factor in whether the baby gets mother's milk or formula. So one of the best things you can do for your baby during the first months of its life is to encourage your wife to continue breastfeeding.

Jealousy or Feeling Left Out

There are fathers who feel left out when they see how close the relationship is between mother and child. It's normal to feel excluded or a little jealous. But even though these feelings are common, don't take it out on your wife by ignoring her or distancing yourself from the family. That will only make things worse.

Your baby needs your partner to survive. There's not a creature on the planet that is as vulnerable as a human newborn. Talk to your wife about how you feel, but without making her feel at fault. Join in when she's breastfeeding the baby or take over with a bottle of her milk. Change the baby, play with him or her. Your baby will recognize you because it's been listening to your voice for the past months from inside your wife's belly.

Relatives and Visits

A relative will likely come to help your family during the first weeks of the baby's life. Or that person may actually move in with you for a while, to give you and your wife time to get back on your feet and back to work. Talk to your partner about what things are important to you both regarding the raising of your child, and tell the relative. Maybe your mother is coming to stay with you. But let your wife make her own decisions. She is learning how to be a mother, and she needs your support.

As far as visits go, no one can protect your wife from unusually long visits as well as you can. You two should agree on a signal that means she is tired and it's time for the company to leave. During the first few weeks it's tough to receive all the guests who would like to come over. Your whole household is tired and not really capable of entertaining. So if you can, it's a good idea to put off accepting visitors for a few weeks, until you and your partner feel better and aren't so worn out.

Sex

Reestablishing a normal sex life with your partner can take a while. A doctor will likely recommend your wife wait at least six weeks. If the delivery was by cesarean, maybe by that time she feels up to it. But if the delivery was vaginal, and there was tearing or an episiotomy, your wife may not have recuperated after six weeks. Plus, if she's breastfeeding, her vagina will be less lubricated than normal. Another thing to consider is her fatigue and the lack of time you both have now that a new baby is in the house.

But the fact you may not be able to have sex with penetration doesn't mean you should forget about all sexual activity until the baby is one year old. In fact, now it's more important than ever for you to reestablish a romantic connection. At least once a week, plan a special time with your wife, even if it's in your own home. Two or three hours to talk or cuddle is the best way to keep things in perspective.

§

Above all, enjoy your new baby as much as you can. Despite the fatigue and the diapers and the sleepless nights, these moments are priceless. It can be a bit difficult for a family to adjust from two to three, but once you've made the change, you won't want it any other way.

12

❧

Pregnancy Myths

"María, don't go in the water, the sea will get angry with you." That's what María Maiz's mother would say every time they went to the beach while she was pregnant. According to the belief *la mar,* the sea, which is a female being in Spanish, gets angry when a pregnant woman goes in the water. The saying goes, the water rises up and tries to suck the baby out of the mother.

Latino culture is full of myths about what can happen to a pregnant woman if she doesn't do *esto o aquello,* this or that, or fails to satisfy a particular *antojo* or craving. These stories have been passed down from grandmother to mother and from mother to daughter for generations. In the past, before doctors had made prenatal care a science, these beliefs were respected and followed to the letter.

María, a modern Latina living in the United States, recalls how she used to tell her mother: "Ay *mamá,* that's just an old wives' tale." But she also remembers how, "*por si acaso,* just in case there's something to it," she would end up spending less time in the water, even though her mother's explanation didn't make any sense. Something similar happened to Ana Miriam La Salle:

"I have a neighbor who told me not to eat papaya because it could cause a miscarriage. I never believed it, and I even asked my brother, who is a doctor. He told me that those were just *cuentos,* stories. Nevertheless, I never ate it . . . *por si acaso,* just in case there is something to it."

Most of these myths don't put the mother or the baby in danger. However, some, if carried out in practice, are nuisances for the mother and for those around her. Husbands searching anxiously for *dulce de leche,* ice cream at four in the morning, so the baby won't be born with its mouth open, will agree with this.

In this chapter, you'll find some of the most common myths about pregnancy in our culture. Some of these myths are shared by different cultures, especially those that have to do with how to determine the sex of the unborn child; others are peculiar to certain Latin American countries. Some relate to things or foods that supposedly can be good for or harm a baby's development; others warn against engaging in certain activities because of their consequences.

Popular beliefs and myths about pregnancy, even if they sometimes can get us a bit concerned, do not determine the outcome of a pregnancy—but they are a lot of fun and a great topic of conversation at baby showers.

BOY OR GIRL?

Before the advent of modern prenatal science, predicting the sex of the baby was all the rage. Today, however, ultrasound imaging and amniocentesis have stolen the magic from the many techniques used to determine whether the baby is a boy or a girl. However, this doesn't stop people from announcing, "By the shape of your belly, I can tell you're going to have a boy."

There is no scientific basis for these predictions, and experience demonstrates that the probabilities of getting it right are precisely the same as in flipping a coin: fifty-fifty. But this doesn't mean it isn't a fun game, especially when the parents already know the baby's sex thanks to a sonogram or an amniocentesis. Here are some of the most popular theories in Latin America for predicting whether you are having a boy or a girl.

1. *Tie a hair from the mother to her wedding ring and hold the hair, with the ring hanging from it, over her belly. If the ring turns in circles, it's a girl; if it goes from side to side, it's a boy.*

2. *Put a spoon under one couch cushion and a fork under another. The pregnant woman enters the room. If she sits on the cushion with the fork, it will be a boy; if she sits on the one with the spoon, it will be a girl.*

3. *If she is carrying high, it will be a boy; if she is carrying low, it will be a girl.*

4. *If the belly is pointy, it will be a boy; if it is more rounded, it will be a girl.*

5. *If the fetus's heart beats fast, it will be a girl; if it beats slower, it will be a boy.*

6. *If the mother gains weight in the hips, it's a girl; if the weight gain is in the belly, it's a boy.*

7. *If the mother gets plump in the face, it's a girl; if she gets plump in the bottom, it's a boy.*

8. *If the mother has hair on her belly, the baby will be a boy.*

9. *If her nipples are dark, it will be a boy.*

10. *If she gets nausea during the pregnancy, it will be a girl.*

FOODS AND THEIR EFFECTS

This group of beliefs links what the mother does or doesn't eat during pregnancy with certain characteristics of the baby. For warnings about certain foods that can actually affect you and your baby, see pages 4–6.

Eating meat during pregnancy will make the baby's head big. Meat is a source of protein, and proteins are a necessary part of the pregnant woman's diet. In fact, doctors recommend that during pregnancy, a woman should increase her protein intake. As long as it is properly cooked and not raw, you can eat all the meat you want.

If you get heartburn frequently during pregnancy, the child will be very hairy. Heartburn during pregnancy is caused by a slowing of the digestive process and by the growing baby pushing stomach juices up toward the esophagus. The amount of hair on the baby has to do with how hairy his or her parents are. Also, there are babies born with thick hair who lose much of it after a few months.

If the mother doesn't satisfy all her cravings, the baby will be born with its mouth open. Babies open their mouths at birth to take in their first breath of air. They also open and close their mouths when they are still inside the amniotic sac. Recent studies have shown that they even suck their thumbs before they are born. For the baby to be born with its mouth open is perfectly normal, and for the mother not to fulfill her every *antojo*, craving—well, that's normal, too.

If you eat too much cheese and dairy products, the baby will get cradle cap. Cradle cap, caused by an excess of oil on the scalp, is very common among newborns and disappears in a few weeks. Cheese has nothing to do with this problem, which is merely cosmetic anyway.

If the mother eats yellow foods, the child will be born yellow. The yellow color that some babies acquire after birth is due to problems in processing a substance called bilirubin. Although it is important to keep an eye on these babies, the problem is quite common and usually clears up very soon. Corn, pumpkins or any other yellow, orange or red foods such as yellow squash, carrots or tomatoes, have a high vitamin A content and are good for mother and baby.

If you eat crab during pregnancy, you will have an active child. Crab, just like beef, fish, poultry, eggs and dairy products, is a good source of protein. The child's personality is determined by its genes and the environment it grows up in, not by what the mother eats during gestation.

Don't eat beets during the final months of pregnancy, because it will cause labor to start. Although many women in their last weeks of pregnancy may have wished this were true, the moment of birth is decided by the baby, not the beet. However, it is worth noting that in more traditional areas of Latin America, this belief has long been a boon to couples who have had to get married in a hurry. They can always blame the baby's early arrival on the beet.

If the mother eats ice, the baby will be born with bronchitis. Bronchitis is an infection and/or inflammation of the bronchi. Before birth, the baby is well insulated inside the mother and stays at a constant temperature. The ice that the mother eats does not produce the supposed "chill" in the baby, nor does it cause any infection or inflammation of the bronchial tubes.

Drinking a lot of liquids will excessively increase the amount of amniotic fluid surrounding the unborn baby. If there is one thing that doctors consistently recommend, it's to drink lots of water during pregnancy—at least eight glasses a day. There is a condition where the amniotic fluid increases, but it is not created by drinking lots of liquids.

You should eat lots of fruits during pregnancy so the baby won't come out dirty. Fruits are a very healthy food before, during and after pregnancy. But even if the expectant mother ate a whole basket of fruits every day, her baby would still come out "dirty." At birth, the baby's skin is covered with mucus and a whitish protective substance known as vernix. As if that weren't enough, along with the baby comes the placenta, the blood-rich organ that has been supplying nourishment to the fetus during the entire pregnancy. A warm bath will give the baby its rosy appearance in a matter of minutes.

MOTHERS' ACTIONS THAT SUPPOSEDLY WILL HARM THE BABY

These myths are related to magical beliefs found in Latin America. They seek to explain that certain physical characteristics or defects in the baby are caused by what the mother did or didn't do. For example, not eating a strawberry when the mother craves it will produce a strawberry birthmark; painting will leave stains on the baby, and so on.

If the pregnant mother sees an eclipse, the baby will get a cleft lip, a cleft palate or a birthmark. To protect against a lunar eclipse, wear a safety pin in your panties. Eclipses are some of the most wondrous phenomena in nature. They terrorized ancient cultures because they couldn't be explained. Aztecs believed that a moon eclipse was a "bite" in the moon and the baby of a pregnant woman would get the same bite in his/her mouth. It's a nice story, but wearing a safety pin will have the same effect as wearing a pink carnation, two-tone shoes, or a green umbrella—that is to say, none. Cleft palate and other defects are related to genes or environmental factors.

If you paint during pregnancy, the baby will be born with a birthmark. The only precaution to take before painting is to make sure that the paint is nontoxic and does not contain lead, and even in those cases the painting would not cause birthmarks.

Anyone who says no to a pregnant woman's request will get spots or moles on his nose. Although some women would love to convince their husbands that this is true, so far there is no evidence of any direct relation between denying the wishes of a pregnant woman and getting a mole. If this belief were true, there would be a lot of husbands walking around with very interesting noses.

If the pregnant mother sees something horrible, the baby will be born ugly. This one has a lot of variations, such as if the mother stares for too long at someone who is cross-eyed, the baby will be born cross-eyed; if she looks at beautiful babies, the baby will be beautiful. The fact is, how the baby looks has mostly to do with the looks of the mother and father. Besides, everyone knows *no hay bebés feos*, there are no ugly babies!

If a pregnant woman lifts her hands over her head, the baby can be strangled by the umbilical cord. The umbilical cord is long enough that the baby won't be strangled by it. The movement of the mother's arms does not affect the tension on the cord. If she likes, the mother can hang out the washing or even perform classical ballet without any danger to the baby's health.

A pregnant woman should not knit, because this can cause the umbilical cord to wrap around the baby's neck. Knitting little garments during pregnancy is a practical and relaxing pastime that the mother-to-be can enjoy without worrying that she is putting the baby's umbilical cord through the same twists and turns as the yarn.

If you cut your hair during pregnancy, you will cut the baby's vision. Hair during pregnancy grows more and looks better because of the changes produced by hormones. You can cut your hair or let it grow. *Esté tranquila*, rest assured it has nothing to do with how your baby's sight is developing.

If you cut cloth on the bed, the baby will be born with a cleft palate or cleft lip. Cleft palate and cleft lip are the result of a defect in which parts of the lip or the palate fail to close. Heredity has much to do with this defect, as do certain medications or a lack of nutrients (folic acid, for example) during pregnancy. Expectant mothers can cut all the cloth they want, on the bed, the table, or whatever surface they like, without worrying that the baby will be born with this condition.

You should play music for the baby so that it won't be born deaf. Babies listen to many things during their stay in the womb: The heartbeat of their mother, the sounds of her intestines, her voice, the voices of the people around her, and other sounds in the environment if they are near enough. The fetus will develop its ear with or without Beethoven. What has been demonstrated in several studies, however, is that babies like classical music better than hard rock. So far they haven't experimented with salsa . . .

Sadness or intense depression in the pregnant mother causes malformations of the fetus's heart. A mother's positive attitude during pregnancy gives the baby a calm environment, but heart problems in the fetus have nothing to do with the mother's emotional state. Such malformations are due to problems in fetal development, genetics or other causes.

If you lift a child (or anything heavy) while you are pregnant, the baby will get a hernia during its first year. Lifting heavy objects during pregnancy isn't a good idea. Pregnant women shouldn't lift anything heavier than twenty-five pounds. Nevertheless, a mother's physical activity doesn't have anything to do with a baby getting a hernia.

If you walk during the last trimester of pregnancy, your stomach will drop and cause the baby to be born prematurely. Under normal circumstances, walking is one of the exercises most recommended during pregnancy, especially in the last three months, when the legs swell due to poor circulation caused by the weight of the baby. Labor begins when the baby is ready (regardless of how ready the mother may already be!).

During the last months of pregnancy, the mother should not lean over the sink to wash dishes because the baby will be born with defects to the head. The baby is protected inside the mother by the amniotic fluid, which acts as a cushion. In the last months of pregnancy, fatigue is the mother-to-be's constant companion. *Es una buena excusa,* it's a tempting excuse, but the truth is, no matter how many dishes the future mother washes while leaning over the sink, baby's head will be just fine.

Having sex during the final months of pregnancy can cause a dent in the baby's skull. The fear that sex during pregnancy can cause injury to the baby is widespread among parents-to-be and fathers in particular. However, under normal circumstances, and if you are in the mood, there is no reason not to enjoy sex during those last weeks of pregnancy.

If you take baths in the bathtub during pregnancy, the dirty water will get on the baby. The only precaution necessary when taking baths is to make sure they aren't too hot (see page 13) because during the first months excessive heat can cause malformations of the spinal column and nervous system. However, the baby is well sealed inside the amniotic sac within the mother's womb. The opening of the uterus has a thick plug of mucus that prevents water or anything else from getting through to the baby.

A woman loses a tooth with each pregnancy. It's important to eat foods rich in calcium during pregnancy in order to protect the bones and teeth of the mother and to provide for the baby's optimum development. However, there is no rule that a pregnancy *le costará un diente*, must cost you a tooth. In fact, there are plenty of women who keep all their teeth even though they have had several children.

THE BIRTH

Birth also has its omens in Latin American folklore, for both mother and child. They are not as numerous as those related to the pregnancy, but they are very interesting too.

If the labor pains are in the belly, it's a boy; if they are in the back, it's a girl. Pain in the back or in the belly is caused by the position in which the baby is descending the birth canal. Unless you do a sonogram, it is difficult to predict by the type of pain if you will have a boy or a girl.

Labor will be brought on by a full moon. Some midwives swear that with a full moon, labor will begin, but there is no statistical evidence whatsoever that this is the case. We do know that the baby itself begins the process of labor, but we still do not know the precise workings of the complex hormonal messages involved.

Babies born with the amniotic sac over the face will be lucky all their lives. When a baby has not fully emerged from the amniotic sac, either because it has not broken or due to other circumstances, the sac can be over its face at birth. According to the myth, this guarantees a lifetime of good luck. It's a nice story, but difficult to prove.

If the baby is born at night, it will be awake at night. In the mother's womb the baby has no notion of when it is day or night, and it sleeps on its own schedule. Babies need several days to adjust to the rhythm of day and night after they are born, but the time of their birth has no bearing on this.

If the pregnant woman sleeps in the daytime, the baby will have swollen eyelids. A newborn's eyelids are swollen due to an excess of water, which goes away after a few days. Certainly, the unborn child can tell if the mother is asleep or awake, but this doesn't affect its eyelids.

Babies born naturally are healthier than those born by cesarean section. Babies born by cesarean have a little bit more water accumulated in the lungs during the first days. One of the advantages of being born through the tight vaginal canal is that the baby's excess liquid is "wrung out." Babies born by cesarean eliminate this liquid later, but there are no studies showing that babies born by cesarean have more problems than those born naturally.

When the baby is born, you should take all the flowers and plants out of the room because they will rob the infant of oxygen at night. Plants give off oxygen when the sun is shining; at night they consume some oxygen and give off CO_2, or carbon dioxide. But even if the baby's nursery looked like the Miami Botanical Gardens this would not be a cause for worry. Either way, with or without plants, it's important to have good ventilation in the baby's room.

BREASTFEEDING

A few days after the birth, the mother's milk appears. The fact that it is a substance that comes from the mother's body and nourishes the baby has made it the subject of many popular beliefs.

As long as you are breastfeeding, it's impossible to get pregnant again. Many are the children who have come into the world thanks to this popular belief. In theory, the hormone that is secreted when the mother is nursing prevents ovulation, but this is by no means an infallible rule. If you want to avoid a possible pregnancy while nursing, it's best to take other precautions.

Babies should not nurse during their first days because the yellowish liquid is dirty. That yellow liquid is called colostrum, and it is one of the marvels of nature. Colostrum contains highly nutritious substances as well as antibodies that protect the baby from diseases. Colostrum is the precursor of the milk and is one of the best foods that you can give the baby until the milk appears.

Women with small breasts produce less milk than women with large breasts. The saying *cuanto más grande mejor,* "bigger is better," doesn't apply in this case. The amount of milk secreted is determined by the frequency and duration of nursing. If the baby wants more milk, the mother will produce more.

If the mother has a cold, the baby will catch it from her milk. The viruses that give rise to colds do not reside in the mother's milk. If the mother has a cold, she can continue nursing without worry. She should, however, wash her hands frequently and take care not to sneeze near the baby to avoid passing on the cold.

If you drink anything cold while nursing, it will cut off the milk supply. The mother's milk can stop flowing due to a variety of causes, including medical conditions and, at times, stress on the mother's part. The temperature of what she is drinking will have no effect on the secretion of milk.

You need to drink milk to make milk. Milk is a wonderful source of calcium for nursing mothers, but drinking more of it doesn't mean you will produce more milk. When nursing, it's important to drink sufficient liquids, which can be water, juice or milk if you like. If this myth were true, mothers who eat a lot of oranges would produce orange juice instead of milk!

THE BABY

Latin American folklore also has lots of advice for the first days, months and years of the baby's life. Like everything related to health, the best source of information is a doctor, and in this case, a pediatrician, a physician who has devoted years of study to the development of children. Here is just a small sampling of these myths.

The baby's umbilical cord should be plugged after birth, because otherwise air can enter and give the baby stomach pain. The umbilical cord dries out a few hours after being cut and falls off in about a week to ten days. Although there is an opening in the abdominal muscles that closes in a few weeks, there is no way for air to get through. If the baby has a stomachache, it should be seen by a doctor.

If the baby's hair is cut before its first birthday, the child will be slow in learning to talk. Any connection between the length of the hair and the speech exists only in the realm of magic. Speech is something that is learned in the first years of life, and every child does it in his or her own time. Whether the baby's hair is cut once a month or not at all will have no bearing on how fast she learns to talk.

Always use your teeth to trim the baby's nails, because using scissors or nail clippers will cause the child to go blind. No relationship exists between the growth of the nails and the functioning of the human eye. The only precaution is to use special round scissors for babies because they move a lot.

If a baby stands on its feet too early, its legs will be bent or twisted. It is normal for a baby's legs to be somewhat bowed, but this changes as he/she grows bigger. Babies know more than we think they do, and they won't stand if they aren't ready, no matter how much we want them to. If they stand when they are only a few months old, it's because they know they can do it. It won't have any effect on the future development of their legs.

CONTACT LIST

Chapter 1

NATIONAL LEAD INFORMATION CENTER
1-800-LEAD-FYI (1-800-532-3398)
http://www.nsc.org/ehc/lead.htm

They will give you information about how to check the lead level in your blood and what you can do if there is lead in your home or workplace.

ORGANIZATION OF TERATOLOGY INFORMATION SERVICES
1-866-626-OTIS (1-866-626-6847)
http://www.otispregnancy.com

They will answer your questions regarding how medicines, drugs and substances you have taken may have affected your baby. Leave your name and number on the answering machine so a counselor can call you back. On their Internet page you'll find the number to call in your area.

Chapter 2

On this list, you'll find telephone numbers you can call to get more information on where and how to obtain health insurance or low-cost prenatal care.

In addition to telephone numbers, you'll find Internet addresses for sites that have a lot of useful information. If you don't have a computer at home, you can log on to the Internet for free at most public libraries. The librarians or their assistants will help.

Organizations That Will Help You Find Health Insurance Before Getting Pregnant

Su Familia
1-866-Su-Familia (1-866-783-2645)
Monday to Friday 9 A.M. to 6 P.M. Eastern Time

Su Familia (Your Family) will tell you the options you have for buying health insurance in your community. This organization can also answer some health questions. All calls are confidential. Su Familia receives a lot of calls, so you might get an answering machine, but leave your name and telephone number and one of their representatives will call you back.

The National Alliance for Hispanic Health
1501 Sixteenth Street, NW
Washington, DC 20036
1-202-387-5000
http://www.hispanichealth.org

This is the organization that sponsors the information program of Su Familia. They can also answer your health questions.

National Committee for Quality Assurance
2000 L Street NW, Suite 500
Washington, DC 20036
1-888-275-7585 (Monday to Friday 8:30 A.M. to 5:30 P.M. Eastern time)
http://www.healthchoices.org

This private nonprofit organization takes a close look at how insurance companies operate and then publishes its findings. Through their Internet page you can see what kind of reputation your insurance company has and which insurance options are available where you live. You can search for insurance companies by state, by zip code or by company name.

Agency for Healthcare Research and Quality
2101 East Jefferson Street
Suite 501
Rockville, MD 20852

1-301-594-1364
http://www.ahcpr.gov/consumer/insuranc.htm

AHRQ is a government agency that has information about the quality of medical services provided by a particular insurance company. You can call this number for help on figuring out which types of insurance are available. The Web page has information on how to choose a health insurance carrier.

NATIONAL ASSOCIATION OF INSURANCE COMMISSIONERS
http://www.naic.org/1regulator/usamap.htm

Every state has its own laws regulating exactly what services health insurance companies are required to provide. The NAIC Web page includes a map of the United States. Just click on the state where you live and you will find information on the rules and regulations that apply to you.

How to Find Prenatal Care When You Don't Have Medical Insurance

NATIONAL HISPANIC PRENATAL HELP LINE
1-800-504-7081 (Monday to Friday 9 A.M. to 6 P.M. Eastern time)

This is one of the best resources to help Latina women find prenatal care. The help line receives hundreds of calls daily, so it's likely you'll get an answering machine when you dial their number. But don't hang up; leave your name and telephone number and a representative will call you back in twenty-four to forty-eight hours. If you don't get a call back, keep trying, because it's worth your effort.

1. They have information about which prenatal caregivers in your area offer services to Latinos.

2. They will send you prenatal information for free by mail. You choose English or Spanish.

3. They will answer most questions you may have about prenatal care.

All telephone conversations are confidential. The only information you have to provide is the general area where you live and your household income.

COMMUNITY HEALTH CENTERS
1-888-ASK-HRSA (1-800-275-4772)
http://www.bphc.hrsa.gov/databases/fqhc/

Community Health Centers offer prenatal and medical services to uninsured women whose incomes are too high to qualify for federal health programs such as Medicaid. There are some three thousand of these centers in all fifty states and Puerto Rico.

You will have to provide the number of people in your family and your household income. Depending on how much money you make, the prenatal care visit can be free or you may have to pay a reduced fee. These centers also provide prenatal care packages that combine prenatal care and childbirth services at a reasonable cost. If those services aren't what you need, the centers' representatives can help you find alternatives. Call the telephone number above for the center nearest you.

The HRSA (Health Resources and Service Administration—the federal department that provides this service) also has a Web site, listed above. Once you've logged on, all you have to do is identify the state you live in and your zip code and the site will list the centers nearest you.

PLANNED PARENTHOOD
1-800-230-PLAN (1-800-230-7526)
http://www.plannedparenthood.org

Planned Parenthood is one of the largest family planning networks in the country. They can also provide prenatal care at reasonable prices, depending on your household income. You can find a center in the area you live by calling their phone number or typing your zip code in on their Web page.

Your yellow pages are another good source of information to search for centers that provide low-cost prenatal care.

MATERNAL AND CHILD BUREAU OF HEALTH RESOURCES AND SERVICES
1-800-311-BABY (1-800-311-2229)

This is a program administered by the Department of Health and Human Services that will help you find prenatal care services. When you call the 800 number, you'll automatically be connected with the appropriate department in your state.

STATE CHILDREN'S HEALTH INSURANCE PROGRAM (SCHIP)
1-877-KIDS-NOW (1-877-5437-669)
http://www.insurekidsnow.gov

When you dial this number you will be connected directly to the department in the state you live. This program offers low-cost health insurance for babies and children of low-income families. But in some states the insurance can be extended to cover the rest of the family, as well as prenatal care. You should keep this program in mind when your baby is born, because you can enroll your baby right away if you don't have any other insurance. SCHIP covers all your child's immunizations and all scheduled and emergency visits to the doctor. You can get also get information on their Web site.

MEDICAID
http://www.hcfa.gov/medicaid/obs5.htm (to look up local phone numbers)
http://www.hcfa.gov/medicaid/stateplan/map.asp (requirements)

The Medicaid telephone number is also in the telephone book's white pages government listings under *County Social Service Office.*

Medicaid is a combined federal and state program that provides free prenatal care for women whose household incomes are below a level determined by the state where you live.

At the first Internet address you will find the number for your state. The second one has the requirements to qualify for Medicaid in the state where you live. It could be confusing, and you might be better off if someone explains it by telephone. Nonetheless, this Web site is a good source of information about Medicaid if you want to investigate further.

WOMEN, INFANTS AND CHILDREN (WIC)
3101 Park Center Drive, Room 819
Alexandria, VA 22302
1-703-305-2747
http://www.fns.usda.gov/wic

This program offers food, nutritional advice and help finding prenatal care to pregnant women, mothers (nursing and non-nursing), babies and children up to five years, who have nutritional deficiencies. WIC, as this program is known in the United States, distributes coupons that can be redeemed for free food. To qualify, women must be below a certain income level.

Your Rights at Work During Pregnancy

If you feel you are being discriminated against on the job because of your pregnancy, you can get more information about exactly what your rights are by calling the following numbers. Calls are confidential.

DEPARTMENT OF LABOR
1-800-959-3652

WOMEN'S BUREAU
U.S. Department of Labor
Washington, DC 20507
1-800-827-5335
1-400-326-2577 (TDD)

LOCAL EQUAL EMPLOYMENT OPPORTUNITY COMMISSION (EEOC)
1-800-669-4000
1-800-669-6820 (TDD)

How to find a Latino or Spanish-speaking doctor

AMERICAN MEDICAL ASSOCIATION
515 N. State Street
Chicago, IL 60610
1-312-464-5000
http://www.ama-assn.org/aps/amahg.htm

Call or log into the AMA Web site for access to its data base to find a local Latino or Spanish-speaking doctor.

AMERICAN COLLEGE OF OBSTETRICIANS AND GYNECOLOGISTS
409 12th St., S.W.
P.O. Box 96920
Washington, DC 20090-6920
1-202-638-5577, extension 2518
http://www.acog.org

Some forty thousand gynecologists and obstetricians are members of this organization. It can put you in touch with local Latino or Spanish-speaking doctors. The Web site can also help you locate a doctor in your area.

Chapter 3

PRAYER FOR EXPECTANT MOTHERS

Father we thank you for your marvelous gift; you have allowed us to share in your divine parenthood. During this time of waiting, we ask you to protect and nurture these first mysterious stirrings of life. May our child come safely into the light of the world and to the new birth of baptism. Mother of God, we entrust our child to your loving heart. Amen. *The Pope's Family Prayer Book*

http://www.catholic-forum.com/saints/saintr09.htm (history)

Here you will find Saint Raymond's history and other prayers.

Chapter 4

Devices to measure your blood sugar with less finger poking

Glucowatch: 1-866-459-2824 Web: http://www.glucowatch.com
Soft-Tact: 1-866-763-8228 Web: http://www.medisense.com
FreeStyle: 1-888-522-5226 Web: http://www.therasense.com

Chapter 5

CDC National Sexually Transmitted Diseases Hotline
1-800-227-8922 or 1-800-342-2437 24 hours a day, 7 days a week

Information about where to get free HIV tests or tests for other sexually transmitted diseases. They will also tell you what to do if a test came out positive.

HIV/AIDS Treatment Information Service (ATIS)
1-800-HIV-0440 (1-800-448-0440) Monday to Friday from 12 P.M. to 5 P.M. Eastern time
http://hivatis.org

Information about HIV/AIDS treatment options in your community. The information is personal and confidential.

Chapter 6

National Association of Genetic Counselors
233 Canterbury Dr.
Wallingford, PA 19086-6617
1-610-872-7608
http://www.nsgc.org/resourcelink.asp

The phone number is an answering machine where you can leave your name and number and a counselor will call you back. The easiest way to find a genetic counselor is through their Web page, providing the state where you live. Genetic counselors will give you information about genetically transmitted disease, where to take a test and what can you do if a test detects any abnormalities in your baby.

NATIONAL DOWN SYNDROME SOCIETY
666 Broadway
New York, NY 10012
1-800-221-4602 Monday to Friday 9 A.M. to 5 P.M. Eastern time
http://www.ndss.org

They will talk to you about life with a Down syndrome child and what kind of help and education these children need. They will also put you in touch with parents in your area that have a Down syndrome child.

Chapter 7

CENTERS FOR DISEASE CONTROL AND PREVENTION INTERNATIONAL TRAVELERS HOTLINE
1-888-232-3228

Information about the vaccines you need to travel to certain countries.

Chapter 8

NATIONAL DOMESTIC VIOLENCE HOTLINE
1-800-799-SAFE (1-800-799-7233) 24 hours a day, 7 days a week
1-800-787-3224 (TDD)
http://www.ndvh.org/

They will listen to you and give you information about where to find the help you need, whether it is a place to go if you have to leave your home, legal help, marriage counselors or support groups for women that have gone through domestic violence themselves. Calls are confidential.

NATIONAL CHILD ABUSE HOTLINE
15757 N. 78th Street
Scottsdale, AZ 85260
http://www.childhelpusa.org
1-800-4-A-CHILD (1-800-422-4453)

This hotline will help you in case you, your children or other children are being abused. A professional counselor will listen to you and will give you advice about what to do and where to find help. Calls are confidential.

Chapter 9

CHILDBIRTH CLASSES

These organizations will help you find childbirth classes and instructors near your area.

LAMAZE INTERNATIONAL
2025 M Street N.W., Suite 800
Washington, DC 20036-3309
1-800-368-4404 or 1-202-857-1128
http://www.lamaze-childbirth.com

BRADLEY METHOD
P.O. Box 5224
Sherman Oaks, CA 91413-5224
1-800-4-A-BIRTH (1-818-788-6662)
http://www.bradleybirth.com

INTERNATIONAL CHILDBIRTH EDUCATION ASSOCIATION (ICEA)
P.O. Box 20048
Minneapolis, MN 55420
1-952-854-8660
http://www.icea.org

AMERICAN ASSOCIATION OF PREMATURE BABIES
P.O. Box 46371
Cincinnati, OH 45246-0371
513-956-4331
http://www.aapi-online.org/

Information about the care premature babies need and the problems they face. You can leave your name and number on the answering machine.

PARENTS OF PREMATURE BABIES
http://www.preemie-1.org/newparents.html

Updated information about the care and problems of premature babies.

DOULAS OF NORTH AMERICA
P.O. Box 626
Jasper, IN 47547
1-888-788-dona (1-888-788-3662) 9 A.M. to 4 P.M. Eastern time
http://dona.org/findingdoula.htm

Will give you a list of the doulas in your area. Here you can find some doulas that will not charge for their services and others that will help you after you give birth. They will also send information to your home about how a doula can help you and the questions you should ask before hiring her.

Chapter 11

LA LECHE LEAGUE
1400 North Meacham Road
Schaumburg, IL 60173-4808
1-800-LA-LECHE (1-800-525-3243)
1-847-519-7730
http://www.lalecheleague.org

La Leche League will answer your questions about breastfeeding and will give you advice on how to overcome difficulties you may encounter in the process. They will put you in contact with groups of breastfeeding mothers in your area. The Web page has a lot of information about breastfeeding.

DEPRESSION AFTER DELIVERY
91 East Somerset Street
Raritan, NJ 08869
1-800-944-4PPD (1-800-944-4473)
http://www.depressionafterdelivery.com

The phone number connects you with an answering machine where you can leave your name and address so they can send you a list of the postpartum depression help you can find in your area.

POSTPARTUM SUPPORT INTERNATIONAL
927 North Kellogg Avenue
Santa Barbara, CA 93111
1-805-967-7636
http://www.postpartum.net

They will get you in contact with people or groups specialized in helping women with postpartum depression.

http://1800therapist.com
1-800-THERAPIST (1-800-843-7274)

This is not a crisis line but a private organization that will give you information about therapists and mental health services in your area. You will be connected with a professional in your area.

NOTES

1. Getting Ready for Bebé

6   *mental development of babies born to mothers with high levels of lead:* Howard Hu, M.D., et al., "Lead Exposure Before Pregnancy May Threaten Infant Development," *Harvard School of Public Health Web Digest* (April 2002).

13   *can cause birth defects in laboratory animals:* K. Shiota, "Induction of Neural Tube Defects and Skeletal Malformations in Mice Following Brief Hyperthermia in Utero," *Biol Neonate* 53 (1998): 86–97.

14   *most important factor in determining when to have a second child:* E. Fuentes-Afflick and N. A. Hessol, "Interpregnancy Interval and the Risk of Premature Infants," *Obstetrics and Gynecology* 95 (2000): 383–390(8).

14   *since 70 percent of such pregnancies have a spontaneous rupture of the amniotic sac:* Agustin Conde-Agudelo and José M. Belizán, "Maternal Morbidity and Mortality Associated with Interpregnancy Interval: Cross Sectional Study," *British Medical Journal* 321 (2000): 1255–1259.

16   *The statistics show the earlier a woman gets prenatal care:* "Entry into Prenatal Care—United States, 1989–1997," *Morbidity and Mortality Weekly Report* 49(18) (2000): 393–8.

3. A Healthy Pregnancy

54   *two of every five Latinas don't exercise regularly:* C. J. Crespo, S. J. Keteyian, G. W. Heath, et al., "Leisure-Time Physical Activity Among US Adults: Results from the Third National Health and Nutrition Examination Survey," *Arch Intern Med* 156(1) (1996): 93–98.

59 *this exercise helps with round ligament pain:* "Pelvic Tilt for Ligament Pain Relief," *Journal of Nurse-Midwifery* 39 (1994): 370–374.

60 *use home remedies to treat health problems:* B. Mikhail, "Hispanic Mothers' Beliefs and Practices Regarding Selected Children's Health Problems," *West J Nurs Res* 16 (1994): 623–38.

67 *Ginger helps to ease the discomfort of nausea:* T. Vutyavanich, T. Kraisarin, and R. Ruangsri, "Ginger for Nausea and Vomiting in Pregnancy: Randomized, Double-Masked, Placebo-Controlled Trial," *Obstetrics and Gynecology* 97 (4) (April 2001): 577–82.

4. Diabetes and Pregnancy

73 *Every year there are more diabetics:* "Self-Reported Prevalence of Diabetes Among Hispanics: United States, 1994–1997," *Morbidity and Mortality Weekly Report* 48 (1999): 8–12.

73 *if a diabetic mother has her blood sugar levels under control:* D. R. Coustan, "Gestational Diabetes." In *Diabetes in America,* 2nd Edition. Edited by M. I. Harris, C. C. Cowie, M. P. Stern, E. J. Boyko, G. E. Reiber, and P. H. Bennett, National Institutes of Health, National Institute of Diabetes and Digestive and Kidney Diseases, 1995, p 703–17.

75 *children of diabetic mothers:* A. Plageman et al., "Overweight and Obesity in Infants of Mothers with Long-Term Insulin-Dependent Diabetes or Gestational Diabetes," *International Journal of Obesity* 21 (1997): 451–56.

75 *can have psychological difficulties:* T. Rizzo et al., "Prenatal and Perinatal Influences on Long Term Psychomotor Development in Offspring of Diabetic Mothers," *American Journal of Obstetrics and Gynecology* 173 (1995): 1753–58.

76 *who have had gestational diabetes:* The National Women's Health Information Center, "Diabetes and Hispanic American Women," The Office on Women's Health. US Department of Health and Human Services (April 2001).

77 *glyburide, a pill commonly taken:* O. Langer, M.D. et al., "A Comparison of Glyburide and Insulin in Women with Gestational Diabetes Melitus," *The New England Journal of Medicine* 343(16) (October 2000): 1134–1138.

81 *Food plan adapted from:* Donna L. Jornsay et al., "Answers About Gestational Diabetes," *Boehringer Mannheim Corporation* (1993).

84 *as little as twenty minutes of exercise:* A. S. Lean et al., "Effects of Partially Home Based Exercise Program for Women with Gestational Diabetes," *Obstetrics and Gynecology* 163 (1990): 93–98.

5. Health Concerns for Latinas During Pregnancy

90 *Although preeclampsia isn't too common:* Margaret T. Johnson, M.D., "Hypertensive Diseases in Pregnancy," *Journal of Obstetrics and Gynecology* 25298(17) (March 2002): 4392–4655.

90 *by a problem in the placenta implantation:* N. M. Page, P. J. Lowry et al., "Excessive Placental Secretion of Neurokinin B During the Third Trimester Causes Pre-eclampsia," *Nature* 405 (2000): 797–800.

90 *The main cause of death among Hispanic mothers:* Centers for Disease Control and Prevention, "Fact Sheet: Increased Risk of Dying from Pregnancy among Hispanic Women in the United States," *Surveillance and Research,* National Center for Chronic Disease Prevention and Health Promotion (March 28, 2000).

91 *Obese women are twice as likely:* Karen Mahler, "Errors in Prenatal Risk Assessment More Likely Among Hispanic Women," *Family Planning Perspectives* 28(3) (1998): 128.

91 *If you were already overweight:* Ibid.

91 *Overweight Latinas have a tendency:* Ibid.

92 *only three suffered from diabetes:* C. Fox, J. Esparza et al., "Plasma Leptin Concentrations in Pima Indians Living in Drastically Different Environments," *Diabetes Care* 22 (1999): 413–7.

92 *Other studies of the Manitoba Indians:* R. Hegele et al., "The Hepatic Nuclear Factor-1∂ G319S Variant Is Associated with Early-Onset Type 2 Diabetes in Canadian Oji-Cree," *Journal of Clinical Endocrinology and Metabolism* 84 (1999): 1077–82.

92 *Another genetic study:* A. Guterson et al., "G protein B₃ subunit 825 TT genotype and post-pregnancy weight retention," *The Lancet* 355 (2000): 1240.

94 *Three of every ten pregnant women:* A. Maringhini et al., "Biliary Sludge and Gallstones in Pregnancy: Incidence, Risk Factors and Natural History," *Ann Intern Med* 119 (1993): 116–20.

94 *In order of danger:* R. Hoffman "Gallbladder Disease," *Conscious Choice,* (January 1999).

103 *these medicines does not harm the baby:* Ruth E. Tuomala, M.D., et al., "Antiretroviral Therapy during Pregnancy and the Risk of an Adverse Outcome," *New England Journal of Medicine* 346(24) (June 13, 2002): 1863–1897.

104 *women who have a new sexual partner:* "Bacterial Vaginosis," National Center for HIV, STD and TB Prevention, Centers for Disease Control and Prevention, September 2000.

104 *Surveys done in 2000 show:* Ibid.

106 *Women get depressed more often:* "Mental Health Among Women of Color,"

Women of Color Health Data Book, National Institutes of Health (1998): 83.

109 *Latino babies are born healthy:* R. Scribner, "Paradox as Paradigm—The Health Outcomes of Mexican Americans," *American Journal of Public Health* 86 (1996): 303.

109 *how Mexican women counted:* Natalia Deeb-Sossa et al., "Measurement of Length of Gestation Among Mexican Immigrants," 129th Annual Meeting of APHA, October 2001, Board 1.

6. Pregnancy Medical Tests

121 *The following table lays out:* E. B. Hook, P. K. Cross, and D. M. Schreinemachers, "Chromosomal Abnormality Rates at Amniocentesis and in Live-Born Infants," *Journal of the American Medical Association* 249(15) (1993): 2034–2038.

124 *is also effective in detecting other types:* D. A. Aitken et al., "Dimeric Inhibin A as a Marker for Down's Syndrome in Early Pregnancy," *New England Journal of Medicine* 334(19) (1996): 1231–1236.

131 *A study showed eighteen jelly beans:* K. L. Boyd et al., "Jelly Beans as an Alternative to a Cola Beverage Containing Fifty Grams of Glucose," *American Journal of Obstetrics and Gynecology,* 176;6 (Dec 1995) 1889–92.

7. The First Trimester

153 *nausea came about millions of years ago:* M. Profet, "Pregnancy Sickness as Adaptation: A Deterrent to Maternal Ingestion of Teratogens," In J. H. Barkow, L. Cosmides, and J. Tooby (eds), *The Adapted Mind. Evolutionary Psychology and the Generation of Culture.* New York, Oxford University Press, 327–365.

153 *women who suffer from nausea:* D. B. Petitti, "Nausea and Pregnancy Outcome," *Birth,* 13 (1986): 4.

172 *One way to prevent these infections:* K. Duddeck, "Randomized Trial of Cranberry-Lingonberry Juice and Lactobacillus GG Drink for the Prevention of Urinary Tract Infections in Women," *British Medical Journal* 332 (June 29, 2001); 1571–1573.

8. The Second Trimester

190 *pregnant women who suffered this disease:* S. Offenbacher et al., "Maternal Periodontitus and Prematurity," *Annals of Periodontology* 6(1) (2001): 164–82.

209 *it presents more risks for the child and the mother:* Jenny W. Y. Pang et al., "Outcomes of Planned Home Births in Washington State: 1989–1996," *Obstetrics and Gynecology* 100(2) (August 2002): 253–259.

216 *studies where women took calcium:* G. Young et al., "Interventions for Leg Cramps in Pregnancy," Cochrane review. In The Cochrane Library, 1, 2002. Oxford: Update Software.

9. The Third Trimester

230 *difficulties with their short-term memory:* C. Janes et al., "Memory Loss During Pregnancy," *Journal of Psychosomatic Obstetrics and Gynaecology* 20 (1999): 80–7.

231 *lack of sleep also worsens:* M. Brett et al., "Motherhood and Memory: A Review," *Psychoneuroendocrinology* 26 (2001): 339–362.

235 *pregnant women who have the support of a doula:* K. D. Scott et al., "The Obstetrical and Postpartum Benefits of Continuous Support During Childbirth," *Journal of Women's Health Gender Based Medicine* 10 (1999): 1257–64.

261 *food, the number of prior pregnancies:* R. Mittendorf et al., "The Length of Uncomplicated Human Gestation," *Obstetrics & Gynecology* 75(6) (1990): 929–932.

10. Labor and Delivery

292 *to prove any significant increase in back pain:* A. Macarthur et al., "Epidural Anaesthesia and Low Back Pain After Delivery: A Prospective Cohort Study," *British Medical Journal* 311(7016) (1995): 1336–9.

293 *women who get an epidural have a greater chance:* C. J. Howell et al., "A Randomized Controlled Trial of Epidural Compared with Non-epidural Analgesia in Labor," *British Journal of Obstetrics and Gynecology* 108 (2001): 27–33.

294 *Latino fathers-to-be speak in sweet terms:* C. M. Khazoyan and N. Anderson, "Latinas' Expectations for Their Partners During Childbirth," *Maternal Child Nursing* 19 (1994): 226–229.

299 *induced labor, especially in the first pregnancy:* J. D. Yeast et al., "Induction of Labor and the Relationship to Cesarean Delivery: A Review of 7001 Consecutive Inductions," *American Journal of Obstetrics and Gynecology* 180 (3 pt 1) (1999): 628–33.

305 *Some doctors feel that it's much easier:* C. W. Nager et al., "Episiotomy Increases Perineal Laceration Length in Primiparous Women," *American Journal of Obstetrics and Gynecology* 185 (2001): 444–50.

11. After Birth

334 *fewer chances of developing cancer:* M. K. Davis et al., "Infant Feeding and Childhood Cancer," *The Lancet* (1988): 365–368.

334 *less likely to die from sudden infant death syndrome (SIDS):* E. A. Mitchel et al., "Results From the First Year of the New Zealand Cot Death Study," *New Zealand Medical Journal,* 104 (1991): 71–76.

334 *fewer respiratory infections:* A. C. Wilson et al., "Relation of Infant Diet to Childhood Health: Seven Year Follow up of Cohort of Children in Dundee Infant Study," *British Medical Journal,* 316 (7124) (1998): 21–5.

334 *Better sight during the first months:* L. J. Horwood et al., "Breastfeeding and Later Cognitive and Academic Outcome," *Pediatrics,* 101(1) (1998): 01–07.

343 *Postpartum Depression Test:* J. L. Cox, J. M. Holden, and R. Sagovsky, Edinburgh Postnatal Depression Scale (EPDS), *British Journal of Psychiatry* 150 (1987).

348 *the support the father gives:* M. Sweeney and C. Guilino, "The Health Belief Mode as an Explanation for Breastfeeding Practices in a Hispanic Population," *Advanced Nursing Science,* 9(4) (1987): 35–50.

SEND YOUR COMMENTS

You can send your comments to the author at **lourdes@waitingforbebe.com** and visit the book's Web site at **http://www.waitingforbebe.com** to share your pregnancy experiences with other Latino mothers.

Index

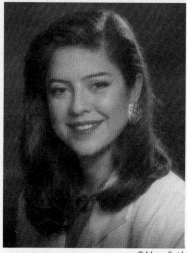

© Merret Smith

ABOUT THE AUTHOR

LOURDES ALCAÑIZ is an award-winning journalist with more than twenty years of experience writing, producing and reporting on health-related subjects. She has worked for Univision, NBC, CNN, CBS-UPI, and Hispanic Radio Network. She is a Fulbright Fellow and the recipient of the Carole Simpson Radio and Television National Directors Foundation Scholarship, the Latino Literary Mariposa Award and a team Emmy Award for her writing at Univision in Los Angeles. She currently writes regularly for several publications dedicated to health issues in the Latino community. She is married and has two daughters, Adriana and Patricia. She is expecting her third baby.